Machine Learning, Medical AI and Robotics

Translating theory into the clinic

Online at: https://doi.org/10.1088/978-0-7503-4637-5

IOP Series in Artificial Intelligence in the Biomedical Sciences

Series Editor

About the Series

The *IOP Series in Artificial Intelligence in the Biomedical Sciences* aims to develop a library of key texts and reference works encompassing the broad range of artificial intelligence, machine learning, deep learning and neural networks within all applicable fields of biomedicine. There is now significant focus in using advancements in the field of AI to improve diagnosis, management, and better therapeutic options of various diseases. Some examples and applications incorporated would be AI in cancer diagnosis/prognosis, implementing artificial intelligence, data mining of electronic health records data, ambient intelligence in hospitals, AI in virus detection, AI in infectious diseases, biomarkers and genomics utilizing machine learning and clinical decision support with augmented reality (AR). These are just a few of the many applications that AI and related technologies can bring to the biomedical sciences. The series contains two broad types of approach. Those addressing a particular field of application and reviewing the numerous relevant artificial intelligence methods applicable to the field, and those that focus on a specific AI method which will permit a greater in-depth review of the theory and appropriate technology.

A full list of titles published in this series can be found here:
https://iopscience.iop.org/bookListInfo/iop-series-in-artificial-intelligence-in-the-biomedical-sciences#series.

Machine Learning, Medical AI and Robotics

Translating theory into the clinic

Edited by
Varut Vardhanabhuti
Department of Diagnostic Radiology, The University of Hong Kong, Hong Kong, China

Ka-Wai Kwok
Department of Mechanical Engineering, The University of Hong Kong, Hong Kong, China

Jason Y K Chan
Department of Otorhinolaryngology, Head and Neck Surgery, Faculty of Medicine, The Chinese University of Hong Kong, Hong Kong, China

Qi Dou
Department of Computer Science and Engineering, The Chinese University of Hong Kong, Hong Kong, China

IOP Publishing, Bristol, UK

ISBN 978-0-7503-4637-5 (ebook)
ISBN 978-0-7503-4635-1 (print)
ISBN 978-0-7503-4638-2 (myPrint)
ISBN 978-0-7503-4636-8 (mobi)

DOI 10.1088/978-0-7503-4637-5

Version: 20231201

IOP ebooks

British Library Cataloguing-in-Publication Data: A catalogue record for this book is available from the British Library.

Published by IOP Publishing, wholly owned by The Institute of Physics, London

IOP Publishing, No.2 The Distillery, Glassfields, Avon Street, Bristol, BS2 0GR, UK

US Office: IOP Publishing, Inc., 190 North Independence Mall West, Suite 601, Philadelphia, PA 19106, USA

We dedicate this book to all those who strive for knowledge, understanding, and growth, in the hope that it may serve as a valuable resource and inspiration for further exploration and discovery.

Contents

Preface

This book serves as a comprehensive compilation of the latest and most innovative artificial intelligence practices being employed in the field of medicine today. By summarizing the cutting-edge theories that are currently being applied and integrated into modern medical practices, this captivating volume offers readers a unique glimpse into the future of healthcare.

Drawing upon the insights and commentaries of numerous experts from a diverse range of specialties, the book distills an extensive body of knowledge into individual chapters, each focusing on a specific area of interest. These include medical imaging, ophthalmology, dentistry, surgery, pathology, wearable technology, robotics, ageing, and longevity, among others. Additionally, the book delves into the more technical aspects of the subject matter, examining the generalizability of deep learning in medicine and its potential to revolutionize the field.

While the scope of this book is undeniably broad, it serves to highlight the most critical areas currently under active research and development. Each chapter is carefully crafted, drawing upon the expertise of leading investigators in their respective fields. It is the author's hope that readers will not only find the content intriguing and informative but that it will also spark their curiosity, inspiring them to delve deeper into the subject matter and perhaps even embark on their own investigative journeys.

Varut Vardhanabhuti
Ka-Wai Kwok
Jason YK Chan
Qi Dou

Editor biographies

Varut Vardhanabhuti

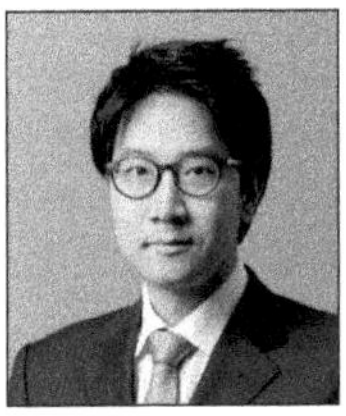

Dr Varut Vardhanabhuti is currently Clinical Assistant Professor at the Faculty of Medicine in the University of Hong Kong. He completed his medical degree at Guy's, King's and St Thomas' School of Medicine in London with subsequent training in London, Oxford, Plymouth, Exeter, and Imperial College London, UK whilst also completing a PhD. His research interests spans the field of medical artificial intelligence with focus on imaging and multi-modality integration using big data with the goal of early clinical translation to benefits patients. He has wide-ranging projects in the AI space including the use of quantitative radiomics in cancer prognostication, using deep learning models as a tool for automatic segmentation and cancer detection, big data using electronic patient records, and longevity medicine etc. He is the author of > 90 published peer reviewed articles, some patented inventions, and is a co-founder of the medical longevity startup, Snowhill Science Ltd. He is passionate about using technology in education. He has previously served as a Microsoft Cloud Research Software Fellow and an Amazon Faculty Ambassador in AWS Educate Cloud Ambassador Program. He previously serves as the Vice Chair for community engagement in the International Society of Radiology.

Ka-Wai Kwok

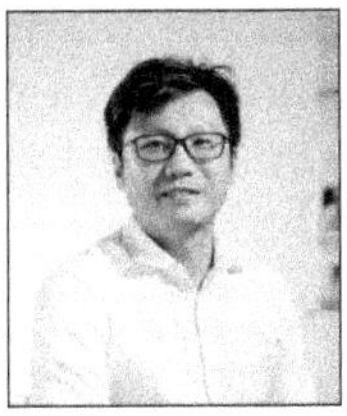

Dr Ka-Wai Kwok currently serves as Associate Professor at the Department of Mechanical Engineering, in the University of Hong Kong (HKU). His research focuses on surgical robotics and intra-operative image guidance. He has participated in various designs of robotic devices/interfaces for endoscopy, and MRI-guided interventions. His multidisciplinary work has been recognized by various (>11) awards in international conferences and journals, e.g. the largest flagship conferences of robotics, ICRA and IROS. He was the recipient of the ICRA Best Conference Paper Award in 2018, and the IROS Toshio Fukuda Young Professional Award in 2020. Moreover, Ka-Wai is the principal investigator of the Interventional Robotic and Imaging Systems (IRIS) group at HKU. The group has (>5) inventions that have been licensed/transferred from university to industry in support of their commercialization. He is a co-founder of Agilis Robotics Ltd., aimed at advancing interventional endoscopy with small, flexible robotic instruments and their intelligent control systems.

Jason Y K Chan

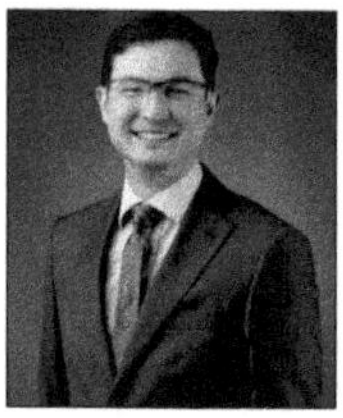

Dr Jason YK Chan is currently an Assistant Dean (Health Systems) and Associate Professor in the Faculty of Medicine at CUHK within the Department of Otorhinolaryngology, Head and Neck Surgery. He is also Deputy director of the CUHK Jockey Club Minimally Invasive Surgical Skills Centre. His research interests center around the application of robotics in minimally invasive surgery and the role of the microbiome in head and neck cancers. In this regard, he has numerous publications, grants and is the co-founder of a robotics startup, Agilis Robotics Ltd. focusing on robot use in endoluminal surgery. He is currently an associate editor of the *Journal of Otolaryngology – Head & Neck Surgery and the Journal for Oto-Rhino-laryngology, Head and Neck Surgery.*

Qi Dou

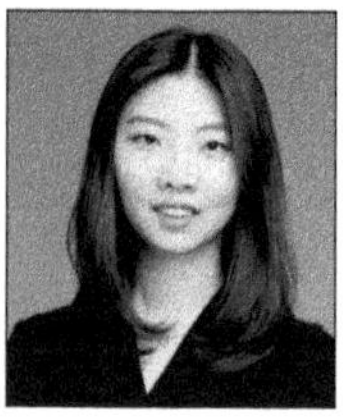

Dr Qi Dou is an Assistant Professor with the Department of Computer Science & Engineering at The Chinese University of Hong Kong. Her research interest lies in the interdisciplinary area of AI for healthcare with expertise in medical image analysis and robot-assisted surgery towards the goal of advancing disease diagnosis and intervention via machine intelligence. She has received the IEEE EMBS Early Career Award, NSFC Excellent Young Scientists Fund (HK & Macau) and a number of best paper awards including the MedIA-MICCA'17 Best Paper Award, and the IEEE ICRA'21 Best Paper Award in Medical Robotics. She served as Program Co-Chair for international conferences of MICCAI, IPCAI, MIDL, and Associate Editor for *journals of Medical Image Analysis and IEEE Transactions on Medical Imaging.*

List of contributors

Ghazal Aarabi
Department of Periodontics, Preventive and Restorative Dentistry, Center for Dental and Oral Medicine, University Medical Center Hamburg-Eppendorf, Hamburg, Germany

Kwok Wai Samuel Au
Multi-Scale Medical Robotics Center Ltd, Department of Mechanical and Automation Engineering, The Chinese University of Hong Kong, Hong Kong Special Administrative Region of China, People's Republic of China

Ronald C K Chan
Clinical Assistant Professor, Department of Anatomical and Cellular Pathology, Faculty of Medicine, Chinese University of Hong Kong, Hong Kong Special Administrative Region of China, People's Republic of China

Cheng Chen
Department of Computer Science and Engineering, The Chinese University of Hong Kong, Hong Kong Special Administrative Region of China, People's Republic of China

Jamie B J Chen
Department of Otorhinolaryngology, Head and Neck Surgery, Faculty of Medicine, The Chinese University of Hong Kong, Hong Kong Special Administrative Region of China, People's Republic of China

Jason Y K Chen
Department of Otorhinolaryngology, Head and Neck Surgery, Faculty of Medicine, The Chinese University of Hong Kong, Hong Kong Special Administrative Region of China, People's Republic of China

Yeow Kuan Chong
Chemical Pathology Laboratory, Department of Pathology, Princess Margaret Hospital, Hong Kong, Hong Kong Special Administrative Region of China, People's Republic of China

Kendrick Co Shih
Department of Ophthalmology, The University of Hong Kong, Hong Kong Special Administrative Region of China, People's Republic of China

Qi Dou
Department of Computer Science and Engineering, The Chinese University of Hong Kong, Hong Kong Special Administrative Region of China, People's Republic of China

Yifeng Hao
Department of Mechanical Engineering, The University of Hong Kong, Hong Kong Special Administrative Region of China, People's Republic of China

Zhuoliang He
Department of Mechanical Engineering, The University of Hong Kong, Hong Kong Special Administrative Region of China, People's Republic of China

Pheng-Ann Heng
Department of Computer Science and Engineering, The Chinese University of Hong Kong, Hong Kong Special Administrative Region of China, People's Republic of China

Joshua W K Ho
School of Biomedical Sciences, Li Ka Shing Faculty of Medicine, The University of Hong Kong, Hong Kong Special Administrative Region of China, People's Republic of China
and
Laboratory of Data Discovery for Health Limited (D24H), Hong Kong Science Park, Hong Kong Special Administrative Region of China, People's Republic of China

Edmond Ho Nang Pow
Restorative Dental Sciences, Faculty of Dentistry, The University of Hong Kong, Hong Kong, Special Administrative Region of China, People's Republic of China

Fan Huang
Department of Diagnostic Radiology, The University of Hong Kong, Hong Kong Special Administrative Region of China, People's Republic of China

Julian Iordachita
Laboratory for Computational Sensing and Robotics (LCSR), Johns Hopkins University, Baltimore, MD, USA

Meirui Jiang
Department of Computer Science and Engineering, The Chinese University of Hong Kong, Hong Kong Special Administrative Region of China, People's Republic of China

Mahdis Khodadadi
Division of Applied Oral Sciences and Community Dental Care, Faculty of Dentistry, The University of Hong Kong, Hong Kong, Special Administrative Region of China, People's Republic of China

James Kit Hon Tsoi
Division of Applied Oral Sciences and Community Dental Care, Faculty of Dentistry, The University of Hong Kong, Hong Kong Special Administrative Region of China, People's Republic of China

Mohamad Koohi-Moghadam
Division of Applied Oral Sciences and Community Dental Care, Faculty of Dentistry, The University of Hong Kong, Hong Kong Special Administrative Region of China, People's Republic of China

and
Department of Diagnostic Radiology, Li Ka Shing Faculty of Medicine, The University of Hong Kong, Pok Fu Lam, Hong Kong Special Administrative Region of China, People's Republic of China

Ka-Wai Kwok
Department of Mechanical Engineering, The University of Hong Kong, Hong Kong Special Administrative Region of China, People's Republic of China
and
Multi-Scale Medical Robotics Center Ltd, Hong Kong Special Administrative Region of China, People's Republic of China

Christopher K C Lai
Department of Microbiology, Faculty of Medicine, Chinese University of Hong Kong, Hong Kong Special Administrative Region of China, People's Republic of China

Nike Kwai Cheung Lau
Chemical Pathology Laboratory, Department of Pathology, Princess Margaret Hospital, Hong Kong, Hong Kong Special Administrative Region of China, People's Republic of China

Alfred L H Lee
Department of Microbiology, Faculty of Medicine, Chinese University of Hong Kong, Hong Kong Special Administrative Region of China, People's Republic of China

Yingqi Li
Department of Mechanical Engineering, The University of Hong Kong, Hong Kong Special Administrative Region of China, People's Republic of China

Jie Lian
Department of Diagnostic Radiology, The University of Hong Kong, Hong Kong Special Administrative Region of China, People's Republic of China

Quande Liu
Department of Computer Science and Engineering, The Chinese University of Hong Kong, Hong Kong Special Administrative Region of China, People's Republic of China

Shichao Ma
School of Biomedical Sciences, Li Ka Shing Faculty of Medicine, The University of Hong Kong, Hong Kong Special Administrative Region of China, People's Republic of China
and
Laboratory of Data Discovery for Health Limited (D24H), Hong Kong Science Park, Hong Kong Special Administrative Region of China, People's Republic of China

Kei Shing Ng
Department of Diagnostic Radiology, The University of Hong Kong, Hong Kong Special Administrative Region of China, People's Republic of China

Russell H Taylor
Laboratory for Computational Sensing and Robotics (LCSR), Johns Hopkins University, Baltimore, MD, USA

Libaihe Tian
Department of Mechanical Engineering, The University of Hong Kong, Hong Kong Special Administrative Region of China, People's Republic of China

Curtis C K To
Department of Anatomical and Cellular Pathology, Faculty of Medicine, Chinese University of Hong Kong, Hong Kong Special Administrative Region of China, People's Republic of China

Varut Vardhanabhuti
Department of Diagnostic Radiology, The University of Hong Kong, Hong Kong Special Administrative Region of China, People's Republic of China

Xiaomei Wang
Department of Mechanical Engineering, The University of Hong Kong, Hong Kong Special Administrative Region of China, People's Republic of China
and
Multi-Scale Medical Robotics Center Ltd, Hong Kong, Hong Kong Special Administrative Region of China, People's Republic of China

Mengjie Wu
Department of Mechanical Engineering, The University of Hong Kong, Hong Kong Special Administrative Region of China, People's Republic of China

Jiayi Xin
School of Biomedical Sciences, Li Ka Shing Faculty of Medicine, The University of Hong Kong, Hong Kong Special Administrative Region of China, People's Republic of China
and
Laboratory of Data Discovery for Health Limited (D24H), Hong Kong Science Park, Hong Kong Special Administrative Region of China, People's Republic of China

Charlene Yat Che Chau
Department of Ophthalmology and Visual Sciences, Prince of Wales Hospital, Hong Kong Special Administrative Region of China, People's Republic of China

Ying Ye
Department of Oral Implantology, Stomatological Hospital and Dental School of Tongji University, Shanghai Engineering Research Center of Tooth Restoration and Regeneration, Shanghai, People's Republic of China

Chun-Yat Yee
School of Biomedical Sciences, Li Ka Shing Faculty of Medicine, The University of Hong Kong, Hong Kong Special Administrative Region of China, People's Republic of China
and
Laboratory of Data Discovery for Health Limited (D24H), Hong Kong Science Park, Hong Kong Special Administrative Region of China, People's Republic of China

Walter Yu Huang Lam
Restorative Dental Sciences, Faculty of Dentistry, The University of Hong Kong, Hong Kong, Special Administrative Region of China, People's Republic of China

Yan Yu
Snowhill Science Limited, Hong Kong Special Administrative Region of China, People's Republic of China

Miaoru Zhang
Department of Diagnostic Radiology, The University of Hong Kong, Hong Kong Special Administrative Region of China, People's Republic of China

Chapter 1

Machine learning in medicine—focus on radiology

Jie Lian, Fan Huang, Miaoru Zhang, Kei Shing Ng and Varut Vardhanabhuti

1.1 Artificial intelligence in radiology imaging

Artificial intelligence (AI) is increasingly being used in a variety of health care applications, including drug development, remote patient monitoring, medical diagnostics and imaging, wearables, virtual assistants, and hospital administration. Many areas that rely on large data are also predicted to gain from the deployment of AI. Medical fields that rely on imaging data, such as radiology, pathology, dermatology, and ophthalmology, have already reaped the benefits of AI applications. Radiologists are trained to visually examine medical imaging and report results to detect, define, and monitor various diseases. Such evaluations are frequently based on education, training, and experience. Over time, radiologists are trained to a diagnose complex constellation of findings with medical insights and reasoning, although as with any human-centric tasks, these may be prone to subjectivity. Emerging now are various AI radiological applications, although these have been mainly targeting certain specific diagnostic tasks. In comparison to human-centric qualitative reasoning, the strength of AI may be to tackle repetitive but straightforward tasks or deliver an automated quantitative extraction of imaging features longitudinally. When AI is integrated into the clinical process as a tool to aid clinicians, more accurate and repeatable radiological assessments may be performed. This section will review the application of AI technologies in the radiology imaging field.

1.1.1 Object segmentation

In diagnostic radiology, the visual interpretation by certificated radiologists is crucial when studying the medical images of patients. However, reading the images and writing radiology reports take time and are frequently subjective, depending

doi:10.1088/978-0-7503-4637-5ch1

on the radiologist's experience. Apart from the diagnostic usage, big data analysis on medical images also received lots of interest. Computed tomography (CT) represents an ideal body imaging modality with vast potential. It is used widely in routine clinical practices and provides robust and objective volumetric data that over the years have standardised acquisition and protocols, making them relatively reproducible and consistent across patients. Moreover, the specific body coverage scanning, such as the abdominal CT scans, contains rich body composition data that can be quantitatively measured. These CT biomarkers, including organ size and attenuation coefficients (Hounsfield unit; HU), muscle mass and density, visceral and subcutaneous fat, and liver fat content, have emerged as additional tools in the radiology armoury to help with various tasks such as the initial disease diagnosis and studying the progression in tumour diseases [1], but they also have paved new quantitative population-based assessments utilising a big data approach [2–4].

To enable large-scale data extraction based on various body regions, automatic medical image segmentation is the first and one of the most important steps toward computer-aided medical image analysis (see figure 1.1). Its objective is to generate a pixel-to-pixel mapping, from the original images to categorical maps. Commonly in the categorical maps, the pixels values of 0 represent the background, and the pixels values of 1, 2, 3, ..., indicate the locations of interests (e.g. liver, kidney, nodule, and fat compartment, etc).

The recent advancement in deep learning (DL) techniques has brought a breakthrough to AI, most notably with the use of convolutional neural networks (CNNs). The CNN models (see figure 1.2) can extract non-handcrafted features from diverse medical images if human annotations are provided. By further processing these deep features, the CNN models can perform a series of tasks, including segmentation, detection, classification, and disease prediction [5–7].

This subsection introduces some of the essential steps for training a neural network for medical image segmentation. We focus on the multi-organ segmentation tasks on abdominal CT scans. We will first introduce some publicly available datasets for various segmentation tasks. Then we will introduce some pre-processing steps before the network training. Finally, several commonly used network architectures will be introduced.

1.1.1.1 Publicly available datasets

The abnormalities in density, shape and textures are commonly assessed on CT scans. Liver cancer, or hepatocellular carcinoma (HCC), is one of the most common cancers in the world and is the main cause of death in all cancers [8]. HCC accounts for about 80% of all primary liver cancers, and most patients with chronic liver disease may develop HCC eventually. Automatic liver tumour segmentation (LiTS) is being applied to improve the interpretation components of medical imaging. Apart from the liver tumour, the liver is also subject to diverse pathologies that could modify its density, namely, attenuation coefficient (HU) and morphological shape and size.

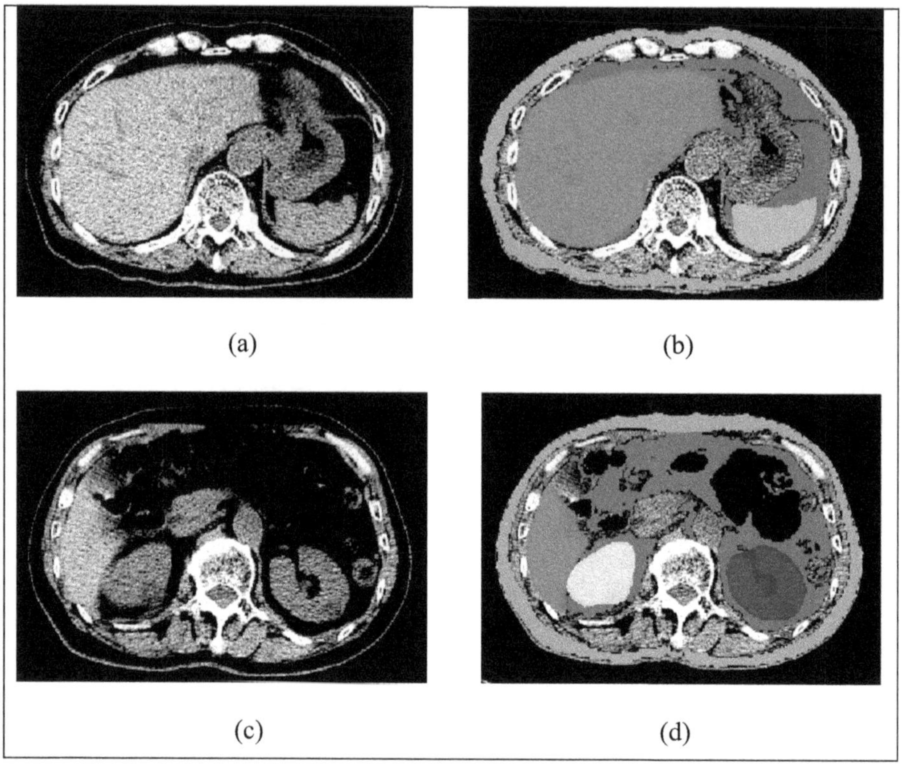

Figure 1.1. Organ segmentation is essential for medical image analysis. Its objective is to generate a binary pixel-to-pixel mapping of the original images. Commonly, the pixel values of 1 are the foreground indicating the location of regions of interest (e.g. organs, tumour, nodule, fat compartment, etc), and the pixel values of 0 are the background. (a) and (c): original non-contrast CT scans; (b) and (d): The segmentations for multiple organs/tissues including liver (red), spleen (green), left kidney (blue), right kidney (yellow), visceral fat (purple), and subcutaneous fat (pink).

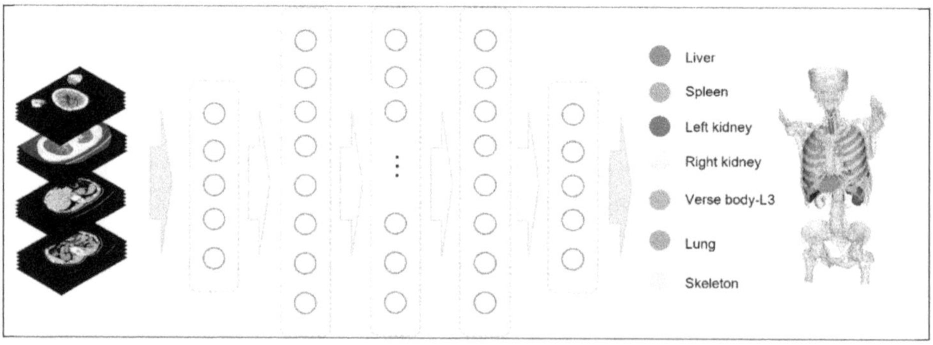

Figure 1.2. A CNN model can extract non-handcrafted features from diverse medical images with human labelled structures.

- Liver and LiTS

  There are multiple publicly available datasets for developing automatic liver and LiTS on abdominal CT scans. Most of the data are contrast-enhanced CT scans in the portal venous phase, which is the most common examination in a standard post-contrast CT abdomen in clinical practice.

  The SLIVER07 dataset was used to compare different algorithms to segment the liver from clinical 3D CT scans on the workshop 'Segmentation in the Clinic: A Grand Challenge' in conjunction with International Conference on Medical Image Computer Assisted Intervention (MICCAI) 2007 [1]. It contains 20 training scans and 10 test scans. The images were contrast-enhanced CT scans acquired in the portal venous phase. The image data are isotropic pixel spacing (approximated $0.8 \times 0.8 \times 0.8$ mm).

  The LiTS dataset contains 200 contrast-enhanced CT scans, in which 130 cases were for training and 70 cases were for evaluation [9]. The image data were from patients with HCC or colorectal cancer; thus, the human annotations include both the liver contour and the liver tumour locations. The CT scans (axial slices) have resolutions of 512×512 pixels with various pixel sizes ranging from 0.625 to 1.0 mm. The slice thickness was variable, between 0.7 and 5 mm.

  The liver data from the Visual Sweden project DROID data consist of 77 CT abdominal examinations taken with contrast in the portal venous phase [10]. All the scans showed liver malignancies. In total, 317 lesions were annotated and reviewed by two radiologists. The livers were not delineated.
- Kidney

  Kidney cancer incidence is growing in both developed countries and developing countries, affecting elderly patients between 60 and 70 years [11]. Automatic kidney and kidney tumour segmentation produce a rich quantitative representation of the organs for various proposed nephrometry scoring systems, e.g. the RENAL system (Radius, Exophytic/endophytic tumor location, Nearness to the renal collecting system, Anterior or posterior location and Location relative to the renal poles) [12], the PADUA system (Preoperative Aspects and Dimensions Used for an Anatomical classification) [13], and the Centrality Index [14].

  To develop automatic kidney and kidney tumour segmentation techniques, the Kidney and Kidney Tumour Segmentation Challenge 2019 and 2021 (KiTS19 and KiTS21) were held in 2019 and 2021 in conjunction with the MICCAI 2019 and 2021 [15], respectively. The KiTS19 dataset consisted of 300 patients (210 were referred to as training set and 90 as the testing set), who underwent partial or radical nephrectomy for suspected renal cancer. Moreover, the KiTS21 dataset consisted of extra 300 patients with the same inclusion/exclusion criteria as the KiTS19.
- Pancreas

  The Pancreas-CT dataset consists of 82 abdominal contrast-enhanced CT scans retrieved from The Cancer Imaging Archive [16], including 53 men and 27 women. Among all the subjects, 17 were healthy kidney donors scanned prior to nephrectomy, and the remaining 65 patients were selected by a radiologist from patients who had neither major abdominal pathologies nor pancreatic cancer lesions. The CT scans have resolutions of 512 × 512 pixels with varying pixel sizes; the slice thickness was between 1.5 and 2.5 mm.

- Spine bone

  Spine bone or vertebral body segmentation is crucial in the automated quantification of spinal morphology and pathology. In addition, it is a robust reference landmark for comparison across subjects. Such as in the work by Pickhardt *et al*, multiple CT biomarkers, including the visceral-to-subcutaneous fat ratio, mean muscle density, and volumetric liver density, were measured on the spine L1 and L3 and the axial slices between the L1 and L4 level [3].

  The Large Scale Vertebrae Segmentation Challenge dataset consisted of 374 scans from 355 patients [17]. This was a multi-centre study, and the image data were acquired using different CT scanners (GE, Siemens, Phillips, and Toshiba). It also consists of a variety of fields of view (e.g. cervical, thoraco-to-lumbar, and cervico-thoraco-lumbar scans) and a mix of sagittal and isotropic reformations. In terms of the human annotations, the labels of 7 cervical bones (C1–C7), 12 thoracic bones (T1–T12), and 5 lumbar bones (L1–L5) are provided. For some of the cases, labels of L6 and T13 were provided due to normal anatomical variations.

- Multi-organ segmentation

  The above mentioned datasets are limited to a single organ. However, a few recent works have explored the feasibility of training a multi-organ segmentation network using multiple datasets with partially labelled data [18]. It is still a challenging task to simply combine all the data together for multi-organ segmentation since this requires consistent labelling of all objects of interest across all the images. Thus, a few datasets provide the human annotations for multiple organs, allowing researchers to train their models for multi-organ segmentation tasks.

  The CT-ORG consists of 140 whole-body CT scans, each of which has 6 organs labelled in 3D [19]. The image data are initially from the LiTS19 challenge and expanded to other organs, including lungs, bladder, kidney, bones, and brain. The data are divided into 119 training volumes and 21 testing volumes, which were annotated to a higher degree of accuracy for certain organs. The data exhibit a wide variety of imaging conditions collected from various medical centres to ensure the generalisability of the trained models.

  The Combined Healthy Abdominal Organ Segmentation (CHAOS) dataset consisted of two subsets: (1) 40 abdominal contrast-enhanced CT scans with liver annotated and (2) 40 magnetic resonance imaging (MRI) scans (T1 and T2 weighted) with liver, spleen, and right/left kidneys annotated. The CT and MRI scans were from different subjects and were not registered [20].

  The Beyond the Cranial Vault dataset comprises 50 abdominal CT scans from patients with metastatic liver cancer or post-operative ventral hernia. Human labels include the spleen, left and right kidney, gallbladder, oesophagus, liver, stomach, aorta, inferior vena cava, portal vein and splenic vein, pancreas, right adrenal gland, and left adrenal gland [21].

1.1.1.2 Internal datasets

Despite publicly available image datasets, researchers would like to create human labelling on their datasets to fine-tune pre-trained models and validation. Normally, the delineations of organs were drawn by students with medical background knowledge, and tumour lesions were drawn by experienced radiologists. Commonly used annotation platforms are 3D Slicer [22] and ITK-Snap [23]. Most of the time, the approach to annotation is to perform them on the axial view slice by slice and further refine on the coronal/sagittal views.

The annotation works can also be done semi-automatically via traditional machine learning (ML) techniques, including intensity thresholding and region growing. For instance, in non-contrast CT images, the pixel density represents the HU scale, which is the linear transformation of the original radiation attenuation coefficient of various materials in the body. For example, the HU of water and air are 0 and −1000, respectively. Therefore, the bone, organs (e.g. liver and kidney), muscle tissues, and fat tissue can be briefly separated by simply threshold the HU scales. On the other hand, the region-growing method partitions the image into separate regions that share the same similarity properties (e.g. pixel density). Thresholding works efficiently for segmenting liver tissue, visceral fat, and muscle tissue, while it requires the foreground to have a sharp boundary. Otherwise the segmentation might not be consistent at the edges and will need further modification.

1.1.1.3 Data pre-processing

Before training the segmentation network, the raw data must be pre-processed. Common pre-processing steps include resampling all the image data's spatial resolution (pixel spacing) to a common resolution. The images were mostly down-sampled to a lower resolution because up-sampling cannot ensure the accuracy of the resultant image and could introduce unexpected artefacts. Additionally, the CT density can be limited to a specific HU range (−1000, +1000) or a preferred window level (e.g. soft-tissue window (−100, 400) to exclude irrelevant organs and objects [24]. For network training, a common approach of image augmentations can be performed. These include scaling (slightly changing the pixel spacing), rotations (with a reasonable degree range (e.g. (−5°, 5°)) along the x-, y-, and z-axis), brightness, contrast, a gamma transformation, and the introduction of Gaussian noise.

1.1.1.4 Deep neural network architecture

In this section, we introduced a few deep neural network architectures that were commonly used in multiple medical image segmentation challenges. Most of the segmentation networks used the U-Net architecture proposed by Ronneberger *et al* [25]. It is a CNN based on the fully convolutional network (FCN) family [26]. It replaces the pooling operations (i.e. contracting path) used in the second half of a regular FCN by up-sampling operators (i.e. expansion path), yielding a symmetric

U-shape architecture. U-Net increases the resolution of the output and allows the network to propagate contextual information to higher resolution layers.

Christ *et al* trained two separated 2D U-Net for liver and LiTS on abdominal axial slices. Afterwards, the U-Net segmentation results were refined by a 3D conditional random fields model, which applies the locality information across adjacent slices [24].

The framework proposed by Tian *et al* integrated both image interpretation and patients' diagnostic reports. It utilised a fully CNN to segment 2D CT slices and a separate long short-term memory (LSTM) language model to generate captions from diagnostic reports, which might be regarded as interpretations accompanying segmentation [27]. This framework won first place in the LiTS task.

The H-Dense U-Net proposed by Li *et al* contains one 2.5D Dense U-Net followed by a 3D Dense U-Net [28]. The 2.5D Dense-U-Net takes three adjacent slices as input and predicts the segmentation for the middle slice. This configuration explored hybrid representative in-plane features and neglected the spatial information along the axial axis. Afterwards, the 2D segmentations were concatenated into 3D volume. A 3D Dense U-Net were trained on the concatenated volume and produced the final liver and LiTS. This model won third place for liver segmentation and first place for LiTS in the LiTS19 challenge.

The MedicalNet, developed by the Tencent YouTu X-Lab, used a pre-trained 3D ResNet [29] as the backbone and re-trained on the medical data with diverse imaging modalities, target organs, and pathologies using the concept of transfer learning [18]. The ResNet architecture was constructed by a sequence of blocks containing convolution layers and pooling layers, reducing the image/feature map resolutions. Afterwards, an up-sampling interpolation is needed to rescale the ResNet output back to the original resolution to provide the segmentation map.

The nnU-Net, proposed by Isensee *et al*, who won first place in the LiTS19 challenge, was designed to deal with the dataset diversity found in the domain. It condenses and automates the critical decisions for designing a successful segmentation pipeline for any given dataset [30]. The framework implemented extensive preprocessing steps to generate diverse training data based on the available data with limited ground truth annotations. The backbone of nnU-Net contains a 2D U-Net, 3D full resolution U-Net, and 3D U-Net cascade (in both low and full resolutions). Therefore, the training period of nnU-Net is much more extended than training a regular FCN, but once the network has been trained, the segmentation results usually outperform the others.

1.1.2 Abnormality detection

Abnormality detection is one of the significant tasks in the diagnostic workflow. It is one of the earliest areas that AI has attempted to tackle within the medical imaging domain, especially radiology. The common radiology modalities include radiography, CT, mammography images, ultrasound images, MRI, nuclear medicine imaging, and positron emission tomography, to name a few. On the other hand, medical images can also be challenging to analyse; in comparison to conventional

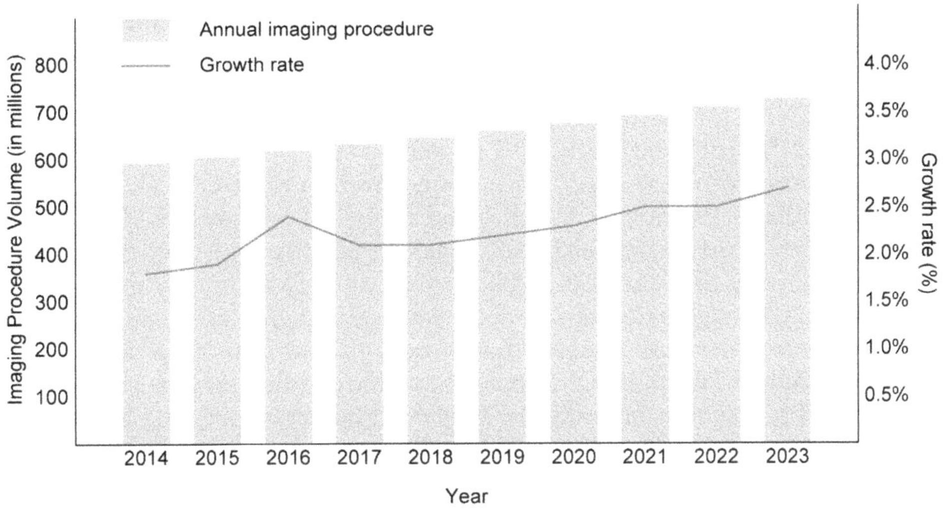

Figure 1.3. Diagnostic imaging procedure volume in the United States.

computer vision tasks, the abnormality can be a small area in a whole imaging stack or volumes, which requires special consideration when training. However, there is a potentially significant benefit as a chronic shortage of radiologists remains a problem despite the ever-increasing workload requiring radiology images interpretation (see figure 1.3).

These problems can be solved by AI. ML is a form of AI which functions without being precisely programmed. It learns from data and makes predictions or decisions based on that data. There are three types of learning in ML, including supervised learning, unsupervised learning, and semi-supervised learning. The selection of significant features for a specific problem requires domain expertise and ML techniques. Features can be selected using DL techniques. DL can be considered as a specific subset of ML, enabling the automatic extraction of essential features from raw input data. DL algorithms (DLAs) are based on cognitive and information theories. There are two basic properties of DL: (1) multiple layers of abstraction that learn distinct features of data and (2) learning whether features are presented unsupervised or supervised.

Different DLAs have been adapted from computer vision and applied to various types of medical image analysis. Recurrent neural networks (RNNs) and CNNs are traditional examples of supervised DLA, although these can also learn in an unsupervised way. Medical image analysis has also investigated unsupervised learning algorithms, such as deep belief networks, restricted Boltzmann machines, autoencoders, and generative adversarial networks (GANs). The DLA can detect an abnormality and classify a specific disease. CNN is an artificial visual neural network structure used for medical image pattern recognition based on convolution operation (see figure 1.2). Regarding medical images, CNNs are ideal for classification, segmentation, object detection, registration, and other tasks.

Researchers have trained various deep neural networks to analyse medical images and detect abnormalities. Chiu *et al* [31] created a DL AI model, called COV19NET, which is designed for the detection of COVID-19 on frontal-view chest x-ray (CXR), with a model pre-trained on ImageNet. Chamberlin *et al* [32] employed a CNN prototype (AI-RAD Companion, Siemens Healthineers) to detect lung nodules and coronary artery calcium on low-dose chest CT. The AI process involves a cardiac segmentation model based on U-Net architecture. Training and validation were based on 660 chest CT scans to identify and crop the region of interest surrounding the heart. Candidate voxels were placed in the cardiac area by thresholding. An image patch of 32 × 32 pixels surrounding each candidate voxel and the corresponding prior likelihood map were employed as image features. The spatial coordinates of the point in the patient-specific coordinate system were utilised as additional features. Furthermore, an AI-RAD also performed lung lobe segmentation for nodule localisation. The AI model for lung nodule detection, localisation, and segmentation was trained on 5000 manually curated chest CT scans and validated against 129 different CT datasets. Chougrad *et al* [33] used transfer learning from raw images to breast cancer images by combining state-of-art architectures such as VGG16, ResNet50, and Inception, which were pre-trained on ImageNet. It aids the radiologist in the classification of mammography mass lesions. Hajabdollahi *et al* [34] introduced the Bifurcated CNN to detect more than one abnormality for common types of gastrointestinal symptoms concurrently with the minimal use of computational resources.

1.1.3 Abnormality characterisation

In recent research, the DLA can accurately identify nine different abnormalities in the brain CT scan [35]. Brain CT is one of the most critical imaging diagnostic methods to evaluate intracranial abnormalities, particularly in acute settings. Brain CT scans can represent several pathologies, allowing for accurate localisation of lesions in terms of number, location, size, contour, density, as well as the presence of intracranial haemorrhage and calcification. The common findings on emergency brain CT include skull fracture, epidural haematoma, subdural haematoma, subarachnoid haemorrhage, hypertensive cerebral haemorrhage, and so on.

Various AI systems have been developed, which have shown high areas under the curve (AUCs) ranging from 0.848 to 0.945 [36, 37], to provide an auxiliary diagnosis for lung nodules and lung diseases. It can replace and assist human eyes intelligently to detect and recognise lung nodules and pneumonia on CT images as well as to detect other suspected lesions. After the lesion is marked, the doctor will perform a second screening to diagnose lung diseases more accurately and quickly, including new pneumonia. At the same time, this system can also assist in screening early images of new pneumonia. The intelligent assisted diagnosis technology in the system can automatically detect and analyse lesions on CT lung images of patients and quickly detect various signs of different types of pneumonia. It has a high detection rate for signs such as patchy shadows, ground-glass opacities, and streaky scarring changes. Another significant research result is from the Google Health team [38], which mainly revealed the difference between DL of normal and abnormal chest radiographs and the generalisation of two diseases that are not obvious causative factors of tuberculosis and COVID-19.

AI algorithms can be used to identify cases that are less likely to be abnormal, helping health care professionals to rule out specific differential diagnoses quickly, and spend more working time in treating the disease. More importantly, it is necessary to conduct an AI evaluation of abnormal CXR that has not been encountered during the development process to verify its robustness to new diseases or manifestations of new diseases. Google researchers [38] pointed out in the paper that, in some cases, their DL model has more significant advantages in radiological detection, which can significantly improve the work efficiency of radiologists.

1.1.4 Outcome prediction

As previously noted, AI-based segmentation, detection, and diagnostic techniques have progressed significantly over the last decade [39–41]. In many cases, their ability has matched or even surpassed human specialists, especially in some specific disease areas. As a result of this success, AI technologies are now being used on more complex decision-making tasks, such as disease prognosis and treatment response prediction.

Biomarkers are commonly employed in the medical field to determine the likelihood of a given disease-related endpoint and the overall risk of patient survival [42]. In terms of survival-related biomarkers, prognostic biomarkers are developed by assessing a patient's risk profile utilising tumour feature information. This helps with risk stratification and could be used to plan treatment strategies. For example, if a patient has a biomarker score indicating high risk, these people can then be directed to clinical trials or receive a more advanced degree of treatment. On the other hand, if cancer is found early, patients with good prognosis may benefit from de-escalated therapy and avoid the physical and financial burden associated with cancer treatment (e.g. omitting chemotherapy after surgery to avoid the risk of treatment-related toxicity). These decision processes must be tailored to an individual patient, but having a more accurate biomarker for prognostication will aid this decision-making process. As a result of rapid advancements in computer vision and pattern recognition, AI-enabled imaging biomarkers have developed in recent years. Radiological biomarkers are derived by extracting quantitative representations of tumour phenotypic features associated with clinical information.

1.1.4.1 AI-enhanced biomarkers

In radiology, AI-enhanced biomarkers are classified into two broad categories: handcrafted radiomics approach [43, 44] and DL approach [45]. Handcrafted radiomic features are created to represent a collection of tumour characteristics shown in medical images captured by radiologists, oncologists, and computer scientists based on a defined region of interest with the extraction of features based on the underlying imaging properties. Following the feature extraction phase, some statistics, ML, or DL models can be used to predict the outcome of an experiment using these image-based biomarkers. While the second technique utilises deep neural network models to produce deep texture features automatically from images and make predictions for individual patients.

- Handcrafted radiomic biomarkers

  With the growing popularity of Python, there have been several well-designed public radiomics toolkits [46, 47] that include the most often used feature computation functions. After inputting the tumour segments images, users may calculate all the relevant characteristics using a single line of Python code. Additionally, users may be able to include some custom-built radiomic features into their work without creating the feature pipeline themselves.

Numerous study findings indicate that a variety of radiomic features are generally effective at predicting outcomes. Those most used radiomic features can be categorised as follows (table 1.1).

In principle, after computing all the above radiomics features, a common first step in this approach is algorithmically filtering down many generated features to only a few that are most appropriate for the study aim. By selecting the most suitable features, predictive performance [51] or enhanced resilience and stability [52] can be obtained. Finally, a statistical ML model or a DL model will be used to predict individuals' clinical outcomes using these selected features [53]. For instance, Xie applied the least absolute shrinkage and selection operator method to reduce

Table 1.1. Radiomic features category.

Feature category	Description
First-order features [48]	Applying commonly used and simple metrics, first-order statistics quantify the distribution of voxel intensities inside the target region designated by the mask, for instance, maximum, minimum, mean, median, 10 percentile, and 90 percentile intensities values.
Shape-based features [48]	This category of characteristics includes descriptions describing the region of interest (ROI)'s 2D and 3D size and shape, which are not dependent on the grey level intensity distribution inside the ROI. Shape features include metrics about tumour volume, surfaces, sphericity, compactness and so on.
Grey level features	There are several grey level metrics that are used for image texture analysis. • **Grey level co-occurrence matrix (GLCM) features** [49]: The second-order joint probability function of an image region bounded by the mask is described by a GLCM. • **Grey level size zone matrix (GLSZM) features** [49]: Images' grey levels can be measured with a GLSZM. A single GLSZM matrix is computed for all directions in the ROI, making it rotation independent. • **Grey level dependence matrix (GLDM) features** [50]: The GLDM tests the correlation with an image's grey levels.

feature dimension and make predictions [53]. Other feature reduction methods such as principal component analysis, Least Absolute Shrinkage and Selection Operator (LASSO), or analysing robustness to resampling; reproducibility between observers; and redundancy methods are also commonly used, followed by a set of prediction models for survival analysis [54, 55]. The approaches for feature reduction and prediction model selection vary, and researchers should carefully assess their options considering their research questions.

1.1.4.2 Deep learning biomarkers

A deep neural network uses non-linear operations to transform input data into a representation that may be used to identify patterns in the data. The input data is further abstracted into a deep representation as successive layers apply modifications to it. Finally, the network's last layer can produce desired outputs, such as the likelihood of a treatment outcome. CNNs are commonly used to derive predictions from imaging data in DL biomarker applications in radiology. In recent years, CNNs have gained a lot of interest because of their ability to understand spatial patterns in the medical vision field and their success in diagnostic tasks. In this case, it is believed that the convolutional layers of a CNN may be taught to distinguish new imaging features that are indicative of a patient's prognosis.

Currently, there are two general methods to apply DL biomarkers for individuals. In the first scenario, researchers construct deep neural networks that can be trained with vast amounts of medical images directly to generate new representations that can be synthesised to make predictions about specific outcomes. In this case, the input of the network will be individual patients' medical images while a prognostic risk score will be generated automatically as output.

DL models require a large quantity of training data, and their performance typically improves as additional data are provided to learn. This is a challenge, however, because it is not always possible to get access to large medical images datasets in the real world. The second technique, inspired by the concept of Transfer Learning, employs pre-trained deep neural networks to generate deep medical image features. These pre-trained models have been extensively trained on publicly available datasets, which include images from both the natural world (e.g. ImageNet [56]) and the medical area (e.g. MedicalNet [18]), and those features can be extracted from the middle of the final layer prior to classification layer. It is assumed that these deep image biomarkers may be applied to perform prognostic analysis using statistical ML or DL models. After generating the above AI-enhanced biomarkers, a prognostic model can be built to predict individual patients' outcomes such as disease-free survival or overall survival or can also be applied to predict individual response to therapy [57]. For instance, Hu extracted DL features from pre-trained ResNet50 and applied SVM to predict treatment response in patients with oesophageal cancer undergoing neoadjuvant chemoradiotherapy prior to surgery, reaching an AUC score of 0.771. While DL-generated features often have a high representation capacity for survival analysis, performance can suffer dramatically in some circumstances due to a scarcity of training data. Whether to use DL-generated features or radiomics-generated features remains an ongoing research subject, and both the research question and the data size should be considered.

1.1.5 Challenges and opportunities

Although AI-enhanced biomarkers have already been widely used in research, there are some challenges, particularly when it comes to the widespread implementation and adoption of such tools. In this section, we will discuss the challenges and opportunities in AI prognostic outcome prediction.

- Data imbalance
  When making predictions for a binary classification task (or even multi-class classification), there is an assumption that both the positive and negative cases are relatively equal in numbers, which is hard to be achieved in clinical practice. For example, when it comes to early-stage lung cancer survival prediction, more than 80% of patients survive after 5 years, which means that conventional models learn extensively from survived cases while overlooking critical information from death cases. Training on such imbalanced data often does not yield satisfactory performance, and researchers have attempted to resolve the issue using various resampling approaches such as ADASYN or SMOTE [58]. However, due to their inherent limitations, it is unknown if those resampling strategies can demonstrate dependable performance in medical practice, and how to cope with unbalanced data distributions remains a concern for researchers.
- Data acquisition and annotation
  Designing an AI-based model from appropriate data is always a challenge, and it becomes even more challenging when developing predictive and prognostic radiology AI tools. Due to the difficulty of obtaining big medical imaging datasets and the need to continually follow strict inclusion/exclusion criteria, this may result in inefficient learning for AI systems. Additionally, certain handcrafted radiomics features require precise tumour segment inputs, which requires the expert radiologist to create masks manually. This is time-consuming and may involve human error when dealing with large datasets. While researchers have attempted to apply GAN models to learn and generate data and labels for dealing with the problems in general, due to the complexity of medical data, it has not been widely used in the medical field yet. As a result, obtaining appropriate training data with annotation masks still presents a challenge for future studies.
- Consistency and replicability
  One of the key obstacles for AI imaging approaches before being adopted in clinical use is reproducibility over a wide range of acquisition processes, institutions, and patient populations. In some research, from training to independent validation, the performance metrics of most radiomic approaches decline precipitously [59, 60]. In this case, developing with more generalised and robust AI-enhanced features to improve models' replicability remains an open problem.

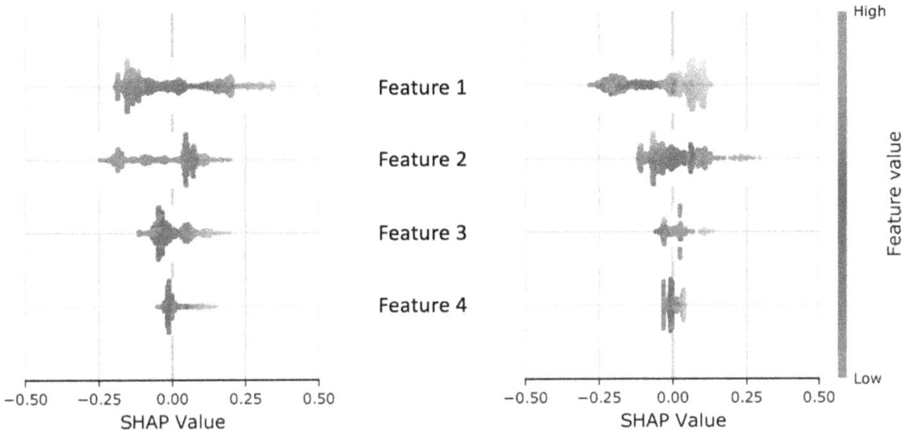

Figure 1.4. An example plot of SHAP values showing the impact of different features in the machine learning model on the output prediction of the model. A high positive SHAP indicates a feature driving the output score higher (increasing risk), and vice versa.

- Interpretability

  AI-enabled biomarkers have an interpretability problem before they can be widely deployed. It is possible to gain some insight into how AI algorithms make their decisions using handcrafted radiomic tools, for example, using Local Interpretable Model-Agnostic Explanations (LIME) technique or SHapley Additive exPlanations analysis (see figure 1.4). However, with DL techniques, it is often not easy to decipher explanation, due to the inherent 'black-box' nature. This is an area of active research. Especially in the medical imaging field, researchers are trying to use visualisation or attribution-based methods to explain the models' prediction [61]. In [62], an approach inspired by DeepDreams [63] was presented for explaining the segmentation of tumours from liver CT images. It assessed the sensitivity of the characteristics by maximising the activity of the target neuron by gradient ascent, that is, finding the function's steepest slope. While it gave some intuition for explaining the medical DL model, it is a long way from fully comprehending its inner workings. Some researchers believe that interpretable models should be developed from the start [64], and it is widely believed that explainable AI should be developed further in this field [65].

1.2 AI in learning radiology reports

1.2.1 Automatic data mining on text report

Data mining in the biomedical document is becoming increasingly important in medical big data analysis. In the medical field, electronic medical records (EMRs) contain patients' medical history and examination measurements. The diagnostic reports written by radiologists after the visual interpretation of patients' medical images, not only summarise their diagnostic findings but also usually include other relevant measurements (e.g. lesion size, the density of organ parts, etc). However, there is often little in the way of standardisation, and only a few EMRs are set up in such a way that data are fully structured. The majority are semi-structured and unstructured data, which are hard to derive useful information from at scale. Therefore, ML-based natural language processing (NLP) techniques were developed to analyse dozens of text documents and extract meaningful information automatically.

Named entity recognition (NER) is one of the most fundamental biomedical text mining tasks, which involves recognising numerous domain-specific proper nouns in a biomedical corpus. The goal for NER is to automatically extract desired information, such as tumour location, size, appearance, and so on, converting an unstructured/semi-structured text document to the structured one.

Another data mining application on EMR is the question answering (QA), a task of answering questions posed in semi-structured/unstructured clinical texts, such as diagnostic reports. In QA, a piece of text and a set of questions were given to an ML model. The model would answer these questions based on the given clinical text, which attempts to discover potential information.

The Bidirectional Encoder Representations from Transformers for Biomedical Text Mining (Bio-BERT) is a pre-trained NLP transformer developed for medical domain–specific language representation. The model used a pre-trained BERT model as the backbone [66], which had been trained beforehand with the general domain texts extracted from BooksCorpus (0.8 billion words) [67] and English Wikipedia (2.5 billion words). The authors of Bio-BERT fine-tuned and re-trained the BERT model using the texts extracted from PubMed abstracts (4.5 billion words) and PMC full-text articles (13.5 billion words), which contain a wide range of terms relevant to the medical field. The Bio-BERT model's performance out-performed the general BERT model on medical text mining tasks. It has been fine-tuned and adapted for multiple tasks such as the mentioned NER and QA problems.

1.2.2 Automatically radiology report generation system

The interpretation of medical images such as CT and MRI is a complex task and requires extensive training. As it is a visual detection and perception task, human errors may exist during this process. With the concern of increasing demands for the accurate interpretation of medical images and increasing time pressure in existing medical practices, an automatic medical imaging report generation model can be helpful to alleviate the labour-intensive task. With the advancement of AI technology, researchers are now attempting to use DL approaches to generate radiology reports automatically. The majority of existing approaches employ similar network architectures, such as a CNN encoder and an RNN decoder [68], with the encoder extracting information from the image and the decoder producing language descriptions (see figure 1.5). Within this structure, to connect the images and semantics selectively, attention algorithms have been widely used in captioning features.

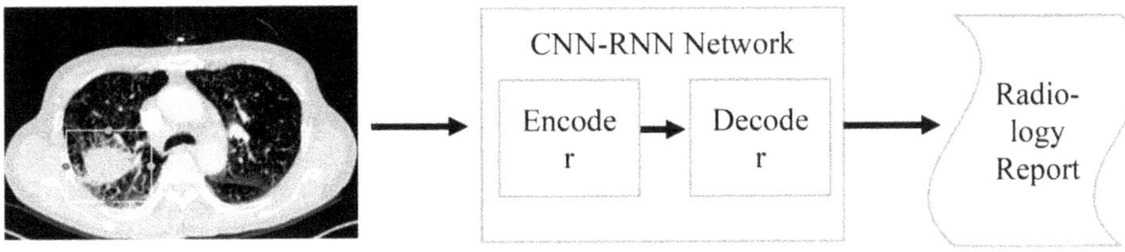

Figure 1.5. Automatically radiology report generation process.

The key question in this topic is to select a proper decoder and design reasonable attention algorithms. Recent studies on the generation of radiological reports have revealed encouraging outcomes. A hierarchical LSTM decoder has been used to construct medical imaging reports [69] that incorporate visual and tag attentions for paragraph-level production. A visual attentions iterative decoder is developed to enforce the sentence coherence [70]. Recently, the NLP community has begun to transition away from recurrent models, which have been found to be slower to train and less able to take advantage of GPU parallelisation than attention-only–based models known as transformers [66, 71, 72]. The NLP community reached the transfer learning phase that computer vision experienced after ImageNet with the widespread usage of transformer-based models. Fine-tuning a pre-trained Transformer model on a large corpus is now the preferred method for most NLP research. Because applying a pre-trained transformer has advantages like quicker training, eliminating the need to define a vocabulary, and already learning word structure and punctuation, it is believed that investigating the utility of applying existing pre-trained transformers on radiology report generation tasks will be the next opportunity for the AI in radiology reports field.

1.3 AI in radiology practice

There has been increasing interest in using AI to improve radiology over the last decade. Numerous AI applications are currently in development, with potential benefits involving all stages of the imaging chain, AI has shown great potential on optimising patient scheduling, improving worklist management, improving image acquisition, and assisting radiologists in the interpretation of diagnostic studies. Furthermore, while the current use of AI in radiology has been focused on clinical applications, some of which are still in the distant future, it is becoming increasingly clear that AI algorithms could be used soon for a variety of non-interpretive and quality improvement purposes.

1.3.1 Improving radiographic workflow

1.3.1.1 Pre-examination assessment of patients

As part of the imaging workflow, radiographers need to check patients' identification and indications of the requested examination and inform patients of related examination potential risks before the start of the scanning procedure. These processes all require radiographers to have direct contact and time-consuming communication with each patient.

AI systems can help with automated approval of patient referral, which could be done by pre-screening a pre-approved list of clinical indications and matching to the appropriate imaging techniques to be used and confirming patient identification by interaction with the hospital's electronic health record system. AI chatbot systems could be utilised in patient communication regarding the pre-procedural preparations and answer any queries regarding potential risks of such procedures. In that case, the interaction time between radiographers and patients can be shortened and lower the potential exposure risk of transmittable diseases, and the scanning procedure and workflow will be more efficient. Thereafter, radiographer oversights are required to match patient electronic health record data and consistent AI decisions [73].

1.3.1.2 Imaging production and quality control

Several recent advances in applying AI to image reconstruction for a variety of image modalities (e.g. CT, PET, and MRI) have been made. Imaging time, radiation dose, and contrast dose have been reduced because of these techniques, while image quality has improved.

- Noise reduction

  DL techniques have been applied to minimise imaging noise and artefacts, improve image contrast, and improve pathology visualisation [74]. In the early stage, DL approaches would have the shortcoming of over-smoothing effect on images, resulting in loss of features and making critical structures less visible [75]. Recently, CNNs and GANs have addressed this issue, which can produce de-noised images without the loss of key information [76, 77].

  AI can either act on the processed image or directly turn the raw sensor scanning data into images to improve image quality, and then a post-processing strategy is added to reduce artefacts and noise [78–80]. Previously developed AI-based algorithms, such as AUTOMAP, may be immediately applied to sensor data to improve performance. AUTOMAP employs DL techniques to generate higher-quality MR images with better noise immunity and fewer reconstruction artefacts than traditional reconstruction algorithms, and no extra information is needed [79].
- Optimisation of scanning protocol

  In recent years, the radiation exposure of increasing CT and PET scanning and wide usage of gadolinium-based contrast agents have attracted much public attention. Nowadays, DL techniques have been used to reduce radiation dose, contrast agents' usage, and scanning time. The most common way to reduce CT radiation exposure is to lower the x-ray tube current, which means that fewer x-ray photons are produced in every scan and noisier images would be produced. DL approaches have recently shown the potential to reduce radiation and contrast dosage while maintaining image quality. Initial dosage reduction methods based on ML produced hazy and over-smoothed images. Currently, algorithms like CNNs and GAN have achieved a good balance between image smoothing and feature retention [81].

It has been reported that one AI model can make high-resolution images from low-dose raw sensor data after training with the imaging features of normal anatomical structures and abnormalities on images with low and standard radiation doses [82]. Such techniques have been applied to help generate high-quality CT and PET images. Residual learning is to study the low-dose CT produced artefacts and remove streak artefacts during the reconstruction of low-dose CT images [83]. Furthermore, DL techniques have been used to create fewer but higher-quality motion artefacts affecting post-contrast MRI images, with only 10% of the standard gadolinium dosage used [84].

Many other aspects of imaging quality control and improvement in CT and MRI have improved with the DL application, including the removal or reduction of CT metal artefact, MRI banding artefact, MRI motion artefact, and enhancement of spatial resolution [85–87]. To shorten the scanning time of MRI, some sacrifices like relative impairment of imaging quality and incomplete k-space sampling in MR sequences might occur. However, these might result in a longer reconstruction time after scanning. CNN has been applied to learn a mapping between zero-filled and fully sampled MR images and used to reconstruct images from undersampled k-space data [88]. DL has also been used to recreate MRI images from clinical multi-coil MRI data, which uses parallel imaging for shortening scan duration [89]. All methods mentioned above can significantly reduce the time to produce MRI images with good quality.

After scanning, the assessment of image quality is commonly done by radiographers immediately after scanning or radiologists on duty, but this is not always the case. In some cases, some significant problems may be missed by the initial screening. There might exist some phenomena such as some processed images may be found to be of poor quality and inadequate for disease diagnosis after the patient has left, which may require repeat scanning and cause increasing radiation exposure, increasing usage of contrast agents, and the delay of disease diagnoses. As a result, the health burden for patients would increase. A recent study has been reported to train an AI model to instantly evaluate imaging quality concerns on abdominal T2-weighted images and allow radiographers to correct the image quality problems before they completed the examination [90].

1.3.2 Improving radiology workflow

- Radiology study protocoling

  Radiology study protocoling is one of the important parts of routine clinical practice because it ensures that patients receive the best and most appropriate study. However, this procedure is time-consuming and prone to human error. Automating this procedure is just getting started, but it is already showing promise. A rule-based ML algorithm was applied to order entry information in one large academic centre. This approach showed promising results, which can help reduce the number of studies manually protocoled and shorten the emergency department turnaround time [91].

The experimental determination of the best pulse sequence for a specific clinical indication is another area investigated for protocol optimisation. Optimal pulse sequences are now chosen after a time-consuming side-by-side assessment of pulse sequences by one or more radiologists. A well-trained CNN can provide an appropriate surrogate for human readers while performing protocol optimisation for the study [91]. On one hand, the application of CNN can make such research less tiresome. On the other hand, it can also significantly increase the number of sequence combinations that could be investigated.

Hanging protocols also play an essential role in radiology workflow. The time between study selection and the radiologist's ability to view the images can be cut in half with a good hanging protocol. The majority of large commercial picture archives and communication systems (PACS) have an automated hanging protocol. PACS vendors, on the other hand, are still striving for more efficient tools, which learn the user's preferences depending on what the user expressly teaches the algorithm. Without explicit user input to the algorithm, AI-based academic work has been conducted to build and adjust hanging protocols based on the user's previously manually corrected hanging protocols [91].

- Disease prioritisation or triage

  Worklist prioritisation is another burgeoning area of AI application in radiologist workflow. DL techniques can help to modify radiologists' worklists with individualised designs on exam type and subspecialty interests. They can also help radiologists by prioritising cases on the worklist that may have anomalies deemed urgent. The application of such prioritisation in the context of screening systems to detect anomalies on chest radiography, abdominal CT, or head CT has been proposed [92–94]. There is an image interpretation component to the AI's activities in these paradigms; however, the AI's function is to alert radiologists to the potential crucial findings and reduce the turnaround time for reporting imaging abnormalities.

  According to a recent study [95], the utilisation rate of CT in emergency rooms in the United States has been rising in recent years. However, in sharp contrast, the number of cases in which emergency room patients are correctly diagnosed and classified through head CT scans and the number of successful rescues are not congruent. Therefore, one of the problems faced by emergency room doctors is how to distinguish the type of head trauma quickly and accurately according to the severity of the disease through a head CT scan. It is worth noting that the AI system prioritises handling abnormal cases in the simulation workflow, and the turnaround time of abnormal cases can be shortened by 7%–28%. Then, the possible causes of abnormalities are grouped for priority review, thereby shortening the turnaround time for testing. In addition, during large-scale disease outbreaks, when clinical demand exceeds the availability of radiologists, this AI system may be used as a front-line point-of-care tool for non-radiologists.

1.3.3 Improving radiology education

In the current radiology residency training system, radiology residents usually draft preliminary radiology reports from the worklist, which are subsequently reviewed by the attending radiologists. The spectrum of disease differs based on hospitals and centres. However, ideally, trainees need to have seen enough of the spectrum of diseases to be deemed competent prior to completing their residency training. An NLP programme has been proposed to use EMRs to follow residents' progress and distribute different cases on more balanced methods for individual residents [96]. This type of application has the potential to assist radiologic residents in identifying knowledge gaps, potentially increasing efficiency in their training time, and help to assist in placing more emphasis where more clinical experience is required.

Assigning cases and preparing teaching materials to radiology residents is also challenging, and we need to consider personalised design according to targeted radiology residents' abilities. NLP tools can be used to address interesting and complicated cases and build a tractable database, correlating the radiology reports with relevant clinical history, lab results, and pathology results, aiming at building a continuous, targeted learning and teaching system. The dynamic difficulty, an AI technique-based video game, can be used by the teachers to prepare individualised teaching materials in real time [97]. AI can also be applied in tracking radiologic residents' performance and help to evaluate competency.

However, there exist some drawbacks of the AI-assisted radiology educational system. Furthermore, AI tools must not take the position of radiologic residents in the interpretive workflow for instructional purposes. Take the widely used lung nodules detecting AI programme, for example. The AI programme can help shorten the time of finding lung nodules and make advice on diagnosis since it is time-consuming and effort-intensive to mark every small lung nodule. Nevertheless, the residents may be over-reliant on the suggested reports produced by the AI system and fail to develop their perspectives. In the future, radiology residency programmes will need to pay close attention to the potential unintended consequences of AI tools.

1.3.4 Challenges, risks, and future of AI in radiology

- AI challenges and risks in radiology

  Although the potential for AI in radiology appears to be nearly limitless, the field is still in its early stages, with many applications still theoretical, in development, or limited to a single institution. Enough data are crucial for the development of AI in radiology, which requires massive patient information and the involvement of clinical care. However, several ethical and legal concerns may exist relating to clinical practices. AI systems should be applied following strict guidelines under the control of medical regulators and in charge of protecting patients. Time-tested, extremely reliable safety measures and perfection of corresponding laws are also required.

The imaging datasets for training an AI system are related to patients' information on electronic health records. Any security breach of relevant clinical information will result in privacy infringement. Before enabling the AI approach, precautionary methods such as data communication protocols and protecting laws should be implemented to protect patients' privacy [98].

- AI future in radiology

  Every year millions of patients have their medical imaging examinations. These imaging data are stored in different health systems worldwide, and their imaging quality varies greatly. Data curation and dataset building remain critical for the development of AI in radiology. It has been proposed that the next generation of AI is data-centric AI rather than model-centric AI, reducing the dependency on big data and making good use of data, even in a small dataset. Data-centric AI focuses on the availability of high-quality data, the so-called good data, through all ML project lifecycle processing stages, with an efficient and systemic approach. It has been shown that significant improvement could be achieved with less than 10 000 examples if the project is tackled with a data-centric approach [99]. Medical facilities worldwide need to upgrade their infrastructure and boost deep collaboration with different research institutes and open the datasets to the public without jeopardising patient privacy so that AI models can be better trained with quality curated data.

  The AI-based automated radiology relevant progress will start from the most prevalent clinical problems with enough data, such as the highly demanding reading of lung screening CT and mammograms. On the other spectrum, the more complicated problems such as improving the inability to address or handle multiparametric MRI may take more time. Thanks to the rapid processing of imaging data and the availability of reports, radiologists and radiographers in the future will be able to make better and more timely medical decisions. This might aid in treating patients in real time, potentially saving lives. Overall, the application of AI in radiology has a promising future in improving human health.

References

[1] Heimann T, Van Ginneken B, Styner M A, Arzhaeva Y, Aurich V and Bauer C *et al* 2009 Comparison and evaluation of methods for liver segmentation from CT datasets *IEEE Trans. Med. Imaging* **28** 1251–65

[2] Weston A D, Korfiatis P, Kline T L, Philbrick K A, Kostandy P and Sakinis T *et al* 2019 Automated abdominal segmentation of CT scans for body composition analysis using deep learning *Radiology* **290** 669–79.

[3] Pickhardt P J, Graffy P M, Zea R, Lee S J, Liu J and Sandfort V *et al* 2020 Automated CT biomarkers for opportunistic prediction of future cardiovascular events and mortality in an

asymptomatic screening population: a retrospective cohort study *Lancet Digit. Health* **2** e192–200
[4] Magudia K, Bridge C P, Bay C P, Babic A, Fintelmann F J and Troschel F M *et al* 2021 Population-scale CT-based body composition analysis of a large outpatient population using deep learning to derive age-, sex-, and race-specific reference curves *Radiol.* **298** 319–29.
[5] Chen H, Qi X, Yu L, Dou Q, Qin J and Heng P-A 2017 DCAN: deep contour-aware networks for object instance segmentation from histology images *Med. Image Anal.* **36** 135–46
[6] Caravagna G, Giarratano Y, Ramazzotti D, Tomlinson I, Graham T A and Sanguinetti G *et al* 2018 Detecting repeated cancer evolution from multi-region tumor sequencing data *Nat. Methods* **15** 707–14.
[7] Du Y, Zhang R, Zargari A, Thai T C, Gunderson C C and Moxley K M *et al* 2018 Classification of tumor epithelium and stroma by exploiting image features learned by deep convolutional neural networks *Ann. Biomed. Eng.* **46** 1988–99
[8] Bosch F X, Ribes J, Díaz M and Cléries R 2004 Primary liver cancer: worldwide incidence and trends *Gastroenterology* **127** S5–16
[9] Bilic P, Christ P F, Vorontsov E, Chlebus G, Chen H and Dou Q *et al* 2019 The liver tumor segmentation benchmark (LiTS) arXiv preprint arXiv:1901.04056
[10] Stadler C B, Lindvall M, Lundström C, Bodén A, Lindman K and Rose J *et al* 2021 Proactive construction of an annotated imaging database for artificial intelligence training *J. Digit. Imaging* **34** 105–15
[11] Capitanio U and Montorsi F 2016 Renal cancer *Lancet* **387** 894–906
[12] Kutikov A and Uzzo R G 2009 The RENAL nephrometry score: a comprehensive standardized system for quantitating renal tumor size, location and depth *J. Urol.* **182** 844–53
[13] Ficarra V, Novara G, Secco S, Macchi V, Porzionato A and De Caro R *et al* 2009 Preoperative aspects and dimensions used for an anatomical (PADUA) classification of renal tumours in patients who are candidates for nephron-sparing surgery *Eur. Urol.* **56** 786–93
[14] Simmons M N, Ching C B, Samplaski M K, Park C H and Gill I S 2010 Kidney tumor location measurement using the C index method *J. Urol.* **183** 1708–13
[15] Heller N, Isensee F, Maier-Hein K H, Hou X, Xie C and Li F *et al* 2021 The state of the art in kidney and kidney tumor segmentation in contrast-enhanced CT imaging: results of the kits19 challenge *Med. Image Anal.* **67** 101821
[16] Clark K, Vendt B, Smith K, Freymann J, Kirby J and Koppel P *et al* 2013 The cancer imaging archive (TCIA): maintaining and operating a public information repository *J. Digit. Imaging* **26** 1045–57
[17] Sekuboyina A, Husseini M E, Bayat A, Löffler M, Liebl H and Li H *et al* 2021 VerSe: a vertebrae labelling and segmentation benchmark for multi-detector CT images *Med. Image Anal.* **73** 102166
[18] Chen S, Ma K and Zheng Y 2019 Med3d: transfer learning for 3D medical image analysis arXiv preprint arXiv:1904.00625
[19] Rister B, Yi D, Shivakumar K, Nobashi T and Rubin D L 2020 CT-ORG a new dataset for multiple organ segmentation in computed tomography *Sci. Data* **7** 1–9
[20] Kavur A E, Gezer N S, Barış M, Aslan S, Conze P-H and Groza V *et al* 2021 CHAOS challenge-combined (CT-MR) healthy abdominal organ segmentation *Med. Image Anal.* **69** 101950

[21] Gibson E, Giganti F, Hu Y, Bonmati E, Bandula S and Gurusamy K *et al* 2018 Automatic multi-organ segmentation on abdominal CT with dense V-networks *IEEE Trans. Med. Imaging* **37** 1822–34

[22] Fedorov A, Beichel R, Kalpathy-Cramer J, Finet J, Fillion-Robin J-C and Pujol S *et al* 2012 3D slicer as an image computing platform for the quantitative imaging network *Magn. Reson. Imaging* **30** 1323–41

[23] Yushkevich P A, Piven J, Hazlett H C, Smith R G, Ho S and Gee J C *et al* 2006 User-guided 3D active contour segmentation of anatomical structures: significantly improved efficiency and reliability *Neuroimage* **31** 1116–28

[24] Christ P F, Elshaer M E A, Ettlinger F, Tatavarty S, Bickel M and Bilic P *et al* (ed) 2016 *Automatic Liver and Lesion Segmentation in CT Using Cascaded Fully Convolutional Neural Networks and 3D Conditional Random Fields* (Berlin: Springer)

[25] Ronneberger O, Fischer P and Brox T 2015 U-Net: convolutional networks for biomedical image segmentation *Int. Conf. on Medical Image Computing and Computer-Assisted Intervention* Lecture Notes in Computer Science 9351 N Navab, J Hornegger, W Wells and A Frangi (Cham: Springer)

[26] Long J, Shelhamer E and Darrell T 2015 Fully convolutional networks for semantic segmentation *Conf. on Computer Vision and Pattern Recognition (CVPR)* pp 3431–40

[27] Tian J, Li C, Shi Z and Xu F (ed) 2018 *A Diagnostic Report Generator from CT Volumes on Liver Tumor with Semi-supervised Attention Mechanism* (Berlin: Springer)

[28] Li X, Chen H, Qi X, Dou Q, Fu C-W and Heng P-A 2018 H-DenseUNet: hybrid densely connected UNet for liver and tumor segmentation from CT volumes *IEEE Trans. Med. Imaging* **37** 2663–74

[29] He K, Zhang X, Ren S and Sun J 2016 Deep residual learning for image recognition *Conf. on Computer Vision and Pattern Recognition (CVPR)* pp 770–8

[30] Isensee F and Maier-Hein K H 2019 An attempt at beating the 3D U-Net arXiv:1908.02182

[31] Chiu W H K, Vardhanabhuti V, Poplavskiy D, Yu P L H, Du R and Yap A Y H *et al* 2020 Detection of COVID-19 using deep learning algorithms on chest radiographs *J. Thorac. Imaging* **35** 369–76

[32] Chamberlin J, Kocher M R, Waltz J, Snoddy M, Stringer N F C and Stephenson J *et al* 2021 Automated detection of lung nodules and coronary artery calcium using artificial intelligence on low-dose CT scans for lung cancer screening: accuracy and prognostic value *BMC Med.* **19** 55

[33] Chougrad H, Zouaki H and Alheyane O 2018 Deep convolutional neural networks for breast cancer screening *Comput. Methods Programs Biomed.* **157** 19–30

[34] Hajabdollahi M, Esfandiarpoor R, Sabeti E, Karimi N, Soroushmehr S M R and Samavi S 2020 Multiple abnormality detection for automatic medical image diagnosis using bifurcated convolutional neural network *Biomed. Signal Process. Control* **57** 101792

[35] Chilamkurthy S, Ghosh R, Tanamala S, Biviji M, Campeau N G and Venugopal V K *et al* 2018 Deep learning algorithms for detection of critical findings in head CT scans: a retrospective study *Lancet* **392** 2388–96

[36] Heuvelmans M A, van Ooijen P M A, Ather S, Silva C F, Han D and Heussel C P *et al* 2021 Lung cancer prediction by deep learning to identify benign lung nodules *Lung Cancer* **154** 1–4

[37] Schwyzer M, Martini K, Benz D C, Burger I A, Ferraro D A and Kudura K *et al* 2020 Artificial intelligence for detecting small FDG-positive lung nodules in digital PET/CT: impact of image reconstructions on diagnostic performance *Eur. Radiol.* **30** 2031–40
[38] Nabulsi Z, Sellergren A, Jamshy S, Lau C, Santos E and Kiraly A P *et al* 2021 Deep learning for distinguishing normal versus abnormal chest radiographs and generalization to two unseen diseases tuberculosis and COVID-19 *Sci. Rep.* **11** 15523
[39] Carmody D P, Nodine C F and Kundel H L 1980 An analysis of perceptual and cognitive factors in radiographic interpretation *Perception* **9** 339–44
[40] Giger M L, Doi K and MacMahon H 1987 Computerized detection of lung nodules in digital chest radiographs *Proc. SPIE* **0767**
[41] Kundel H L and Hendee W R 1985 The perception of radiologic image information. Report of an NCI Workshop on April 15–16, 1985 *Invest. Radiol.* **20** 874–7
[42] Bera K, Braman N, Gupta A, Velcheti V and Madabhushi A 2022 Predicting cancer outcomes with radiomics and artificial intelligence in radiology *Nat. Rev. Clin. Oncol.* **19** 132–46
[43] Aonpong P, Iwamoto Y, Wang W, Lin L and Chen Y-W 2020 Hand-crafted and deep learning-based radiomics models for recurrence prediction of non-small cells lung cancers *Innovation in Medicine and Healthcare* (Berlin: Springer) pp 135–44
[44] Chung A G, Shafiee M J, Kumar D, Khalvati F, Haider M A and Wong A 2015 Discovery radiomics for multi–parametric MRI prostate cancer detection arXiv:1509.00111
[45] Zhu Y, Man C, Gong L, Dong D, Yu X and Wang S *et al* 2019 A deep learning radiomics model for preoperative grading in meningioma *Eur. J. Radiol.* **116** 128–34
[46] Pfaehler E, Zwanenburg A, de Jong J R and Boellaard R 2019 RaCaT: an open source and easy to use radiomics calculator tool *PLoS One* **14** e0212223
[47] Van Griethuysen J J, Fedorov A, Parmar C, Hosny A, Aucoin N and Narayan V *et al* 2017 Computational radiomics system to decode the radiographic phenotype *Cancer Res.* **77** e104–e7
[48] Zwanenburg A, Leger S, Vallières M and Löck S 2016 Image biomarker standardisation initiative arXiv:1612.07003
[49] Haralick R M, Shanmugam K and Dinstein I H 1973 Textural features for image classification *IEEE Trans. Syst. Man Cybern.* **6** 610–21
[50] Sun C and Wee W G 1983 Neighboring gray level dependence matrix for texture classification *Comput. Vis. Graph. Image Process.* **23** 341–52
[51] Wilcoxon F 1992 Individual comparisons by ranking methods *Breakthroughs in Statistics* (Berlin: Springer) pp 196–202
[52] Chirra P, Leo P, Yim M, Bloch B N, Rastinehad A R and Purysko A *et al* 2019 Multisite evaluation of radiomic feature reproducibility and discriminability for identifying peripheral zone prostate tumors on MRI *J. Med. Imaging* **6** 024502
[53] Xie C, Ng M-Y, Ding J, Leung S T, Lo C S Y and Wong H Y F *et al* 2020 Discrimination of pulmonary ground-glass opacity changes in COVID-19 and non-COVID-19 patients using CT radiomics analysis *Eur. J. Radiol. Open* **7** 100271
[54] Du R, Lee V H, Yuan H, Lam K-O, Pang H H and Chen Y *et al* 2019 Radiomics model to predict early progression of nonmetastatic nasopharyngeal carcinoma after intensity modulation radiation therapy: a multicenter study *Radiol. Artif. Intell.* **1** e180075
[55] Hu Y, Xie C, Yang H, Ho J W K, Wen J and Han L *et al* 2020 Assessment of intratumoral and peritumoral computed tomography radiomics for predicting pathological complete

response to neoadjuvant chemoradiation in patients with esophageal squamous cell carcinoma *JAMA Network Open* **3** e2015927
[56] Deng J, Dong W, Socher R, Li L-J, Li K and Fei-Fei L 2009 ImageNet: a large-scale hierarchical image database *IEEE Conf. on Computer Vision and Pattern Recognition* (Piscataway, NJ: IEEE)
[57] Hu Y, Xie C, Yang H, Ho J W K, Wen J and Han L *et al* 2021 Computed tomography-based deep-learning prediction of neoadjuvant chemoradiotherapy treatment response in esophageal squamous cell carcinoma *Radiother. Oncol.* **154** 6–13
[58] Xie C, Du R, Ho J W K, Pang H H, Chiu K W H and Lee E Y P *et al* 2020 Effect of machine learning re-sampling techniques for imbalanced datasets in 18 F-FDG PET-based radiomics model on prognostication performance in cohorts of head and neck cancer patients *Eur. J. Nucl. Med. Mol. Imaging* **47** 2826–35
[59] Le E P V, Rundo L, Tarkin J M, Evans N R, Chowdhury M M and Coughlin P A *et al* 2021 Assessing robustness of carotid artery CT angiography radiomics in the identification of culprit lesions in cerebrovascular events *Sci. Rep.* **11** 1–14
[60] Roberts M, Driggs D, Thorpe M, Gilbey J, Yeung M and Ursprung S *et al* 2021 Common pitfalls and recommendations for using machine learning to detect and prognosticate for COVID-19 using chest radiographs and CT scans *Nat. Mach. Intell.* **3** 199–217
[61] Singh A, Sengupta S and Lakshminarayanan V 2020 Explainable deep learning models in medical image analysis *J. Imaging* **6** 52
[62] Couteaux V, Nempont O, Pizaine G and Bloch I 2019 Towards interpretability of segmentation networks by analyzing deepDreams *Interpretability of Machine Intelligence in Medical Image Computing and Multimodal Learning for Clinical Decision Support* ed K Suzuki, M Reyes, T Syeda-Mahmood, E Konukoglu, B Glocker, R Wiest, Y Gur, H Greenspan and A Madabhushi (Berlin: Springer) Lecture Notes in Computer Science 11797 pp 56–63
[63] Mordvintsev A, Olah C and Tyka M 2015 Inceptionism: going deeper into neural networks
[64] Rudin C 2019 Stop explaining black box machine learning models for high stakes decisions and use interpretable models instead *Nat. Mach. Intell.* **1** 206–15
[65] Holzinger A, Langs G, Denk H, Zatloukal K and Müller H 2019 Causability and explainability of artificial intelligence in medicine *Wiley Interdiscip. Rev.: Data Min. Knowl. Discov.* **9** e1312
[66] Devlin J, Chang M-W, Lee K and Toutanova K 2018 BERT: pre-training of deep bidirectional transformers for language understanding arXiv preprint arXiv:1810.04805
[67] Zhu Y, Kiros R, Zemel R, Salakhutdinov R, Urtasun R and Torralba A *et al* 2015 Aligning books and movies: towards story-like visual explanations by watching movies and reading books *Int. Conf. on Computer Vision (ICCV)* pp 19–27
[68] Vinyals O, Toshev A, Bengio S and Erhan D 2015 Show and tell: a neural image caption generator *Proc. of the IEEE Conf. on Computer Vision and Pattern Recognition*
[69] Jing B, Xie P and Xing E 2017 On the automatic generation of medical imaging reports arXiv:1711.08195
[70] Xue Y, Xu T, Long L R, Xue Z, Antani S and Thoma G R *et al* (ed) 2018 Multimodal recurrent model with attention for automated radiology report generation *Int. Conf. on Medical Image Computing and Computer-Assisted Intervention* (Berlin: Springer)
[71] Radford A, Wu J, Child R, Luan D, Amodei D and Sutskever I 2019 Language models are unsupervised multitask learners *Open AI Blog* **1** 9

[72] Vaswani A, Shazeer N, Parmar N, Uszkoreit J, Jones L and Gomez A N *et al* 2017 Attention is all you need *Advances in Neural Information Processing Systems*
[73] Hardy M and Harvey H 2020 Artificial intelligence in diagnostic imaging: impact on the radiography profession *Br. J. Radiol.* **93** 20190840
[74] Higaki T, Nakamura Y, Zhou J, Yu Z, Nemoto T and Tatsugami F *et al* 2020 Deep learning reconstruction at CT: phantom study of the image characteristics *Acad. Radiol.* **27** 82–7
[75] Dong C, Loy C C, He K and Tang X 2016 Image super-resolution using deep convolutional networks *IEEE Trans. Pattern Anal. Mach. Intell.* **38** 295–307
[76] Jiang D, Dou W, Vosters L, Xu X, Sun Y and Tan T 2018 Denoising of 3D magnetic resonance images with multi-channel residual learning of convolutional neural network *Jap. J. Radiol.* **36** 566–74
[77] Yang Q, Yan P, Zhang Y, Yu H, Shi Y and Mou X *et al* 2018 Low-dose CT image denoising using a generative adversarial network with Wasserstein distance and perceptual loss *IEEE Trans. Med. Imaging* **37** 1348–57
[78] Wang G, Ye J C, Mueller K and Fessler J A 2018 Image reconstruction is a new frontier of machine learning *IEEE Trans. Med. Imaging* **37** 1289–96
[79] Zhu B, Liu J Z, Cauley S F, Rosen B R and Rosen M S 2018 Image reconstruction by domain-transform manifold learning *Nature* **555** 487–92
[80] Quan T M, Nguyen-Duc T and Jeong W-K 2018 Compressed sensing MRI reconstruction using a generative adversarial network with a cyclic loss *IEEE Trans. Med. Imaging* **37** 1488–97
[81] Lakhani P, Prater A B, Hutson R K, Andriole K P, Dreyer K J and Morey J *et al* 2018 Machine learning in radiology: applications beyond image interpretation *J. Am. Coll. Radiol.* **15** 350–9
[82] Chen H, Zhang Y, Kalra M K, Lin F, Chen Y and Liao P *et al* 2017 Low-dose CT with a residual encoder-decoder convolutional neural network *IEEE Trans. Med. Imaging* **36** 2524–35
[83] Xie S, Zheng X, Chen Y, Xie L, Liu J and Zhang Y *et al* 2018 Artifact removal using improved GoogLeNet for sparse-view CT reconstruction *Sci. Rep.* **8** 6700
[84] Gong E, Pauly J M, Wintermark M and Zaharchuk G 2018 Deep learning enables reduced gadolinium dose for contrast-enhanced brain MRI *J. Magn. Reson. Imaging* **48** 330–40
[85] Kim K H and Park S H 2017 Artificial neural network for suppression of banding artifacts in balanced steady-state free precession MRI *Magn. Reson. Imaging* **37** 139–46
[86] Hauptmann A, Arridge S, Lucka F, Muthurangu V and Steeden J A 2019 Real-time cardiovascular MR with spatio-temporal artifact suppression using deep learning-proof of concept in congenital heart disease *Magn. Reson. Med.* **81** 1143–56
[87] Zhang Y and Yu H 2018 Convolutional neural network based metal artifact reduction in X-ray computed tomography *IEEE Trans. Med. Imaging* **37** 1370–81
[88] Wang S, Su Z, Ying L, Peng X, Zhu S and Liang F *et al* 2016 Accelerating magnetic resonance imaging via deep learning *Proc. IEEE Int. Symp. Biomed. Imaging* **2016** 514–7
[89] Hammernik K, Klatzer T, Kobler E, Recht M P, Sodickson D K and Pock T *et al* 2018 Learning a variational network for reconstruction of accelerated MRI data *Magn. Reson. Med.* **79** 3055–71
[90] Esses S J, Lu X, Zhao T, Shanbhogue K, Dane B and Bruno M *et al* 2018 Automated image quality evaluation of T2-weighted liver MRI utilizing deep learning architecture *J. Magn. Reson. Imaging* **47** 723–8
[91] Richardson M L, Garwood E R, Lee Y, Li M D, Lo H S and Nagaraju A *et al* 2021 Noninterpretive uses of artificial intelligence in radiology *Acad. Radiol.* **28** 1225–35

[92] Rajpurkar P, Irvin J, Ball R L, Zhu K, Yang B and Mehta H *et al* 2018 Deep learning for chest radiograph diagnosis: a retrospective comparison of the CheXNeXt algorithm to practicing radiologists *PLoS Med.* **15** e1002686

[93] Winkel D J, Heye T, Weikert T J, Boll D T and Stieltjes B 2019 Evaluation of an AI-based detection software for acute findings in abdominal computed tomography scans: toward an automated work list prioritization of routine CT examinations *Invest. Radiol.* **54** 55–9

[94] Prevedello L M, Erdal B S, Ryu J L, Little K J, Demirer M and Qian S *et al* 2017 Automated critical test findings identification and online notification system using artificial intelligence in imaging *Radiology* **285** 923–31

[95] Drescher F S and Sirovich B E 2016 Use of computed tomography in emergency departments in the United States: a decade of coughs and colds *JAMA Intern. Med.* **176** 273–5

[96] Chen H, Gangaram V and Shih G 2019 Developing a more responsive radiology resident dashboard *J. Digit. Imaging* **32** 81–90

[97] Yanan H, Suoju H, Junping W, Xiao L, Jiajian Y and Wang H 2010 Dynamic difficulty adjustment of game AI by MCTS for the game Pac-Man *6th Int. Conf. on Natural Computation*

[98] Saba L, Biswas M, Kuppili V, Cuadrado Godia E, Suri H S and Edla D R *et al* 2019 The present and future of deep learning in radiology *Eur. J. Radiol.* **114** 14–24

[99] Andrew N 2021 MLOps: from model-centric to data-centric AI. Deep learning AI

IOP Publishing

Machine Learning, Medical AI and Robotics
Translating theory into the clinic
Varut Vardhanabhuti, Ka-Wai Kwok, Jason Y K Chan and Qi Dou

Chapter 2

Machine learning: applications in ophthalmology

Charlene Yat Che Chau and Kendrick Co Shih

2.1 Introduction

Deep learning (DL) technology has revolutionised the screening, diagnosis, and management of eye diseases. Pattern recognition, through direct and indirect visualisation of the eye and adjacent structures via clinical examination and technological adjuncts, forms the cornerstone of ophthalmology [1]. The image-centric nature of ophthalmology makes it the perfect candidate to benefit from DL algorithms and as a test bed for clinical incorporation and advancement of intelligent algorithms within clinical medicine.

Machine learning (ML) refers to pattern-recognition algorithms trained on datasets that are labelled (as in supervised learning), unlabelled (unsupervised learning), or contain a mixture of both (reinforcement learning). DL is a subset of ML; it mimics the hierarchical neural networks of the human cortex to learn the input with multiple levels of abstraction and generate predictions automatically [2]. Compared to traditional techniques, DL has demonstrated superiority in image recognition, classification, and segmentation [3]. Traditional techniques necessitate manual extraction of a set of features that are unique to each image within the training set in a step known as 'feature extraction' (figure 2.1) [3]. This requires expert analysis and lengthy fine-tuning. In addition, the accuracy and applicability of the model would be undermined by variability in human anatomy and clinical presentation, as well as technological complications such as motion or reflection artefacts, and discrepancies in lighting conditions. On the other hand, DL utilises a stack of nonlinear hidden layers to complete an end-to-end learning process with an annotated dataset and the classification as the input and output, respectively (figure 2.1). The automatic feature extraction, transformation, and decoding mitigate the problem of overfitting data points and unconscious biases granted that the DL models are well trained with various diverse datasets of adequate size [4].

doi:10.1088/978-0-7503-4637-5ch2

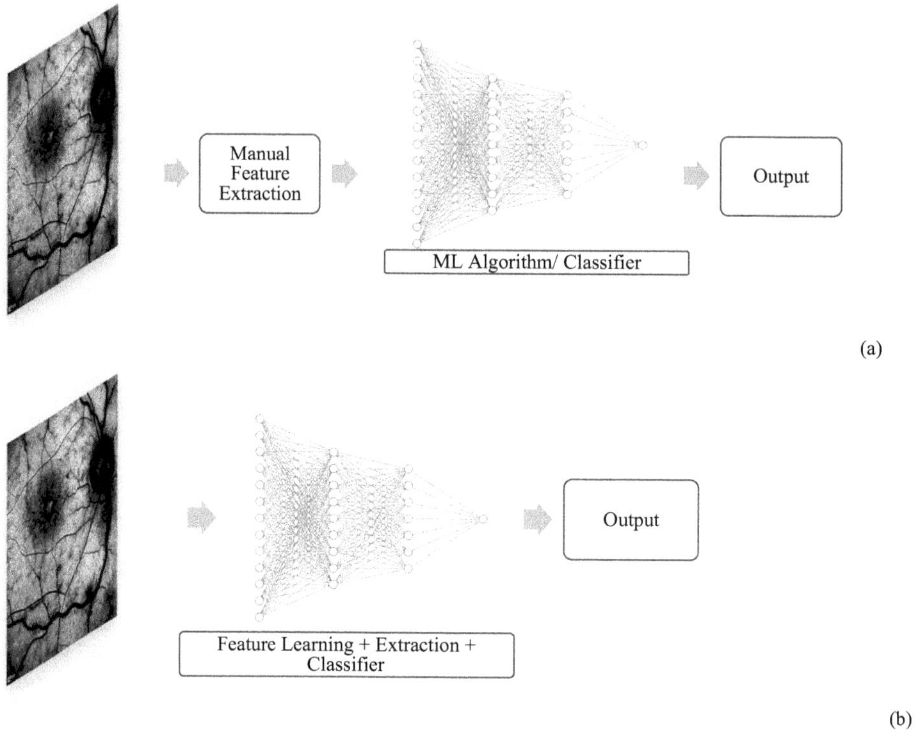

Figure 2.1. Workflows of (a) machine learning (b) deep learning algorithms. Retina image reprinted with permission from Retina Image Bank, American Society of Retina Specialists Neural network architecture schematics created via NN-SVG [5].

2.2 Convolutional neural networks—basic architecture

Amongst the various DL architectures, convolutional neural networks (CNNs) are most commonly used for applications requiring image analysis and interpretation. To understand its usability and limitations in ophthalmology, an understanding of the basic architecture of a CNN is pivotal. The generic architecture of CNNs consists of an input layer, hidden layers, and an output layer. These hidden layers are composed of permutations of a stack of convolution layers and a pooling layer, followed by one or more fully connected layers.

2.2.1 Convolution layers

A convolution layer is key to feature extraction. It involves passing the outputs of a linear convolution operation through a nonlinear activation function. Briefly, a convolution involves sliding a filter kernel (a small matrix of numbers with weights of zeros and ones) across an input image (a larger matrix of pixels) (figure 2.2). Within the image sub-region (or receptive field) in which the filter kernel convolves, the product of the kernel weights and pixel values in the respective overlapped position are summed together to form the output value in the corresponding position

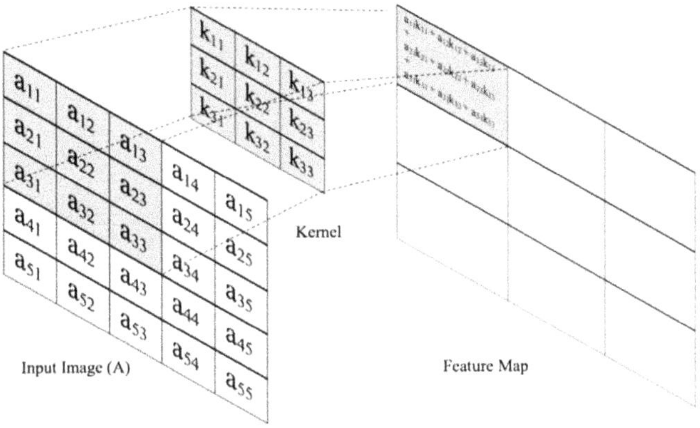

Figure 2.2. An example of a convolution operation with an input image $A_{5 \times 5}$, convolved with a filter $k3 \times 3$ and no padding, mapping onto a feature map. The receptive field of the input image and the corresponding position on the feature map are highlighted in blue. A_{ij} and k_{ij} represent the number located in line I and column j in the respective location of the matrix.

of the output image (or the feature map). The application of multiple kernels on the input will generate feature maps that extract discriminative features of the image. Whether there is reduced dimensionality of the convolution layer compared to the input will depend on user-defined parameters such as padding or stride. Padding adds rows and columns of zeros to the borders of the image in order to retain the dimensions of the output image and to ensure equal representation of the outermost elements of an image. The stride controls the number of pixels the filter window shifts over the input image per step. This determines the degree of overlap between receptive fields and the spatial dimensions of the feature map.

Prior to submission to the next layer of the network, a nonlinear transformation of the output from the convolution layer is achieved via activation functions. The choice of activation layer depends on the type of layer. For instance, rectified linear unit functions [6] are commonly used for convolutional layers, whilst Softmax activation functions [7] are reserved for the final layer in order to convert the output into categorial probabilities.

2.2.2 Pooling layers

A pooling layer functions to down-sample the feature maps from the convolution layers. Through merging semantically similar characteristics into one, pooling reduces the number of parameters for processing in subsequent layers of the network whilst retaining key information [2]. Amongst all pooling operations, max pooling is widely used. Similar to the convolution layer, a filter size, stride, and padding are key hyperparameters. Max pooling outputs the maximum value within each filter and discards the other values. Average pooling (outputs the average value within each filter) and global average pooling can also be used (figure 2.3).

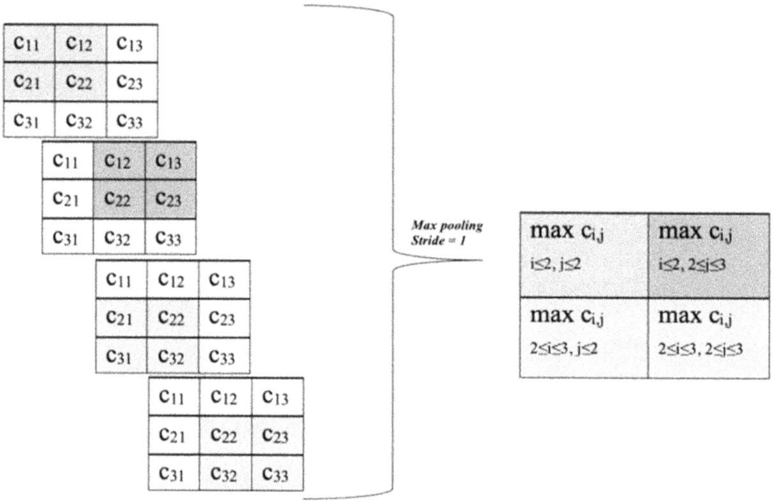

Figure 2.3. An example of a max pooling operation on feature map $C_{3\times3}$ that has passed through the activation function from a convolution layer. This operation uses a filter size of 2 × 2, with no padding and a stride of 1. C_{ij} represents the number located in line i and column j in the respective location of the matrix.

2.2.3 Fully connected layers

Prior to the fully connected layers, the output feature maps are flattened into a one-dimensional array of numbers via global average pooling. The fully connected layers are then mapped to the final output nodes of the network. In image classification tasks, these output nodes would correspond to the probabilities for each class.

2.2.4 Network training

The performance of an artificial intelligence (AI) system can be improved by training iteratively on larger and more varied datasets. The backpropagation algorithm is a commonly used method for training neural networks. The initially random parameters of the neural network will be modified throughout the training process. The loss function measures the extent of inconsistency between the output predictions of the network and the true value of the model. The kernels in convolution layers and weights in fully connected layers are then updated according to the loss value through backpropagation with gradient descent optimisation algorithm [8]. A validation set monitors the performance of the model during the training process, performing a crucial role in fine-tuning hyperparameters and the selection of models. The final model performance will be evaluated by a test set.

2.3 Current applications of DL in ophthalmology

2.3.1 Retinal disorders/fundus images

2.3.1.1 Inherited retinal disorders

Retinopathy of prematurity

The incidence of childhood blindness secondary to retinopathy of prematurity (ROP) is rising rapidly due to improvements in neonatal care. Whilst avoidable with appropriate primary, secondary, and tertiary preventions, major challenges pertaining to the clinical diagnosis remain. The short supply of adequately trained ophthalmologists and interobserver variability in ROP grading undermines timely treatment [9, 10]. In an attempt to achieve a reliable and cost-effective adjunct, various automated ROP detection systems have been built with a focus on the detection and grading of ROP [11–14]. Without the need to explicitly extract features from retinal fundus images, deep neural networks are particularly useful in ROP due to the incomplete understanding of ROP symptomatology [12]. Of note, two DL screening programmes, DeepROP and Imaging and Informatics in ROP (i-ROP), have demonstrated high performance and model to the expert agreement. Wang *et al*'s DeepROP approach utilises two CNN classifiers trained on 20 795 images: an identification network identifies the presence or absence of ROP features, whilst a grading network indicates the severity of ROP cases as either 'minor' or 'severe' using clinical features of plus disease, stages, and zones [12]. The i-ROP Research consortium also developed a two-CNN system trained on 5511 retinal images with the main aim of classifying plus disease of ROP. The first CNN utilises a U-Net architecture for vessel segmentation, the second for diagnosis of plus disease, which serves as indicators for both treatment and prognosis [14]. A quantitative severity score based on the i-ROP DL classifier has demonstrated good performance for the detection of type 1 ROP (area under the receiver operating curve [AUROC] 0.96), clinically significant ROP (AUROC 0.91), and plus disease (AUROC 0.99) [15]. Retrospective studies have demonstrated the clinical utility of the severity score in predicting disease progression, the need for treatment, and treatment failure [16, 17]. High external validity is also demonstrated in a retrospective study that used the I-ROP DL classifier in an Indian population of premature infants for treatment-requiring ROP [10]. Nonetheless, it is important to note that whilst plus disease is a critical feature of severe ROP and an indicator of treatment, it alone does not define ROP [12]. More clinical features should be considered when developing deep neural network models. Going forward, the potential for AI in ROP may not only be limited to objective disease classification systems but can also be used as a decision support tool for initiation of treatment. Standardised treatment thresholds, modelled with other risk factors such as demographics and comorbidities, could be incorporated into evidence-based guidelines [9]. This will also facilitate resource allocation of high-quality neonatal care units with strict oxygen monitoring in low- and middle-income countries [10].

Inherited retinal diseases

Inherited retinal diseases (IRDs) are a clinically and genetically diverse set of conditions that constitute a major cause of blindness in developed countries amongst working-age adults [18]. Whilst they are rare Mendelian disorders individually, the aggregate clinical, administrative, and patient burden is substantial. They are typically classified by disease progression—stationary or progressive—or by the cell types of the retina and pigment epithelium primarily involved in the pathogenesis [19]. However,

IRDs pose a diagnostic challenge given the genotypic and phenotypic heterogeneity. Mutations in the same gene can exhibit a range of phenotypes, as demonstrated in ABCA4 and PRPH2 mutations [20, 21]. Conversely, IRDs can share substantially overlapping clinical features, thus precluding diagnoses made solely on clinical grounds, as exemplified by the similarities shared by retinitis pigmentosa, Leber congenital amaurosis, cone-rod dystrophy, and congenital stationary night blindness [22].

The advent of molecular diagnostics has refined the assessment of IRDs. It allows accurate confirmation of diagnosis and the development of novel genetics-based therapeutics and guides genetic counselling and prognosis. However, significant knowledge gaps remain, specifically pertaining to (1) the integration of molecular genetics diagnostic testing into routine clinical care and (2) improving access, affordability, and accuracy of genetic testing methodologies [23]. DL-guided prediction has been used to facilitate clinical and genetic diagnoses given that IRD exhibits strong gene-characteristic retinal features [24]. Miere *et al* demonstrated the feasibility of using a CNN to automate the diagnostic classification of three IRDs (retinitis pigmentosa, Best disease, Stargardt disease) using fundus autofluorescence (FAF) images with an overall diagnostic accuracy of 0.95 [25]. In another study, Fujinami-Yokokawa *et al* utilised fundus photography and FAF imaging to predict causative IRD genes. Using clinical and genetic data from 1302 subjects, the algorithm was able to identify retinopathies caused by three predefined IRD genes (ABCA4, EYS, RP1L1) with a mean overall sensitivity and specificity of 85.0% and 95.3% [24]. Whilst the application can facilitate early genetic testing and reduce the cost of referrals, the applicability in clinical practice may be limited. With more than 3000 causative IRD genes, other novel gene diagnoses and other retinal disease-associated gene diagnoses would be missed. Owing to the low prevalence of individual disorders amongst IRDs, both studies had a small dataset and selected more common IRDs for algorithm training. This limits the external validity and accuracy of outcome predictions. This is complicated by interindividual and intra-individual variations in genetic expression, fundus abnormality, and media opacities, thus making assessing the classifier within the clinical setting challenging [25].

2.3.1.2 Acquired retinal disorders/systemic causes of retinopathy

Diabetic retinopathy

With the increasing prevalence of diabetes mellitus worldwide, diabetic retinopathy (DR) remains a leading cause of vision loss. The nuanced nexus of genetic, socioeconomic, and environmental factors have more than tripled the number of adults with diabetes, with the 2019 estimate being 463 million and a projected increase to 700 million by 2045 [26]. DR is the commonest microvascular complication [27]. Nearly 100% of patients with type 1 diabetes and >60% of patients with type 2 diabetes will develop DR within the first two decades of the disease [28].

The insidious nature and asymptomatic progression until vision-threatening stages make routine screening of DR essential. Current DR screening protocols employ manual assessment and retinal fundus photography. Such screening programmes are often complicated by the availability of healthcare professionals, logistical barriers, and financial issues. Teleretinal screening programmes have been proposed to increase accessibility for remote and resource-poor communities and improve cost-effectiveness. However, the latter is influenced by a multitude of patient factors (e.g. adherence to post-screening recommendations) and screening logistics (e.g. time lag between imaging and ophthalmologic evaluation and cost considerations) [29]. These drawbacks may be solved with the introduction of an automated grading system which would aid risk stratification and referral decisions.

Automated image analysis of DR has evolved from simple fundus image pre-processing to advanced algorithms which classify DR lesions and stages [30]. A meta-analysis including 24 studies that evaluated the performance of neural networks in the detection of referable DR or diabetic macular oedema (DME) using retinal fundus images revealed a pooled sensitivity of 91.9% (95% CI: 89.6%–94.3%) and specificity of 91.3% (95% CI: 89.0%–93.5%) [31]. The results were superior to pooled sensitivity and specificity derived from meta-analyses on computer-aided diagnoses of melanoma and breast cancer [31]. It is worth noting that Diabetes UK recommends a minimum of 95% specificity for any screening programme [32]. Low specificity causing false-positive referrals may translate to significant consumption of secondary care resources and erode patient trust in the long term. Current AI screening programmes may not have sufficient specificity as a standalone screening tool; notwithstanding, the point-of-care access may allow enhanced patient engagement [33]. Showcasing DR features marked by AI to patients may create an opportunity to discuss the risk of vision impairment and the importance of glycaemic control. A subgroup analysis by Wang *et al* also revealed a non-significant difference between the performance of four CNN models (Inception, EyeArt, VGGNet, and netB) and IDx-DR, an AI algorithm that was first to be approved by the US Food and Drug Administration for DR identification, highlighting their potential in future clinical application [31, 34]. Of note, Wang *et al* 2020 found no significant association between image resolution and the diagnostic accuracy of neural networks. This lends support to the observation that there may be an optimal threshold for image resolution, beyond which does not lead to better diagnostic accuracy. This may minimise the trade-off required to balance amongst image resolution, signal-to-noise ratio, acquisition time, and cost [35]. However, the overlapped samples in the included studies due to duplicated data sources, as well as the high or unclear risk of bias in most studies, preclude a definitive conclusion. More research is required to evaluate the influence of image resolution and the optimum threshold to achieve maximum diagnostic accuracy.

2.3.2 Optical coherence tomography images

Optical coherence tomography (OCT) has transformed the clinical management of many retinal diseases, notably age-related macular degeneration (AMD), glaucoma, DME, and retinal vein occlusions (RVO). Using near infra-red light, the ability to image retinal structures *in vivo* in three dimensions without ionising radiation makes OCT a popular diagnostic procedure [36].

2.3.2.1 AI algorithms in AMD

AMD is a chronic progressive macular disease that affects the geriatric population and is a leading cause of irreversible blindness worldwide. Its bilateral involvement of the macula, 4% of the retinal area that is responsible for central vision and the majority of photopic vision, reflects the profound physical and psychosocial impact [37]. The clinical course and severity of visual impairment depend on the type of advanced AMD, 'dry' or 'wet' AMD based on the absence or presence of neovascularisation. Dry AMD is characterised by drusen (subretinal deposits) and retinal pigment epithelium (RPE) changes in the early or intermediate stages and geographic atrophy (GA) in the advanced stages [38]. Wet AMD is typified by choroidal neovascularisation (CNV) and related features such as serous or haemorrhagic detachment of RPE and/or neurosensory retina and disciform scarring [38].

OCT has largely superseded colour fundus photography for the clinical diagnosis and management of AMD due to the three-dimensional (3D) cross-sectional anatomical information that it provides. The substantial time cost of manual OCT analysis owing to the extensive image data volume has accentuated the clinical need for automated solutions. To date, DL algorithms have demonstrated high accuracy in the detection, prognostication, and assessment of treatment response in AMD.

Convolution neural networks have allowed the automated classification of AMD, which allows monitoring of disease progression and guides the use of anti-vascular endothelial growth factor (VEGF) therapy. Lee *et al* used U-Net to segment, detect, and quantify features of wet AMD on OCT, including intraretinal fluid, subretinal fluid (SRF), pigment epithelial detachment, and subretinal hyperreflective material [39]. The automatic segmentation of lesions may allow better monitoring and prediction of treatment outcome using quantitative data [39]. Nonetheless, the approach to automatic segmentation can affect the precision (reflected by the Dice coefficients), particularly given the unclear boundaries of the basement membrane of RPE. Apart from segmentation algorithms, other methods can be used to classify non-exudative versus exudative AMD. The CNN model developed by Motozawa *et al* utilised a transfer learning model [40]. Transfer learning refers to the use of a pre-trained neural network on a larger unrelated dataset, allowing retention of already optimised lower level convolution layers and allowing higher levels to be fully retrained via back propagation [41]. Such use of transfer learning to train a CNN achieved a stable and more rapid performance (98.4% sensitivity, 88.3% specificity, and 93.9% accuracy) with a smaller dataset (721 exudative AMD + 661 non-exudative AMD). In addition, they used class activation mapping as a heat map to identify the discriminative region on OCT images. This differs from prior models that automatically detects neovascular AMD based on the detection of presence or absence of fluid, as the heat maps allow visualisation of distribution and extent [42, 43]. These heat maps may also prevent overlooking of features and streamline future follow-up. Alternatively, Schlegl *et al* developed a model that allowed localisation and quantification of macular fluid using DL-based pixel-wise and volume-wise segmentation [43]. The automated and manual localisation and quantification of fluid had a high level of concordance: the mean Pearson's correlation coefficient of 0.90 for intraretinal cystoid fluid and 0.96 for SRF. The ability to detect different types of macular fluid also showed high accuracy (mean area under the curve [AUC] 0.94) in detecting other prevalent exudative macular diseases, namely, DME and RVO.

For dry AMD, there has been no proven treatment to halt the progression and development of irreversible GA. Identification of patients with a high risk of progression at the early and intermediate stages will allow optimal clinical monitoring and intervention. Several studies have proposed the use of DL to identify OCT biomarkers that signal the risk of AMD progression. Examples of promising biomarkers include higher drusen volume, the presence of reticular pseudodrusen, and the presence, quantity, and internal reflectivity of intraretinal hyperreflective foci [44–47]. A 2017 systematic review on the algorithms for automated analysis of AMD biomarkers on OCT revealed 27 and 8 algorithms for quantitative and qualitative analysis, respectively [48]. Of note, the samples used to assess the quality of quantitative algorithms were small in size and were preselected for a particular biomarker. This hinders comparison amongst identified algorithms and assessment of external validity since typical AMD patients will most likely present with multiple AMD biomarkers simultaneously [48]. Schmidt-Erfurth *et al* proposed an ML-based predictive model that combines different AMD biomarkers, coupled with demographic and genetic parameters. The model had AUC of 0.68 and 0.8 of individual risk of progression from intermediate AMD to CNV and GA, respectively [49]. Saha *et al* also developed an algorithm that combined multiple early AMD biomarkers (reticular pseudodrusen, intraretinal hyperreflective and hyporeflective foci) with an overall accuracy of 87% [50]. Looking forward, high-quality and standardised validation procedures would have a significant translational value [48].

As for wet AMD, ML has the potential for evaluating treatment outcomes and guiding individualised treatment regimens. Intravitreal injections of anti-VEGF agents are recommended as first-line treatment, but it is clinically difficult to determine an individualised dosing regimen *a priori*. Historically landmark trials established the gold standard of a continuous regimen whereby anti-VEGF was administered at regularly spaced intervals [51, 52]. A discontinuous regimen was proposed to mitigate treatment burdens; the two most commonly used approaches are pro re nata (PRN) and treat-and-extend regimens, both requiring continuous OCT monitoring to inform regimen choice. Bogunović *et al* described an ML model that utilised the spatiotemporal features on a longitudinal series of OCT images acquired during the treatment initiation phase to predict low or high anti-VEGF requirements in a PRN treatment [53]. This study demonstrated the promising prospect of ML for precision medicine, which would not only improve disease outcomes but also reduce the socioeconomic burden of pharmacological therapies. Future work would require more research into sensitive and robust imaging biomarkers, and other non-imaging data such as genetic markers, that would guide retreatment [53, 54].

2.3.2.2 AI algorithms in glaucoma

ML strategies have revolutionised solutions for glaucoma diagnosis and prognosis. Early diagnosis is key to preserving visual function and related quality of life at a sustainable cost, especially given the asymptomatic presentation in the early stage and irreversible visual loss at late stages, and confers better prognosis [55]. Coupled with the expanding disease burden due to the ageing population, with a projected prevalence of 111.8 million in 2040, novel models of glaucoma care delivery are required to address the demand-capacity burden [56]. Structural measures obtained via fundus photography and OCT, and functional measures by automated perimetry, form the basis of glaucoma diagnosis and monitoring in current clinical practice. Fundus photographs are widely used as input datasets for glaucoma detection either through optic disc segmentation and structured learning of retinal clinical indicators (e.g. cup disc ratio, neuroretinal rim) [57–60], or using image texture analyses via DL strategies for pattern identification [61–63]. Despite the high accuracies of these DL algorithms, the subjective interpretation of two-dimensional fundus photographs has been reported to have poor interobserver agreement or risk of under-/over-estimation, which undermines the reliability of ground truth labelling as input [4]. In addition, the two-dimensionality only offers a surface view of the retina and optic nerve head (ONH). On the other hand, OCT images allow a 3D and micro-resolution visualisation, quantification, and topographical measurement of structural changes in anterior (e.g. anterior chamber angle/depth/width) and posterior (e.g. ONH) ocular segments in OCT images [4, 64]. The retinal nerve fibre layer remains the parameter of focus in ML algorithms using OCT images. However, major limitations to date remain to be the generalisability of these algorithms to real-world patient populations. The algorithms that are trained and validated on highly curated cohorts and disc photographs may differ from input data with variable patient characteristics and image quality.

Besides the potential of AI algorithms in screening and diagnosis, personalised predictions of visual field (VF) progression may also be possible for real-world implementation. VF measurements via static automated perimetry remain the clinical standard; ML models have utilised longitudinal VF data to detect glaucoma progression [65–68]. Notwithstanding, predicting progression remains challenging. This is attributable to anatomical factors such as the structure-function discordance in glaucoma and technical factors such as variations in the physiological sensitivity of VF measurements, which increases with a deteriorating VF [69, 70]. As such, more research has identified the predictive role of structural parameters via DL models using SD-OCT images. DL models used retinal nerve fibre layer thickness maps and en face images [71], as well as thickness of the ganglion cell complex, outer segment, and RPE [72]. A combination of both structural and functional measurements via joint modelling strategies (e.g. Bayesian hierarchical models) can also be considered in future models [73].

2.3.2.3 AI algorithms in DME

Several modalities to diagnose DME include indirect ophthalmoscopy, colour retinal photography, fluorescein angiography (FA), and OCT. Whilst the former two are predominantly used, they may miss early or mild DME particularly if the central retinal thickness is <300 μm [74]. OCT has largely supplanted FA in the detection of macular oedema due to its non-invasive nature and its superiority in identifying and quantifying certain diabetic structural changes in the fovea [75]. Whether incorporation of macular OCT as part of DR screening is beneficial from a cost-effectiveness and medical standpoint has been addressed by several studies. Prescott *et al* 2014 demonstrated that the use of OCT in scenarios where fundus photographs suggestive of the presence of macular oedema resulted in cost savings of 16%–17% without reduction of health benefits. For universal OCT screening in conjunction with fundus photographs, a cost-effectiveness study in Hong Kong revealed a potential eight-fold reduction of false-positive results whilst improving sensitivity and long term cost-effectiveness [76]. Contrastingly, O'Halloran and Turner compared the referral rates in DR screening with the use of a standard colour fundus photography versus a combined fundus camera and OCT instrument in an Aboriginal population and concluded no added benefit of OCT [77]. However, this may be dependent on the specific instrument chosen for the study and the higher rate of inadequate fundus photographs obtained by the combined fundus/OCT instrument. Studies investigating smartphone ophthalmoscopy have emerged over recent years, with an increasing interest in smartphone retinal imaging technology in the screening of DR and DME [78]. The low memory and energy footprint requires a different solution to computer-based AI models that require computer systems containing advanced graphic processing units [79]. Hwang *et al* developed an offline smartphone-based CNN architecture (MobileNet), with a diagnostic accuracy of 90.02% in detecting DME, comparable to that of established AI models such as VGG16 and Inception V3 [79]. MobileNet contains three main layers (convolution, pooling, and fully connected layers) but separated the convolution layer into two separate layers, depth-wise and point-wise, to reduce model burden and calculation resource [79]. AI-based smartphone screening holds great clinical potential, particularly for patients in remote areas or underdeveloped countries. Further studies should aim to verify the reliability and feasibility in real-world clinical settings and evaluate potential integration with e-cloud technology.

2.3.2.4 AI algorithms in retinal vein occlusions

RVO is the second most common sight-threatening retinal vascular disease after DR [80]. Classified according to the site of obstruction, RVO is divided into branch RVO (BRVO) and central retinal vascular occlusion, with BRVO being more common. Untreated eyes with RVO have poor visual prognosis, with significant ocular complications being macular oedema, retinal bleeding, and retinal ischaemia [81]. Recent years have seen an increase in DL algorithms for automated detection of nonperfusion areas (NPAs) caused by RVO using optical coherence tomography angiography (OCTA) images. OCTA has been shown to have higher acquisition speed and safety due to its non-invasive nature, as well as better resolution and contrast than the FA, which is the gold standard for evaluation of retinal vasculature [82]. Nagasato *et al* compared the ability to detect NPA in RVO of a VGG-16 DNN, which automatically learns local features of OCTA images with RVO and generates a classification model, with support vector machine and ophthalmologist assessment [81]. The DNN showed significantly better performance than SVM in all parameters (mean AUC, sensitivity, specificity, and the average time required to distinguish RVO + NPA from normal OCTA images) and in AUC and specificity ($p < 0.01$) when compared with ophthalmologist assessment. The heat maps created also illustrated the pixels responsible for the predictions in DNN, which was focused on foveal avascular zone and NPA, thus allowing better interpretability. Automatic quantification of NPA in OCTA images have also been utilised for DR since NPA of the superficial capillary complex of the retina is a crucial indicator of DR stage and progression [83]. Nonetheless, the cost and limited field of view in currently available commercial devices may limit the potential OCTA technologies and related AI algorithms have in diagnosing vascular disorders. Potential solutions may include translating structural images taken by the more widely available OCT into functional flow images as suggested by Lee *et al* [84]. They proposed an AI model that was trained with OCTA images to generate en-face projection flow maps on OCT images, showing similar fidelity to OCTA and significantly better performance than expert clinicians ($p < 0.00001$).

2.3.2.5 Challenges in clinical translation of automated OCT image analysis
Despite the robust AI-based detection systems with high performance, methodological challenges persist thus limiting the translation from bench to bedside.

(i) ***Training dataset: limitations in quantity, availability, and quality***
A major barrier to the clinical application of OCT image analysis is the limited number, quality, and availability of large-image datasets from multiple OCT devices. Deep CNN are reliant on big datasets to avoid overfitting, a phenomenon whereby a network learns a function with high variance and low bias to model the training dataset but fails to generalise for subsequent training sets [85]. Current datasets are lacking in either the quantity of normal and pathological scans or the availability for public use [86]. The option of data sharing between different hospitals is limited by patient consent, institutional review board concerns, and geographical data regulations. Fortunately, several techniques of data augmentation may combat OCT data scarcity. The first would be conventional modifications of the images, such as scaling, translation, and rotation. Devalla *et al* compared the performance of the CNN on OCT images of glaucoma subjects with and without data augmentation (rotation, horizontal flipping, nonlinear intensity shift, additive white noise, multiplicative speckle noise, elastic deformations, and occluding patches) [87]. The CNN trained with data augmentation had better performance (both validation accuracy and training loss) owing to less overfitting and better convergence. Similarly, Kuwayama *et al* trained a CNN for automated detection of chorioretinal

diseases with a dataset augmented from 1100 to 59 400 B-scan images through horizontal flipping, rotation, and shifting [88]. The CNN demonstrated high prediction and recall for wet AMD, DR, and epiretinal membranes, as well as rare diseases such as Vogt–Koyanagi–Harada disease. Such data augmentation techniques are applicable for OCT images, because they, unlike fundus photographs, have small individual variations, stable magnification, and image quality [88]. Moreover, image modifications may parallel true variations that occurred during OCT image capture. Nonetheless, OCT images with minimal pathological findings may still be misidentified. A second technique would be enhanced methods such as transfer learning. It is worth noting that the performance of algorithms would be highly dependent on the weights of pre-trained models. In other words, pre-trained models trained with large datasets would be more effective in enhancing the performance of algorithms. Thirdly, an anatomical data augmentation that was originally exploited for computed tomography liver slices may be applied for OCT images [89]. Unlabelled B-scans adjacent to the training image within the same volume may be utilised as additional examples due to anatomical similarities [86]. Lastly, a novel technique—generative adversarial network (GAN)—has been advocated. This unsupervised ML relies on the synthesis of new OCT images from a training dataset using a generator and a discriminator subnetwork. Zheng *et al* demonstrated GAN was able to synthesise realistic OCT images for use in DL training algorithms; the CNN trained on all-synthetic OCT images achieved a similar AUC as the model trained on all real OCT images (AUC 0.98 vs 0.99) [90]. In addition to data augmentation, GAN may be used as a preprocessing step to remove artefacts, prediction tool for post-therapeutic OCT images, and establishment of shared feature space between two image modalities [91–93].

In addition, certain datasets only contain images from a limited number of manufacturers. OCT manufacturers have proprietary software packages for visualisation and calculation of image-related parameters such as signal quality, retinal thickness, and volume [94]. The difficulty of generalisation as a result of a lack of standardisation of acquisition and processing protocols is further exacerbated by the intradevice variability in image quality due to noise and motion artefacts [86]. Several studies have attempted to propose one single model that can be generalisable to new devices without substantial loss of performance. De Fauw *et al* devised a two-step framework of a device-dependent segmentation network followed by a device-independent classification network [95]. The segmentation network would be separately retrained on different OCT imaging devices, whilst keeping the classification network unmodified. Apart from the easy adaptability to different devices and thus the ease of clinical workflow integration, the readily viewable derivative after the first step of OCT segmentation allows a visual representation of the scan for clinicians and mitigates the 'black box' problem common in DL [95]. It may also act as a proxy for quality control. Other techniques include standardisation of image size and intensities, or the creation of separate CNNs [86]. Further research is required for standardisation protocols which would allow generalisable multivendor OCT image analyses.

(ii) ***Retinal segmentation***

OCT images remain subjected to segmentation artefacts, more frequently particularly in eyes with pathologies. Current research has focused on developing automatic segmentation algorithms. However, designing a system that works well in the clinical setting may be challenging. First, the differences of various intraretinal layers in normal and pathological states often render algorithms unreliable. Pathological changes may alter the structures required as reference value for automatic segmentation [96]. The second relates to the intrinsic noisy structure of OCT images. Since OCTs are generated by detecting interference signals between the reflected signals from the reference mirror and the backscattering signals from biological tissues, OCT images are susceptible to speckle noise [97]. Speckle noise, a phenomenon common in scattering media such as biological tissue, limits image quality and thus the accuracy of segmentation of retinal layers. Denoising AI algorithms and algorithms using 3D contextual information are at their infancy [98, 99]. There remains an urgent need for a device- and pathology-independent DL segmentation algorithm [99].

Apart from methodological challenges, key practical challenges must be addressed. Existing DL algorithms follow the ethos of 'one DL system, one eye disease'. This stems from the nature of DL systems, which typically follows an end-to-end training to generate an output directly from an input image [100]. Within a DL system for a particular eye disease, patient selection criteria and choice of device vary. This highlights the challenges for alternating between the different DL systems, not to mention potential technical and software hurdles. More research has focused on developing and validating DL systems in the classification of multiple eye diseases [100, 101]. In addition, standardised systems to manage misclassified patients (e.g. false positives and false negatives) are yet to be addressed [102].

2.4 Conclusions

There is robust evidence supporting the efficacy of DL systems in ophthalmology, particularly in the screening, diagnosis, and management of macula diseases, glaucomatous optic neuropathy, and retinal manifestations of systemic disease. The key advantage of a DL system for disease recognition and prognostication lies in its high accuracy and consistency of results, comparing favourably to well-trained clinicians. Despite significant advances in ML technology, current limitations remain in the quality and resolution of ophthalmic images obtained, as well as the number of training datasets available. With availability and expertise in AI technologies becoming more commonplace in healthcare industries worldwide, it is only a matter of time before these limitations are overcome.

References

[1] Grewal P S *et al* 2018 Deep learning in ophthalmology: a review *Can. J. Ophthalmol.* **53** 309–13
[2] LeCun Y, Bengio Y and Hinton G 2015 Deep learning *Nature* **521** 436–44
[3] O'Mahony N *et al* 2019 *Deep Learning vs. Traditional Computer Vision* (Berlin: Springer)
[4] Ran A R *et al* 2021 Deep learning in glaucoma with optical coherence tomography: a review *Eye* **35** 188–201
[5] LeNail A 2019 NN-SVG: Publication-ready neural network architecture schematics *J. Open Source Software* **4** 747
[6] Nair V and Hinton G E 2010 Rectified linear units improve restricted Boltzmann machines *Proc. of the 27th Int. Conf. on Machine Learning (ICML)* pp 807–14
[7] Bishop C M 2006 *Pattern Recognition and Machine Learning* (Berlin: Springer)
[8] Yamashita R *et al* 2018 Convolutional neural networks: an overview and application in radiology *Insights Imaging* **9** 611–29
[9] Gensure R H, Chiang M F and Campbell J P 2020 Artificial intelligence for retinopathy of prematurity *Curr. Opin Ophthalmol.* **31** 5
[10] Campbell J P *et al* 2021 Applications of artificial intelligence for retinopathy of prematurity screening *Pediatrics* **147** e2020016618
[11] Worrall D E, Wilson C M and Brostow G J 2016 Automated retinopathy of prematurity case detection with convolutional neural networks *Deep Learning and Data Labeling for Medical Applications* (Cham: Springer) pp 68–76
[12] Wang J *et al* 2018 Automated retinopathy of prematurity screening using deep neural networks *EBioMedicine* **35** 361–8
[13] Mulay S *et al* 2019 Early detection of retinopathy of prematurity stage using deep learning approach *Proc. SPIE* **10950** 109502Z
[14] Brown J M *et al* 2018 Automated diagnosis of plus disease in retinopathy of prematurity using deep convolutional neural networks *JAMA Ophthalmol.* **136** 803–10
[15] Redd T K *et al* 2019 Evaluation of a deep learning image assessment system for detecting severe retinopathy of prematurity *Br. J. Ophthalmol.* **103** 580–4
[16] Taylor S *et al* 2019 Monitoring disease progression with a quantitative severity scale for retinopathy of prematurity using deep learning *JAMA Ophthalmol.* **137** 1022–8
[17] Gupta K *et al* 2019 A quantitative severity scale for retinopathy of prematurity using deep learning to monitor disease regression after treatment *JAMA Ophthalmol.* **137** 1029–36
[18] Liew G, Michaelides M and Bunce C 2014 A comparison of the causes of blindness certifications in England and Wales in working age adults (16–64 years), 1999–2000 with 2009–2010 *BMJ Open* **4** e004015
[19] Cremers F P M *et al* 2018 Special issue introduction: inherited retinal disease: novel candidate genes, genotype-phenotype correlations, and inheritance models *Genes* **9** 215
[20] Chen T-C *et al* 2021 Genetic characteristics and epidemiology of inherited retinal degeneration in Taiwan *NPJ Genomic Med.* **6** 16
[21] Kohl S *et al* 1997 RDS/peripherin gene mutations are frequent causes of central retinal dystrophies *J. Med. Genet.* **34** 620–6

[22] Gao F-J *et al* 2019 Genetic and clinical findings in a large cohort of Chinese patients with suspected retinitis pigmentosa *Ophthalmology* **126** 1549–56
[23] Duncan J L *et al* 2018 Inherited retinal degenerations: current landscape and knowledge gaps *Trans. Vis. Sci. Technol.* **7** 6
[24] Fujinami-Yokokawa Y *et al* 2021 Prediction of causative genes in inherited retinal disorder from fundus photography and autofluorescence imaging using deep learning techniques *Br. J. Ophthalmol.*
[25] Miere A *et al* 2020 Deep learning-based classification of inherited retinal diseases using fundus autofluorescence *J. Clin. Med.* **9** 10
[26] International Diabetes Federation 2019 *IDF Diabetes Atlas* 9th edn (International Diabetes Federation)
[27] Arcadu F *et al* 2019 Deep learning algorithm predicts diabetic retinopathy progression in individual patients *NPJ Digit. Med.* **2** 92
[28] Fong D S *et al* 2004 Retinopathy in diabetes *Diabetes Care* **27** s84
[29] Jones S and Edwards R T 2010 Diabetic retinopathy screening: a systematic review of the economic evidence *Diabet. Med.* **27** 249–56
[30] Li B and Li H K 2013 Automated analysis of diabetic retinopathy images: principles, recent developments, and emerging trends *Curr. Diab. Rep.* **13** 453–9
[31] Wang S *et al* 2020 Performance of deep neural network-based artificial intelligence method in diabetic retinopathy screening: a systematic review and meta-analysis of diagnostic test accuracy *Eur. J. Endocrinol.* **183** 41–9
[32] Scanlon P H 2017 The English National Screening Programme for diabetic retinopathy 2003–2016 *Acta Diabetol.* **54** 515–25
[33] Cuadros J 2021 The real-world impact of artificial intelligence on diabetic retinopathy screening in primary care *J. Diabetes Sci. Technol.* **15** 664–5
[34] He J *et al* 2019 The practical implementation of artificial intelligence technologies in medicine *Nat. Med.* **25** 30–6
[35] Thapa D *et al* 2014 Comparison of super-resolution algorithms applied to retinal images *J. Biomed. Opt.* **19** 056002
[36] Swanson E A and Fujimoto J G 2017 The ecosystem that powered the translation of OCT from fundamental research to clinical and commercial impact [Invited] *Biomed. Opt. Express* **8** 1638–64
[37] Gehrs K M *et al* 2006 Age-related macular degeneration–emerging pathogenetic and therapeutic concepts *Ann. Med.* **38** 450–71
[38] Kramer S G *et al* 1995 Perfluorocarbon liquids in ophthalmology *Surv. Ophthalmol.* **39** 375–95
[39] Lee H *et al* 2018 Automated segmentation of lesions including subretinal hyperreflective material in neovascular age-related macular degeneration *Am. J. Ophthalmol.* **191** 64–75
[40] Motozawa N *et al* 2019 Optical coherence tomography-based deep-learning models for classifying normal and age-related macular degeneration and exudative and non-exudative age-related macular degeneration changes *Ophthalmol. Ther.* **8** 527–39
[41] Kermany D S *et al* 2018 Identifying medical diagnoses and treatable diseases by image-based deep learning *Cell* **172** 1122–31.e9
[42] Chakravarthy U *et al* 2016 Automated identification of lesion activity in neovascular age-related macular degeneration *Ophthalmology* **123** 1731–6

[43] Schlegl T *et al* 2018 Fully automated detection and quantification of macular fluid in OCT using deep learning *Ophthalmology* **125** 549–58
[44] Ouyang Y *et al* 2013 Optical coherence tomography–based observation of the natural history of drusenoid lesion in eyes with dry age-related macular degeneration *Ophthalmology* **120** 2656–65
[45] Nassisi M *et al* 2018 Quantity of intraretinal hyperreflective foci in patients with intermediate age-related macular degeneration correlates with 1-year progression *Invest. Ophthalmol. Vis. Sci.* **59** 3431–9
[46] Abdelfattah N S *et al* 2016 Drusen volume as a predictor of disease progression in patients with late age-related macular degeneration in the fellow eye *Invest. Ophthalmol. Vis. Sci.* **57** 1839–46
[47] Marsiglia M *et al* 2013 Association between geographic atrophy progression and reticular pseudodrusen in eyes with dry age-related macular degeneration *Invest. Ophthalmol. Vis. Sci.* **54** 7362–9
[48] Wintergerst M W M *et al* 2017 Algorithms for the automated analysis of age-related macular degeneration biomarkers on optical coherence tomography: a systematic review *Trans. Vis. Sci. Technol.* **6** 10
[49] Schmidt-Erfurth U *et al* 2018 Prediction of individual disease conversion in early AMD using artificial intelligence *Invest. Ophthalmol. Vis. Sci.* **59** 3199–208
[50] Saha S *et al* 2019 Automated detection and classification of early AMD biomarkers using deep learning *Sci. Rep.* **9** 10990
[51] Brown D M *et al* 2006 Ranibizumab versus verteporfin for neovascular age-related macular degeneration *New Engl. J. Med.* **355** 1432–44
[52] Rosenfeld P J *et al* 2006 Ranibizumab for neovascular age-related macular degeneration *New Engl. J. Med.* **355** 1419–31
[53] Bogunović H *et al* 2017 Prediction of anti-VEGF treatment requirements in neovascular AMD using a machine learning approach *Invest. Ophthalmol. Vis. Sci.* **58** 3240–8
[54] Schmidt-Erfurth U and Waldstein S M 2016 A paradigm shift in imaging biomarkers in neovascular age-related macular degeneration *Prog. Retin. Eye Res.* **50** 1–24
[55] Society E G 2017 European glaucoma society terminology and guidelines for glaucoma, 4th edition – Chapter 3: Treatment principles and options *Br. J. Ophthalmol.* **101** 130–95
[56] Tham Y C *et al* 2014 Global prevalence of glaucoma and projections of glaucoma burden through 2040: a systematic review and meta-analysis *Ophthalmology* **121** 2081–90
[57] Wong D *et al* 2008 Level-set based automatic cup-to-disc ratio determination using retinal fundus images in ARGALI *30th Annual Int. Conf. of the IEEE Engineering in Medicine and Biology Society* (IEEE) pp 2266–9
[58] Joshi G D, Sivaswamy J and Krishnadas S 2011 Optic disk and cup segmentation from monocular color retinal images for glaucoma assessment *IEEE Trans. Med. Imaging* **30** 1192–205
[59] Das P, Nirmala S R and Medhi J P 2015 Diagnosis of glaucoma using CDR and NRR area in retina images *Netw. Model. Anal. Health Inform. Bioinforma.* **5** 3
[60] Das P, Nirmala S and Medhi J P 2016 Diagnosis of glaucoma using CDR and NRR area in retina images *Netw. Model. Anal. Health Inform. Bioinforma.* **5** 3
[61] Abbas Q 2017 Glaucoma-deep: detection of glaucoma eye disease on retinal fundus images using deep learning *Int. J. Adv. Comput. Sci. Appl.* **8** 41–5

[62] Orlando J I *et al* 2017 Convolutional neural network transfer for automated glaucoma identification *Proc. SPIE* **10160** 101600U

[63] Sreng S *et al* 2020 Deep learning for optic disc segmentation and glaucoma diagnosis on retinal images *Appl. Sci.* **10** 4916

[64] O'Neill E C *et al* 2014 Glaucomatous optic neuropathy evaluation project: factors associated with underestimation of glaucoma likelihood *JAMA Ophthalmol.* **132** 560–6

[65] Wen J C *et al* 2019 Forecasting future Humphrey visual fields using deep learning *PLoS One* **14** e0214875

[66] Berchuck S I, Mukherjee S and Medeiros F A 2019 Estimating rates of progression and predicting future visual fields in glaucoma using a deep variational autoencoder *Sci. Rep.* **9** 1–12

[67] Yousefi S *et al* 2018 Detection of longitudinal visual field progression in glaucoma using machine learning *Am. J. Ophthalmol.* **193** 71–9

[68] Brigatti L *et al* 1997 Automatic detection of glaucomatous visual field progression with neural networks *Arch. Ophthalmol.* **115** 725–8

[69] De Moraes C G, Liebmann J M and Levin L A 2017 Detection and measurement of clinically meaningful visual field progression in clinical trials for glaucoma *Prog. Retin. Eye Res.* **56** 107–47

[70] Malik R, Swanson W H and Garway-Heath D F 2012 'Structure-function relationship' in glaucoma: past thinking and current concepts *Clin. Experimental Ophthalmol.* **40** 369–80

[71] Christopher M *et al* 2020 Deep learning approaches predict glaucomatous visual field damage from OCT optic nerve head en face images and retinal nerve fiber layer thickness maps *Ophthalmology* **127** 346–56

[72] Xu L *et al* 2020 Predicting the glaucomatous central 10-degree visual field from optical coherence tomography using deep learning and tensor regression *Am. J. Ophthalmol.* **218** 304–13

[73] Medeiros F A *et al* 2011 Combining structural and functional measurements to improve detection of glaucoma progression using Bayesian hierarchical models *Invest. Ophthalmol. Vis. Sci.* **52** 5794–803

[74] Virgili G *et al* 2007 Optical coherence tomography versus stereoscopic fundus photography or biomicroscopy for diagnosing diabetic macular edema: a systematic review *Invest. Ophthalmol. Vis. Sci.* **48** 4963–73

[75] Ozdek S C *et al* 2005 Optical coherence tomographic assessment of diabetic macular edema: comparison with fluorescein angiographic and clinical findings *Ophthalmologica* **219** 86–92

[76] Wong I Y H *et al* 2020 Incorporating optical coherence tomography macula scans enhances cost-effectiveness of fundus photography-based screening for diabetic macular edema *Diabetes Care* **43** 2959

[77] O'Halloran R A and Turner A W 2018 Evaluating the impact of optical coherence tomography in diabetic retinopathy screening for an Aboriginal population *Clin. Exp. Ophthalmol.* **46** 116–21

[78] Tan C H *et al* 2020 Use of smartphones to detect diabetic retinopathy: scoping review and meta-analysis of diagnostic test accuracy studies *J. Med. Internet Res.* **22** e16658

[79] Hwang D-K *et al* 2020 Smartphone-based diabetic macula edema screening with an offline artificial intelligence *J. Chin. Med. Assoc.* **83** 12

[80] Rogers S L *et al* 2010 Natural history of branch retinal vein occlusion: an evidence-based systematic review *Ophthalmology* **117** 1094–101.e5

[81] Nagasato D *et al* 2019 Automated detection of a nonperfusion area caused by retinal vein occlusion in optical coherence tomography angiography images using deep learning *PLoS One* **14** e0223965

[82] Mc Grath O *et al* 2021 Clinical utility of artificial intelligence algorithms to enhance wide-field optical coherence tomography angiography images *J. Imaging* **7** 32

[83] Guo Y *et al* 2018 MEDnet, a neural network for automated detection of avascular area in OCT angiography *Biomed. Opt. Express* **9** 5147–58

[84] Lee C S *et al* 2019 Generating retinal flow maps from structural optical coherence tomography with artificial intelligence *Sci. Rep.* **9** 5694

[85] Shorten C and Khoshgoftaar T M 2019 A survey on image data augmentation for deep learning *J. Big Data* **6** 60

[86] Yanagihara R T *et al* 2020 Methodological challenges of deep learning in optical coherence tomography for retinal diseases: a review *Trans. Vis. Sci. Technol.* **9** 11

[87] Devalla S K *et al* 2018 DRUNET: a dilated-residual U-Net deep learning network to segment optic nerve head tissues in optical coherence tomography images *Biomed. Opt. Express* **9** 3244–65

[88] Kuwayama S *et al* 2019 Automated detection of macular diseases by optical coherence tomography and artificial intelligence machine learning of optical coherence tomography images *J. Ophthalmol.* **2019** 6319581

[89] Ben-Cohen A *et al* 2018 Anatomical data augmentation for CNN based pixel-wise classification *IEEE 15th Int. Symp. on Biomedical Imaging (ISBI)* (IEEE) pp 1096–9

[90] Zheng C *et al* 2020 Assessment of generative adversarial networks model for synthetic optical coherence tomography images of retinal disorders *Trans. Vis. Sci. Technol.* **9** 29

[91] Liu Y *et al* 2020 Prediction of OCT images of short-term response to anti-VEGF treatment for neovascular age-related macular degeneration using generative adversarial network *Br. J. Ophthalmol.* **104** 1735

[92] Cheong H *et al* 2020 DeshadowGAN: a deep learning approach to remove shadows from optical coherence tomography images *Trans. Vis. Sci. Technol.* **9** 23

[93] Tavakkoli A *et al* 2020 A novel deep learning conditional generative adversarial network for producing angiography images from retinal fundus photographs *Sci. Rep.* **10** 21580

[94] Huang Y *et al* 2012 Signal quality assessment of retinal optical coherence tomography images *Invest. Ophthalmol. Vis. Sci.* **53** 2133–41

[95] De Fauw J *et al* 2018 Clinically applicable deep learning for diagnosis and referral in retinal disease *Nat. Med.* **24** 1342–50

[96] Enders C *et al* 2019 Quantity and quality of image artifacts in optical coherence tomography angiography *PLoS One* **14** e0210505

[97] Tomlins P H and Wang R K 2005 Theory, developments and applications of optical coherence tomography *J. Phys.* D **38** 2519

[98] Devalla S K *et al* 2019 A deep learning approach to denoise optical coherence tomography images of the optic nerve head *Sci. Rep.* **9** 14454

[99] Devalla S K *et al* 2020 Towards label-free 3D segmentation of optical coherence tomography images of the optic nerve head using deep learning *Biomed. Opt. Express* **11** 6356–78

[100] Son J *et al* 2020 Development and validation of deep learning models for screening multiple abnormal findings in retinal fundus images *Ophthalmology* **127** 85–94

[101] Ting D S W *et al* 2017 Development and validation of a deep learning system for diabetic retinopathy and related eye diseases using retinal images from multiethnic populations with diabetes *JAMA* **318** 2211–23

[102] Gunasekeran D V and Wong T Y 2020 Artificial intelligence in ophthalmology in 2020: a technology on the cusp for translation and implementation *Asia-Pac. J. Ophthalmol.* **9** 61–6

[103] Prescott G *et al* 2014 Improving the cost-effectiveness of photographic screening for Diabetic Macular Oedema: A prospective, multi-centre, UK study *Br. J. Ophthalmol.* **98** 1042–9

Chapter 3

Artificial intelligence clinical applications of wearable technologies

Shichao Ma, Chun-Yat Yee, Jiayi Xin and Joshua W K Ho

3.1 Wearable devices: healthcare sensors blended into everyday life

Wearable devices are electronic gadgets which are lightweight and portable enough to be worn on the body or embedded into clothing. Many sensors are integrated into wearable devices which allows signals from the human body to be constantly logged and analyzed. Because wearable devices blend automatic monitoring of health and activity into people's everyday life, their popularity has continued to grow in the past 5 years. One representative example of wearable devices is a smartwatch. CCS Insight reported a strong upward trajectory of shipments of smartwatches and fitness trackers worldwide in the past 5 years (2016–2020) and forecasted that the shipments will continue to rise in the next 4 years (figure 3.1). Analysts believe that the recent global pandemic has further enhanced people's awareness of their health, and it will cause the continuous boom of the adoption of wearables [1].

Wrist-worn devices including smartwatches and fitness trackers have gained widespread popularity because these products have been able to maturely combine usability and functionality to target a wide user base. Apart from wrist-worn devices, there are many other commercial wearables that aim to accomplish specialized monitoring tasks. Seneviratne *et al* surveyed current wearable products and classified them into three categories: (1) accessories including wrist-worn devices like smartwatches and head-mounted devices like smart eyewear and headsets, (2) e-textiles including smart garments and foot or hand-worn devices, and (3) e-patches including sensor patches, e-tattoo and e-skin [2].

The invention and integration of portable sensors give rise to an opportunity to acquire useful data from the human body constantly, which makes data collected from wearable devices different from medical data produced in hospitals and medical centers. Wearable devices trade off the multitude of health information they obtained for the accessibility of it.

doi:10.1088/978-0-7503-4637-5ch3

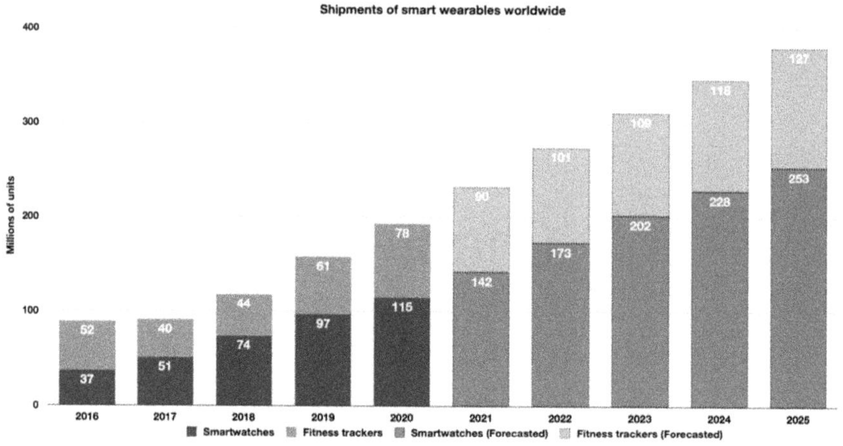

Figure 3.1. Real (2016–2020) and projected (2021–2025) number of shipments of smartwatches and fitness trackers worldwide, reproduced with permission from [1].

Wearable devices usually consist of standard electronic components including random-access memory unit and central processing unit to store and process data. However, wearables naturally need to compromise the capability of computing for portability, which implies that wearable devices vastly rely on connectivity with other digital computing systems such as smartphones, personal computers, or cloud-based computing systems. The concept of Wearable Internet of Things was proposed by Hiremath *et al* to illustrate the connectivity-demanding characteristic of wearable devices [3], which can be characterized by having (1) wearable body area sensors, (2) Internet-connected gateways, and (3) cloud and big data support.

Sensors equipped in wearable devices play the role of making the device unique and being capable of handle specific tasks. Hiremath *et al* categorized sensors into on-body contact sensors and peripheral non-contact sensors; different types of sensors are listed in table 3.1.

As one of the common tests used to evaluate the heart, a conventional 12-lead electrocardiogram (ECG) is usually conducted by placing 10 electrodes at certain spots on the patient's limbs and the chest. These electrodes are wired with an ECG machine to form closed circuits so that the electrical activity of the heart can be measured and recorded. An ECG generated by a smartwatch, on the other hand, typically involves fewer electrodes. For example, an Apple Watch is snug onto the wrist of one upper limb, and users are required to hold one finger of another upper limb on the crown of the watch to form a closed circuit. Two electrodes positioned on the case back of the watch and the digital crown receive electrical signal to form a single-lead ECG. A 12-lead ECG often contains more details than a single-lead ECG. Nonetheless, performing a single-lead ECG in wrist-worn devices predominates the wearable device market because of its practicality. This enables ECG measurement from wrist-worn devices to gain widespread popularity, which in turn may become useful in widespread disease screening, such as atrial fibrillation [5].

Table 3.1. Different types of wearable body area sensors [3].

Category	Main purpose	Types of sensors and example application	Target wearable device
On-body contact sensors	Monitoring	Physiological (electrocardiogram, electromyogram, electroencephalogram)	Wrist-worn devices for electrocardiogram, e-textiles/e-patch for electromyography and head-mounted devices for electroencephalography
		Chemical (sweat, glucose, saliva)	E-patch
		Optical (oximetry, tissue properties, photoplethysmogram)	Wrist-worn devices and other accessories
	Therapeutic[a]	Medication (drug delivery patches)	E-patch
		Stimulation (chronic pain relief)	
		Emergency (defibrillator)	E-textiles
Peripheral non-contact sensors[b]	Fitness and wellness	Motion (physical activity, calorie count)	Accessories
		Location (GPS, indoor localization)	
	Behavioral[c]	Activity (fall, sleep, exercise)	
		Emotion (anxiety, stress, depression)	
		Diet (calorie intake, eating habits)	
	Rehabilitation	Speech (language development)	
		Camera (technology for blinds)	

Notes[a] Electronic component with therapeutic potential is more about delivering something instead of sensing something, but they can still be integrated into wearable devices for therapeutic purposes.
[b] Notably, the above-mentioned peripheral non-contact sensors in wearable devices are still usually in contact with skins, but the contact may not be compulsory to receive corresponding data.
[c] Behavioral data like the emotion of the user may be analyzed from other forms of health data collected by common sensors, e.g. Shu *et al* conducted a study about recognizing emotion through heart rate data from a smart bracelet [4].

Apart from making medical impact from its widespread availability, data from wearable devices are also effective because of wearable devices' ability to collect continuous, medium- to long-term longitudinal data. Implementing wearable devices into the study of estimating sleep parameters is an example. Polysomnography is usually adopted in a hospital or a sleep center to diagnose sleep disorders by recoding multiple physiological signals, and numerical sensor data including electroencephalography

(EEG; which is a recording of brain waves), electrooculography (which can measure eye movements), electromyography (EMG; which can measure muscle movements and contractions), oxygen level of blood, heart rate, etc [6]. Comparatively, actigraphy monitors people's rest and activity cycles during sleep and only very limited electronic units, mainly an accelerometer, are required. Polysomnography is comprehensive and reliable, and it has been regarded as a gold standard for sleep assessment; however, more sleeping-relevant studies [7, 8] are carried out nowadays by analyzing actigraphy data collected from wearable devices, and more consumer-grade wearable monitors that implement actigraphy to assess sleep are being created because actigraphy is a less expensive, demanding, and cumbersome way to monitor people's sleep. A large amount of actigraphy data can be gathered through wearables 24/7, which can be used to understand sleeping patterns through processing and algorithms, even though the method is completely different from polysomnography.

3.2 Deep learning enables artificial intelligence applications of wearable devices

The acquisition of data is just the end of the beginning. For most people, these data are not easy to understand even though the data are reflections of their own health status. Even for physicians, having to interpret a large amount of data during a clinical consultation is not feasible. Besides asking for interpretation from professionals, artificial intelligence (AI) algorithms, especially machine learning techniques, provide insights into health data.

Before developing the algorithm, it is necessary to clearly formulate the specific machine learning tasks in which data generated by wearable devices can be used. Many healthcare tasks can be formulated as supervised machine learning tasks, such as classification and regression. Classification tasks involve prediction of discrete class labels and can be further split into binary classification, such as distinguishing between normal activities of daily living and fall activities [9], and multi-classes classification, such as discriminating the ECG data of myocardial infarction from healthy samples, samples with other chronic heart conditions, and noisy samples [10]. A regression task aims to predict a continuous outcome, for instance, estimating the energy expenditure from physiological signals collected from wearable devices and other information [11]. Generally, classification problems are more common in the domain of wearable AI. (As of December 2021, there are around 145 thousand results on Google Scholar with keywords *classification* and *wearable devices* and there are only around 50 thousand results with keywords *regression* and *wearable devices.*)

Developing a supervised machine learning system using data collected from wearable devices is not easy. Most raw sensor data collected are continuous and large, which requires careful extraction and discovery of useful features for machine learning development. It is challenging for researchers and developers to identify the best feature representation of the data, which may be a high-dimensional feature space. These signals contain both useful information and noise; feature extraction is one of the significant methods to extract useful parts and ignore unwanted parts. For example, time-domain features such as mean absolute value, root mean square, and wavelength and frequency domain features like mean frequency and median frequency are widely regarded as important features for EMG signal classification [12]. Apart from turning raw signals into features through calculation, there are other common techniques including low variance filter, high correlation filter, principal component analysis, independent component analysis, and so on, to do dimensionality reduction.

Once discriminative features are extracted from raw data, some traditional machine learning classifiers which rely on handcrafted feature learning including logistic regression (LR), *k*-nearest neighbors, decision tree and random forest, support vector machine, and so on, may be implemented to learn patterns from features (i.e. update parameters in model based on feedback) and make a prediction (i.e. output result based on the input and tuned parameters) in a relatively short time.

Nevertheless, extraction of important features is often not easy for sensor data collected from wearable devices, as they are often noisy and large. In recent years, neural networks, especially deep neural networks, have become increasingly popular methods to skip the burdensome stage of feature extraction and turn raw health data into comprehensions accurately through training.

Deep neural networks are artificial neural networks that consist of multiple hidden layers of inter-connected neurons. It is the backbone of the field of deep learning. Deep learning methods like convolutional neural networks (CNNs) and recurrent neural networks (RNNs) differ from other machine learning classifiers and regular neural networks not only in the number of parameters and the depth of structure but also in the fact that CNNs and RNNs implement special layers and architectures to process specific kinds of data. Deep learning method is believed to be a highly effective way to process sensor data [13], and there have already been many implementations in wearable devices.

CNN is a deep neural network utilizing a mathematical operation called convolution to learn the features from input. This kind of neural network uses convolution in place of general matrix multiplication in at least one of its layers, and these special layers are called convolutional layers [14]. Pooling layers are usually included in CNN as well to reduce the dimensionality of data (figure 3.2). Then, fully connected layers are attached to compute the flattened matrix outputted from previous layers to produce outputs. The CNN is very popular in computer vision and widely used to classify image data, and it is also a great choice to recognize patterns from physiological signals like ECG through one-dimensional (1D) convolution [15] because image data and ECG data are both continuous, sparse in information, and involving much noise, even though their dimensionalities are different. Moreover, heat map–like spectrograms are generated after applying time–frequency analysis such as short-time Fourier transform (STFT) into signals, and these 2D spectrograms are even more like images in normal computer vision tasks. Amoh *et al* presented a system called DeepCough which used a CNN to detect coughs through a wearable acoustic sensor. They preprocessed the sensor data by performing STFT on it to create 2D spectral segments from 1D signals [16].

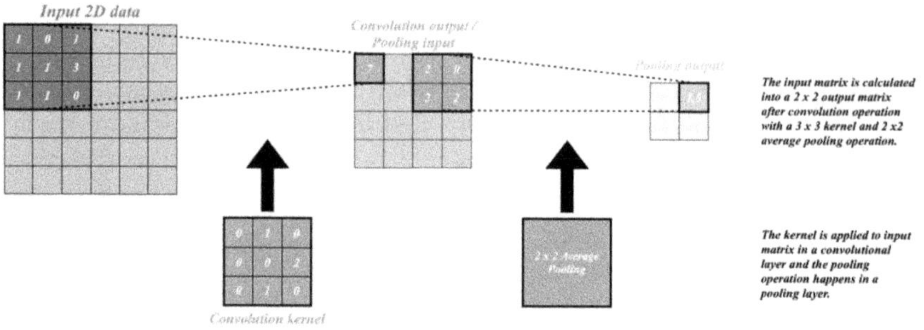

Figure 3.2. Simple illustrations of 2D convolution and 2 × 2 average pooling. The kernel as a parameter in a CNN is updated during the backpropagation to better extract important features from the input matrix. Apart from the average pooling method, the max pooling method is also widely used to reduce dimensionality. All convolutional layers and pooling layers are important parts of a CNN.

Unlike CNNs, which are most suitable for images and 2D spectral data, RNNs including long short-term memory and gated recurrent unit are particularly suitable for processing temporal and sequential data. This kind of neural network can extract information from a sequence by recurrently feeding the results of a segment back into the network and relating segments in the sequence. RNNs have been widely applied to natural language processing (NLP) and proved to be effective, and there is an increasing number of studies about implementing RNNs on the classification of data collected from wearables because many sensor data contain segments that are related temporally. RNNs have been implemented to recognize hand gesture [17] and human activity [18] through data collected from wearable sensors.

Transformer is a recent groundbreaking advance in deep learning and introduced from the highly cited paper *Attention is All You Need* [19]. A transformer model was initially introduced as a sequence-to-sequence model which consists of a group of encoders and a group of decoders, and both encoder and decoder contain multi-head attention layers. Multi-headed attention mechanism implemented in these layers is an imitation of cognitive attention. Another important part of the model is the positional encoding, which introduces positional information into the input sequence so that the model does not have to process the data in order like an RNN does. All these components and mechanisms of transformer make the model capable of sequential processing; in fact, transformers have outperformed RNNs in many NLP tasks [20]. The model is now being modified and implemented to process image data on a large scale [21–23], but many works are very recent and still in the stage of open review as of December 2021. Although the number of studies is small, some researchers have already implemented the model into tasks of classifying data from wearable sensors; for example, Behinaein *et al* applied transformer architecture to detect stress from ECG data collected by wearable devices [24]. They designed an architecture that consisted of convolutional layers to extract features, a transformer encoder, and fully connected layers to do classification. The proposed model achieved strong results in their experiments.

It is foreseeable that there will be an upcoming trend in implementing transformers in research on health data and data from wearable sensors because of a transformer's capability of processing various kinds of data and its outstanding general performances in various tasks.

Deep learning methods are saving a lot of trouble from manually extracting and selecting features, but they are data hungry. Lin *et al* showed that their handcrafted features outperformed CNN features in the classification of hepatobiliary phase magnetic resonance images when the size of the training dataset was small, while CNN features achieve better classification results as the size of training data is expanded [25].

3.3 Federated and transfer learning boost performance of health AI applications

Healthcare-related data collected from wearable devices can potentially contain sensitive and confidential information like other medical data. It is often not easy to gather huge amount of medical data to train a deep neural network. There are several innovative paradigms of training deep neural networks, and these methods could be the solution to tackle the dilemma about medical data.

Federated learning is a distributed machine learning method which trains a machine learning algorithm including a deep neural network across multiple edge nodes that hold data without gathering data together. Edge nodes in the federated learning network are usually edge devices such as smartphones and wearable devices or side servers. All data will be kept locally and will not be exposed to either the central server or other edge nodes. During the training process, each edge node trains the downloaded machine learning model locally based on its exclusive dataset, then the update of the model resulting from training is uploaded to the central server for the later aggregation (figure 3.3). The model in the central server is updated with consensus after aggregation. The process is repeated until the model is well trained. In medical AI, edge nodes can be wearable devices that constantly collect data from people or hospitals, medical centers, and institutions that own medical data. This paradigm is able to train a machine learning model without breaching the confidentiality of data no matter what kinds of participants are involved as nodes. Can and Ersoy implemented a federated learning strategy in the task of detecting mental stress levels with the heart activity data collected from wrist-worn devices through a multilayer perceptron [26]. Surprisingly, the result of privacy-preserved federated learning even slightly exceeded the accuracy achieved by combining all data in a traditional way.

Transfer learning is also a potential option to address the shortage issue of medical data for machine learning training. The idea of transfer learning is about immigrating the knowledge learned from task A into a relevant task B so that the learning procedure does not need to start from scratch. More specifically, when the pre-trained parameters including weights and biases from the EMG classification neural network are used for the initialization of the network rather than a random parameters initialization for EEG classification, and vice versa, the accuracy of

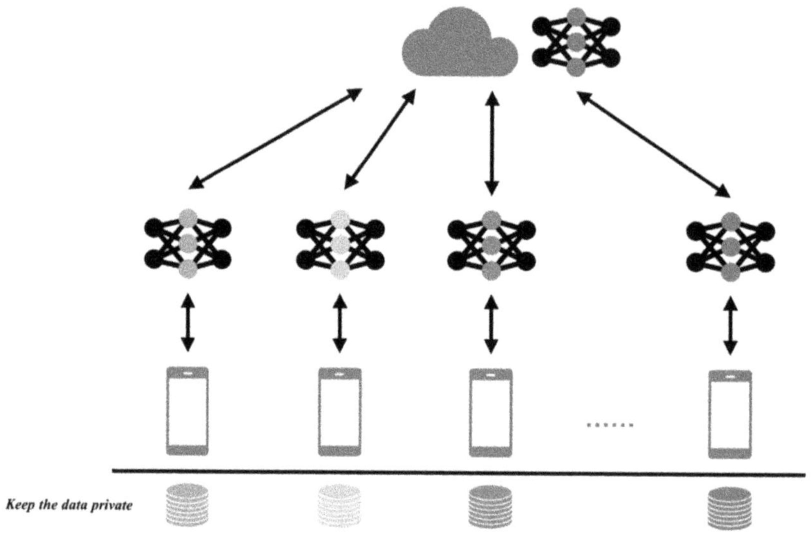

Figure 3.3. This figure shows the idea of federated learning. The machine learning models, or the updates of models, instead of the data are transmitted over the network, which avoids the exposure of data.

classification is improved because of the similar physical natures between EMG and EEG [27]. Transfer learning provides the possibility of reducing both the need for large amount of training data and the need for long training time for training a complicated machine learning classifier if it can be pre-trained from a related task (figure 3.4).

Both above-mentioned approaches aim to solve problems in wearable healthcare so that wearable devices and state-of-the-art machine learning algorithms can help people to monitor their health status and prevent disease without sacrificing any privacy or security, and the efficiency of the learning process can be enhanced. There have already been some interesting attempts of implementing these methods into real healthcare applications. For instance, FedHealth is a framework that proposes a learning procedure as presented in Algorithm 3.1 to start with training a CNN with a limited public dataset and achieve more accurate as well personalized classification at edge nodes based on federated learning and transfer learning [28]. They firstly implemented the framework in a Parkinson's disease auxiliary diagnosis task in which the data was activity signal collected from acceleration and gyroscope sensors in smartphones.

Algorithm 3.1. The learning procedure of FedHealth.

Input: Data from different users $\{\mathscr{D}_1, \mathscr{D}_2, \mathscr{D}_3, \ldots\mathscr{D}_N\}, \eta$
Output: Personalized user model f_u
1: Construct an initial cloud model f_S with public datasets
2: Distribute f_S to all users
3: Train user models locally

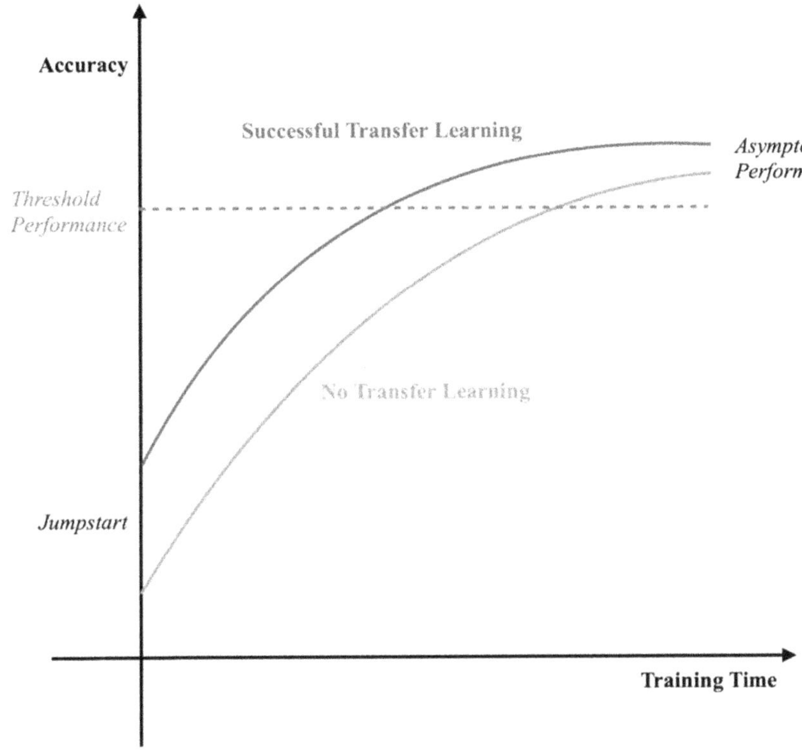

Figure 3.4. An illustrative learning curve of successful transfer learning. As shown in this example, less training time is required for transfer learning to reach the threshold performance.

4: Update all user models to the server using homomorphic encryption. Make models aggregation by averaging all models. Then the server takes this aggregation model as the updated cloud model f'_S
5: Distribute f'_S to all users, then perform transfer learning on each user to get their personalized model f_u
6: Repeat the above procedures with the continuously emerging user data

3.4 Current healthcare applications of AI and wearable technology

The combination of wearable devices and AI has been implemented in many fields, including telemedicine, health monitoring, and disease prediction. Most wearables take advantage of the wireless data transmission technology to transfer data from the devices to users' smartphones or other platforms. One major advantage of these devices is that sensor data can be collected constantly. As long as the wearable device is being worn, data can be collected around the clock. This contrasts with most clinical measurements in the current healthcare setting, where they are only performed during each visit. In addition, these devices enable scalability in their deployment in a healthcare system. Most wearable devices are smart devices that can collect physiologically relevant data with little human input, as well as advanced data processing and digital storage functions. In most cases, the cost of data generation, processing, storage, and retrieval can be significantly reduced at the population scale. Furthermore, data can be collected unobtrusively. Patients may have psychobiological reaction during clinical measurements. The most notable example is white coat hypertension, in which 15%–30% of patients have elevated blood pressure when visiting a doctor in a clinic. Such a phenomenon can result in non-representative blood pressure measurements [29]. On the contrary, wearable devices enable data collection from patients without them noticing and without restriction to location, thus avoiding such response.

Telemedicine has become more popular since the COVID-19 pandemic in early 2020. Many physicians and patients around the world have been experimenting with this new model of healthcare delivery. In the United States, a six-fold increase in telemedical consultations was observed following the pandemic [30]. Compared to traditional face-to-face consultations, the major limitation of telemedicine consultations is the inability to make routine clinical measurements across the monitors. Wearable devices can fill this gap by a remote collection of real-time physiological data from patients like heart rate, ECG readings, blood oxygen saturation, and blood glucose and send them to physicians to provide additional real-time information to facilitate the consultation [31].

Wearable technology is not only helping people cope with the pandemic through remote medical consultation but also providing the detection of COVID-19 and the assessment of physical conditions during the infection with the help of AI technology. Quer *et al* used wearable sensor data such as resting heart rate, sleep data, activity data, demographic data such as gender and age, and a multivariate LR model to detect COVID-19 [32]. An area under the curve of 0.80 was achieved when both sensor data and self-reported symptom data were involved. Similar research was published by Mishra *et al* even earlier to use wearable sensor data like heart rate, number of steps, and sleep time to detect pre-symptomatic cases of COVID-19 [33]. However, it is also stated that one limitation of the aforementioned research is that they are not capable of differentiating COVID-19 specifically from other viral infections [34]. On the other hand, the authors of the same article believed that these problems could be solved by involving more wearable devices and more kinds of sensor data to make more comprehensive predictions. Apart from detecting the infection, Natarajan *et al* made an assessment of physical conditions including physiological signs and self-reported symptoms of actively infective subjects through machine learning to predict the need for hospitalization and the illness of on a specific day [35]. Moreover, COVID-19 is making an impact on people not just pathologically, but behaviorally as well. Sun *et al* analyzed data from smartphones and wearable devices to monitor people's behavioral changes under non-pharmaceutical interventions like social distancing and lockdown during the pandemic [36]. Besides application to screening of infectious diseases such as COVID-19, the combination of wearable technology and AI technology can help people to prevent and monitor disease extensively.

Earlier detection and treatment of a disease is often preferred. One of the strengths of wearables is the ability to establish individualized baseline levels.

Deviations from baseline can be utilized as potential signals of early disease detection, instead of using population-based reference intervals. Individualized baseline allows disease screening algorithms to account for normal biological variations within the population. For instance, a large-scale study in the United States using Fitbit wearable identified that elevation of resting heart rate and longer sleep time by 0.5 to 1 standard deviations of baseline are significant predictors of influenza-like illnesses, indicating that the potential of using wearable-based physiological data to predict disease state individually and even influenza outbreak within a population [37].

Patients with chronic conditions like hypertension and diabetes need regular checking of their health status. Conventionally, many patients need to use logbooks to record their daily health status, like blood pressure and blood glucose in the case of patients with hypertension and diabetes, respectively. The major drawback of this practice is the assumption that patients are compliant enough to keep a daily habit to record their health regularly at a specific time. Through leveraging the unique characteristics of wearables to collect continuous and unobstructed data, hundreds or even thousands of data samples can be collected without the patients noticing, be they awake or asleep. Also, wearables enable the detection of real-time dynamic changes of physiological parameters, such as changes in blood glucose level after a meal for diabetic control [38]. Altogether, studies found out that continuous glucose monitoring (CGM) promotes better glycemic and weight controls and induces behavioral changes in diabetic patients [39]. In recent literature, the use of CGM has also demonstrated the early and more sensitive detection of impaired glucose homeostasis [40]. For example, severe glucose variability was present in 25% of normoglycemic individuals, and within this subgroup, glucose reached prediabetic or diabetic glucose levels 15% and 2% of the time, respectively. Different 'glucotypes' could be uncovered revealing more understanding about the disease.

3.5 Practical considerations, challenges, and future of wearable technologies in healthcare

There are many factors that determine the successful application of wearable devices in practical healthcare settings. An important consideration of incorporating wearable devices into an existing healthcare system is to ensure the devices are used by patients in a sustained manner. Studies have shown that the more patients understand their own conditions, the more likely they will be to change their behavior in a positive way [41]. Wearable devices offer an opportunity for patients to visualize and monitor their real-time health data, instead of physicians recording them in patients' medical records. As a result, patients can have a better understanding of their current health status, which translates to more incentives to improve their health by actively changing their health behaviors [41].

Switching to physicians, how to streamline the use of wearable devices into their existing clinical practice is the focus. Continuous and scalable data from wearables implies a high volume of data, which may lead to information overload. Without a way to reliably identify clinically meaningful signals, the sheer volume of data can be a source of burden to physicians in their clinical decision-making process. Hence, a smart system is invaluable here to highlight parts of the data that are of potential yield to reduce the time spent by physicians to analyze the entire dataset [42]. Another direction is to consider whether to accept wearable device findings as a part of the electronic health records (EHR) of patients. An integrated EHR is increasingly implemented to facilitate better communication and retrieval of a patient's medical record among healthcare providers. If local health authorities grant permission to include wearable device records as part of the routine entries, it enables viewing and use of wearable device data by multiple health centers when patients go from one clinic or hospital to another, thus facilitating long-term continuous care [43].

In designing any system that involves sharing of wearable device data, privacy issues must be considered carefully. The concept of decentralized blockchain was initially proposed by Nakamoto together with the digital currency Bitcoin [44]. A blockchain can be simplified as a growing chain of records which is designed to be immutable and timestamped, and identical copies of the chain are owned by each node in the network. This decentralized and distributed structure and the cryptographic way of appending content to the chain can achieve an equivalence among all participants as well as the preservation of privacy. Azaria *et al* applied blockchain technology into their decentralized EHR management system MedRec to manage sensitive medical information under cryptographic protocols [45]. They explored a blockchain-based structure to attain confidentiality, immutability, and transparency of the communication in the system. Apart from data management, implementing cryptographic technologies in the decentralized machine learning has also been brought to the fore as the recent introduction of Swarm Learning [46]. Similar to federated learning, parameters of machine learning models are transmitted in the system to alleviate the need of explicit data sharing. Moreover, Swarm Learning introduces blockchain into the system to equalize all nodes in the network and secure the communication, accordingly excluding the need for a central custodian.

Currently, many health-related wearable devices or related applications are listed under the umbrella group of 'wellness' or 'fitness', rather than 'medical'. One of the main driving forces of such phenomenon is 'wellness' or 'fitness' applications face lower regulatory barriers compared to 'medical' applications, which leads to an easier path to the market. Loose regulations in the long run may cause misuse of such products, which may result in unintended harmful consequences to the user. For example, some individuals may overinterpret the so-called abnormal findings generated by these applications, leading to unnecessary anxiety and medical check-up. The World Health Organization and the UK National Institute for Health and Care Excellence have seen this threat and established guidelines on digital health interventions [47].

On the other hand, physicians may not be prepared for consultations based on 'abnormal' findings from a wearable device, because wearable technology is not a standard part of the medical school curriculum. Whether to consider these findings as clinically relevant and how to interpret these results can be a great challenge to physicians without prior knowledge and experience. Technology companies may have to provide more clinically relevant guides for physicians to understand the piece of technology and incorporate it in clinical practice. Performing rigorous analytical, test–retest repeatability, robustness and clinical validation from regulatory authorities like the Food and Drug Administration can enhance the confidence of both patients and physicians.

The high volume of data presents a challenge to storage, security, and privacy. Traditionally, patients' sensitive information is safely stored and managed within by the healthcare sector. However, in the case of wearable technology, a third party, usually a health technology company, may be involved in data transfer and management. It is possible that sensitive information can be leaked along any part of the data transfer pipeline, should there be any loopholes in data security or if the relevant technology companies lack creditability and transparency. A small-scale survey done in the United States showed that half of the respondents did not acknowledge the associated privacy risks when using wearable devices [48]. More public education in this aspect would be necessary.

It is of concern that wearables may be a source of health inequality. A commercial-grade smartwatch can cost a few hundred US dollars, and around half of the mobile health apps do not come free of charge [49]. Also, since the use of wearable technology requires stable access to the Internet and a moderate level of technological literacy, users of these smart devices tend to be younger, having higher educational levels and socioeconomic status. This implies that disadvantaged groups like the elderly and those of lower socioeconomic status are less likely to benefit from wearables, and the inverse care law may set in to exacerbate health inequality, that is, individuals who are more in need of healthcare resources tend to receive fewer.

Optimal incorporation of wearables in the clinical setting requires multidisciplinary collaboration between healthcare and technology experts to foster more standardized guidelines and regulations to improve the acceptance, usability, and interpretability of wearable technology in clinical practice. As a rule of thumb, healthcare practitioners shall always observe the 'do no harm' principle to decide how best to incorporate AI-enabled wearable technology into any healthcare setting. Regardless, there are enormous opportunities ahead.

Acknowledgment

This work was supported by AIR@InnoHK administered by Innovation and Technology Commission.

References

[1] Koytcheva M and Gebbie L 2021 Good times for the smart wearables market (available at: https://my.ccsinsight.com/reportaction/D22615/Toc)

[2] Seneviratne S, Hu Y, Nguyen T, Lan G, Khalifa S and Thilakarathna K *et al* 2017 A survey of wearable devices and challenges *IEEE Commun. Surv. Tutor.* **19** 2573–620

[3] Hiremath S, Yang G and Mankodiya K 2014 Wearable Internet of Things: concept, architectural components and promises for person-centered healthcare *Proc. of the 4th Int.*

Conf. on Wireless Mobile Communication and Healthcare – 'Transforming Healthcare through Innovations in Mobile and Wireless Technologies' (ICST) pp 304–7
[4] Shu L, Yu Y, Chen W, Hua H, Li Q and Jin J *et al* 2020 Wearable emotion recognition using heart rate data from a smart bracelet *Sensors* **20** 718
[5] Perez M V, Mahaffey K W, Hedlin H, Rumsfeld J S, Garcia A and Ferris T *et al* 2019 Large-scale assessment of a smartwatch to identify atrial fibrillation *N. Engl. J. Med.* **381** 1909–17
[6] Rundo J V and Downey R 2019 Polysomnography *Handbook of Clinical Neurology* (Amsterdam: Elsevier) pp 381–92
[7] Sadeh A 2011 The role and validity of actigraphy in sleep medicine: an update *Sleep Med. Rev.* **15** 259–67
[8] Morgenthaler T, Alessi C, Friedman L, Owens J, Kapur V and Boehlecke B *et al* 2007 Practice parameters for the use of actigraphy in the assessment of sleep and sleep disorders: an update for 2007 *Sleep* **30** 519–29
[9] Nyan M N, Tay F E H and Murugasu E 2008 A wearable system for pre-impact fall detection *J. Biomech.* **41** 3475–81
[10] Lui H W and Chow K L 2018 Multiclass classification of myocardial infarction with convolutional and recurrent neural networks for portable ECG devices *Inf. Med Unlocked* **13** 26–33
[11] O'Driscoll R, Turicchi J, Hopkins M, Horgan G W, Finlayson G and Stubbs J R 2020 Improving energy expenditure estimates from wearable devices: a machine learning approach *J. Sports Sci.* **38** 1496–505
[12] Phinyomark A, Phukpattaranont P and Limsakul C 2012 Feature reduction and selection for EMG signal classification *Expert Syst. Appl.* **39** 7420–31
[13] Jin C Y 2019 A review of AI technologies for wearable devices *IOP Conf. Ser. Mater. Sci. Eng.* **688** 044072
[14] Goodfellow I, Bengio Y and Courville A 2016 *Deep Learning* (Cambridge, MA: MIT Press) Adaptive Computation and Machine Learning
[15] Cheikhrouhou O, Mahmud R, Zouari R, Ibrahim M, Zaguia A and Gia T N 2021 One-dimensional CNN approach for ECG arrhythmia analysis in fog-cloud environments *IEEE Access* **9** 103513–23
[16] Amoh J and Odame K 2015 DeepCough: a deep convolutional neural network in a wearable cough detection system *IEEE Biomedical Circuits and Systems Conf. (BioCAS)* (IEEE) pp 1–4
[17] Shin S and Sung W 2016 Dynamic hand gesture recognition for wearable devices with low complexity recurrent neural networks *IEEE Int. Symp. on Circuits and Systems (ISCAS)* (IEEE) pp 2274–7
[18] Mutegeki R and Han D S 2020 A CNN-LSTM approach to human activity recognition *Int. Conf. on Artificial Intelligence in Information and Communication (ICAIIC)* (IEEE) pp 362–6
[19] Vaswani A, Shazeer N, Parmar N, Uszkoreit J, Jones L and Gomez A N *et al* 2017 Attention is all you need *31st Conf. on Neural Information Processing Systems (NIPS)* 11 p
[20] Devlin J, Chang M-W, Lee K and Toutanova K 2019 BERT: pre-training of deep bidirectional transformers for language understanding *Proc. of NAACL-HLT* pp 4171–86
[21] Dosovitskiy A, Beyer L, Kolesnikov A, Weissenborn D, Zhai X and Unterthiner T *et al* 2021 An image is worth 16x16 words: transformers for image recognition at scale arXiv:2010.11929

[22] Bao H, Dong L and Wei F 2021 BEiT: BERT pre-training of image transformers arXiv:2106.08254

[23] He K, Chen X, Xie S, Li Y, Dollár P and Girshick R 2021 Masked autoencoders are scalable vision learners arXiv:2111.06377

[24] Behinaein B, Bhatti A, Rodenburg D, Hungler P and Etemad A 2021 A transformer architecture for stress detection from ECG *Int. Symp. on Wearable Computers* (ACM) pp 132–4

[25] Lin W, Hasenstab K, Moura Cunha G and Schwartzman A 2020 Comparison of handcrafted features and convolutional neural networks for liver MR image adequacy assessment *Sci. Rep.* **10** 20336

[26] Can Y S and Ersoy C 2021 Privacy-preserving federated deep learning for wearable IoT-based biomedical monitoring *ACM Trans. Internet Technol.* **21** 1–17

[27] Bird J J, Kobylarz J, Faria D R, Ekart A and Ribeiro E P 2020 Cross-domain MLP and CNN transfer learning for biological signal processing: EEG and EMG *IEEE Access* **8** 54789–801

[28] Chen Y, Qin X, Wang J, Yu C and Gao W 2020 FedHealth: a federated transfer learning framework for wearable healthcare *IEEE Intell. Syst.* **35** 83–93

[29] Franklin S S, Thijs L, Hansen T W, O'Brien E and Staessen J A 2013 White-coat hypertension: new insights from recent studies *Hypertension* **62** 982–7

[30] Mann D M, Chen J, Chunara R, Testa P A and Nov O 2020 COVID-19 transforms health care through telemedicine: evidence from the field *J. Am. Med. Inform. Assoc.* **27** 1132–5

[31] Mobbs R J, Ho D, Choy W J, Betteridge C and Lin H 2020 COVID-19 is shifting the adoption of wearable monitoring and telemedicine (WearTel) in the delivery of healthcare: opinion piece *Ann. Transl. Med.* **8** 1285

[32] Quer G, Radin J M, Gadaleta M, Baca-Motes K, Ariniello L and Ramos E *et al* 2021 Wearable sensor data and self-reported symptoms for COVID-19 detection *Nat. Med.* **27** 73–7

[33] Mishra T, Wang M, Metwally A A, Bogu G K, Brooks A W and Bahmani A *et al* 2020 Pre-symptomatic detection of COVID-19 from smartwatch data *Nat. Biomed. Eng.* **4** 1208–20

[34] Ates H C, Yetisen A K, Güder F and Dincer C 2021 Wearable devices for the detection of COVID-19 *Nat. Electron.* **4** 13–4

[35] Natarajan A, Su H-W and Heneghan C 2020 Assessment of physiological signs associated with COVID-19 measured using wearable devices *NPJ Digit. Med.* **3** 156

[36] Sun S, Folarin A A, Ranjan Y, Rashid Z, Conde P and Stewart C *et al* 2020 Using smartphones and wearable devices to monitor behavioral changes during COVID-19 *J. Med. Internet Res.* **22** e19992

[37] Radin J M, Wineinger N E, Topol E J and Steinhubl S R 2020 Harnessing wearable device data to improve state-level real-time surveillance of influenza-like illness in the USA: a population-based study *Lancet Digit. Health* **2** e85–93

[38] American Diabetes Association 2021 7. Diabetes technology: standards of medical care in diabetes—2021 *Diabetes Care* **44** S85–99

[39] Taylor P J, Thompson C H and Brinkworth G D 2018 Effectiveness and acceptability of continuous glucose monitoring for type 2 diabetes management: a narrative review *J. Diabetes Invest.* **9** 713–25

[40] Hall H, Perelman D, Breschi A, Limcaoco P, Kellogg R and McLaughlin T *et al* 2018 Glucotypes reveal new patterns of glucose dysregulation *PLoS Biol.* **16** e2005143

[41] Greiwe J and Nyenhuis S M 2020 Wearable technology and how this can be implemented into clinical practice *Curr. Allergy Asthma Rep.* **20** 36

[42] Dinh-Le C, Chuang R, Chokshi S and Mann D 2019 Wearable health technology and electronic health record integration: scoping review and future directions *JMIR MHealth UHealth* **7** e12861

[43] Smuck M, Odonkor C A, Wilt J K, Schmidt N and Swiernik M A 2021 The emerging clinical role of wearables: factors for successful implementation in healthcare *NPJ Digit. Med.* **4** 45

[44] Nakamoto S 2009 *Bitcoin: a peer-to-peer electronic cash system* 1–9

[45] Azaria A, Ekblaw A, Vieira T and Lippman A 2016 MedRec: using blockchain for medical data access and permission management *2nd Int. Conf. on Open and Big Data (OBD) (IEEE)* pp 25–30

[46] Warnat-Herresthal S, Schultze H, Shastry K L, Manamohan S, Mukherjee S and Garg V *et al* 2021 Swarm learning for decentralized and confidential clinical machine learning *Nature* **594** 265–70

[47] Gordon W J, Landman A, Zhang H and Bates D W 2020 Beyond validation: getting health apps into clinical practice *NPJ Digit. Med.* **3** 14

[48] Cilliers L 2020 Wearable devices in healthcare: privacy and information security issues *Health Inf. Manag. J.* **49** 150–6

[49] Aydin G and Silahtaroglu G 2021 Insights into mobile health application market via a content analysis of marketplace data with machine learning *PLoS One* **16** e0244302

IOP Publishing

Machine Learning, Medical AI and Robotics
Translating theory into the clinic
Varut Vardhanabhuti, Ka-Wai Kwok, Jason Y K Chan and Qi Dou

Chapter 4

Artificial intelligence in dentistry and oral health

Mahdis Khodadadi, Ying Ye, Ghazal Aarabi, Edmond Ho Nang Pow, Walter Yu Hang Lam, James Kit Hon Tsoi and Mohamad Koohi-Moghadam

Recent years have seen an increase in interest in the advancement of artificial intelligence (AI) across all fields of science. AI is a general term that refers to the ability of a machine to learn and react in the same way that a human does. AI-based systems are trained to perform a variety of tasks rationally without the need for specific programming. These intelligent platforms are widely used in real-world applications like image processing, text mining, and voice recognition [1]. Moreover, by incorporating AI into healthcare, we can improve the performance of disease diagnosis, treatment planning, and development of new drugs or protocols [2]. Disease diagnosis and treatment planning using AI may become less expensive and more widely available in the near future. Through AI, machines can learn from big patient data samples to determine the fundamental characteristics of each patient, allowing clinicians to diagnose disease in early stages. Some eye-catching examples of AI in healthcare include brain tumor detection via MRI, retinopathy detection via eye images, and cardiac health assessment via electrocardiograms [3].

Dentistry and oral health, like other healthcare fields, have benefited from AI. AI has made strides in improving the efficiency of diagnosis and treatment of oral diseases. With the emergence of advanced dental equipment like intraoral and extraoral x-ray, cone beam computed tomography (CBCT), three-dimensional (3D) facial scanning, and intraoral scanner, each patient now has such a large amount of medical data that manually processing these data is a difficult task. Dentists may consider a wide range of patient factors when formulating a treatment plan, including previous medical records, current oral health, and post-treatment conditions. In some cases, their knowledge and experience might be limited in processing all of these data to make the best decision. Here, AI can assist dentists in making more precise clinical decisions. When applied to dentistry, AI has the potential to significantly improve patient care and transform the oral healthcare industry. In recent years, AI models have been proposed to better understand the

doi:10.1088/978-0-7503-4637-5ch4

interaction between humans and digital technology in the clinical setting, emphasizing their adaptive and supplementary roles for dental professionals. These automatic approaches are expected to improve the accuracy of diagnosis and treatment, leading to an efficient workflow for dentists to deal with big digital data. Therefore, it is critical to maintain a proactive approach to AI to ensure its positive role in efficient clinical trials.

Machine learning (ML) and deep learning (DL), two major subsets of AI, help in providing automatic solutions for these applications. ML is a subset of AI that focuses on the development of intelligent systems via the application of statistical learning techniques. Without being explicitly coded, ML systems can self-learn and improve. The term 'DL' refers to a subset of ML methods inspired by the human brain. DL iteratively learns from data by applying successive layers of neural networks (NNs). DL is particularly advantageous when attempting to learn patterns from unstructured data like medical images. The primary distinction between ML and DL is that ML requires some hand-crafted features to operate, whereas DL extracts all required features from the input data automatically. With the help of ML and DL, dentists will be able to improve their decision-making in diagnosis and provide a better treatment plan. These methods contribute to the advancement of dental and oral health quality in a variety of ways, including image classification, image segmentation, disease diagnosis and prognosis, operation assessment through speech recognition, and automatic treatment planning [4]. However, to date, very few applications of AI has been used in real clinical practice, but its role will grow in the near future.

4.1 Automatic tooth segmentation

A crucial step in any dental diagnosis and treatment is tooth segmentation to identify tooth type and location. For example, tooth segmentation is a key step in computer-aided design (CAD) and computer-aided manufacturing systems for virtual treatment planning. Manual tooth segmentation is a time-consuming task that completely relies on specialist expertise, and it is also prone to human error. Several automated techniques for segmenting and classifying teeth have been introduced to improve efficiency and accuracy by minimizing manual intervention. AI appears to be useful in automatic segmentation and numbering of teeth from dental medical images. The use of AI, particularly ML and DL, has sparked a significant interest in this field. Optical intraoral scans (IOS), 3D CBCT, and 2D panoramic images are the input clinical data that can be used to train such AI models (figure 4.1). For example, Zanjani *et al* introduced a 3D semantic segmentation of individual teeth and gingiva based on the PointCNN DL [5]. They used 120 IOS from 60 patients to train the model. The model will help to segment 3D intraoral scan images automatically with a precision of 0.93, a recall of 0.90, and an intersection over union (IoU) score of 94%. Also, they employed a Monte Carlo convolutional network with some modifications to segment tooth instances in the 3D point cloud on the same dataset [6]. Similarly, Tian *et al* used 600 3D scans from dentition plaster models to train a DL model using sparse

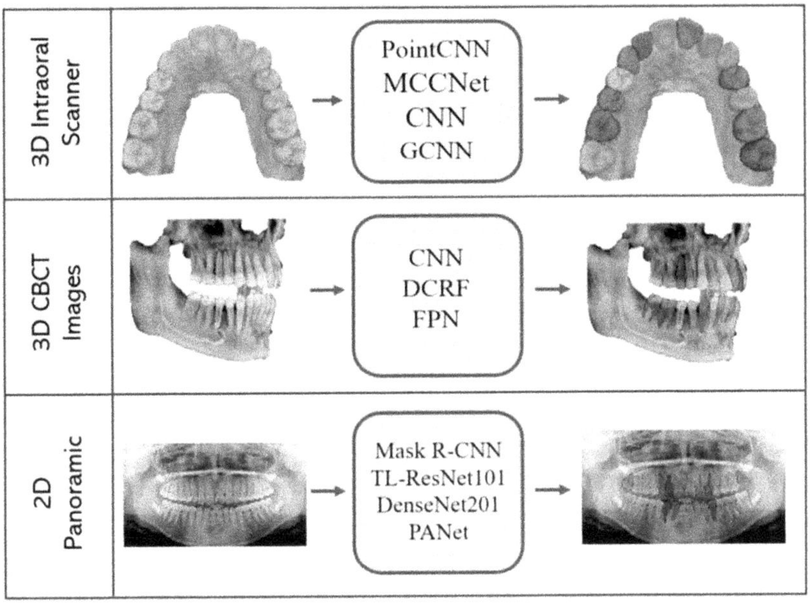

Figure 4.1. Tooth segmentation using deep learning model. The input of the models can be IOS, CBCT, or 2D panoramic images (DCRF: dynamic conditional random field model, CNN: Convolutional Neural Network, FPN: Feature Pyramid Networks).

voxel octree and 3D convolution neural networks (CNNs) [7]. A two-level CNN was utilized for classification, and a three-level CNN was used for segmentation. The average classification accuracy at levels one and two was 95.96% and 88.06%; the average tooth segmentation accuracy is stated to be 89.81%. Also, a graph convolutional neural network (GCNN) has been used to perform segmentation on the IOS images. Zhang *et al* acquired 80 3D dental models by intraoral scanners to perform the segmentation [8]. They implemented a two-stream graph CNN to be able to learn more discriminative features from the models. These two streams, namely, C-stream and N-stream, are used parallelly to obtain the features from coordinates and normal vectors of the dental shape, respectively. Their model achieved a mean IoU of 88.99%, which outperforms the state-of-the-art methods.

Besides, CBCT is a powerful voxel-based computer tomography (CT) that is very commonly used and is being taught at undergraduate-level dentistry at some schools [9]. Xu *et al* developed an automatic approach to perform segmentation on the 3D CBCT scans [10]. They used 1200 3D CBCT images to train a hierarchical DL model. Following deep CNN segmentation, graph-based label optimization and edge refinement with an improved version of fuzzy clustering were performed. Similarly, Cui *et al* used deep convolutional neural networks (DCNNs) to perform two-stage tooth identification and segmentation on 3D CBCT [11]. The first stage involves the extraction of an edge map from 20 CBCT images. The second stage involves delivering the edge maps to the 3D region proposal network for identification and segmentation. Also, a UNet-based model [12] has been used to perform segmentation on the 3D CBCT images. Lee *et al* [13] used 102 CBCT images and trained the model in three phases: first with the teeth sub-volume, then with teeth-containing slices, and finally with the entire CBCT image. They obtained a dice value of 0.93 on their test dataset. Furthermore, Lahoud *et al* developed a feature pyramid network (FPN) DL approach to segment 3D CBCT images [14]. They used 433 CBCT images, including single- and double-rooted teeth, to train their model. Manual annotation of the training set was performed in MeVisLab [15].

Also, DL models have been used to perform dental segmentation on 2D panoramic images. Koch *et al* used 1500 panoramic images from Lahoud *et al* [16] and Silva *et al* [17] to train a UNet model. Jader *et al* employed mask Region-based convolutional neural network (R-CNN) to perform the semantic segmentation on 2D panoramic images [18]. They trained the model using 1500 panoramic radiographs including ten different categories of buccal images. They used a transfer-learning approach using a ResNet101 model to build an FPN, and regions of interest (ROIs) are extracted. Finally, they used a fully connected network to segment the images pixel-wise. They achieved a 98% accuracy, 88% *F*1-score, 94% precision, 84% recall, and 99% specificity. Similarly, R-CNN with DenseNet and ResNeSt have been used in multiple research to perform instance segmentation and detection of teeth on panoramic radiographs [19–23].

There are still some challenges to performing tooth segmentation using ML/DL models. One of the biggest difficulties with these models is that a tooth viewed from different angles may look like a completely different shape. Also, sometimes a tooth can be obstructed by other teeth, which makes it difficult to identify and label using DL models. Therefore, a sufficient number of training samples is necessary to cover different viewpoints. To use IOS images as input of the models, it should be noted that the common file type of IOS is Standard Tessellation Language (stl), which is a file format that has used multiple triangles to generate a 3D surface geometry of an object under a 3D Cartesian coordinate system with arbitrary unit without scale and contrast. Thus, applying a conversion of stl to voxel (and vice versa) commonly generates error and deformation, whereas a correction is deemed necessary [24]. The error between the file format translation should not be neglected, and apparently many studies have focused on the ML/DL algorithm development but ignored the error terms, which can be detrimental for any digital translation into clinical practice [25, 26]. Anyhow, DL approaches showed promise in performing tooth segmentation in both 3D and 2D images. However, it is still possible to develop more accurate models by aggregating data from two different sources to build an ensemble segmentation model [27].

4.2 AI in designing dental crown and dental inlay surface

ML can be used to predict the best structure for the dental crown figure 4.2 [28–30]. Hwang *et al* used a generative ML approach to predict the crown structure [31]. They used a 3D IOS of the missing and opposite side teeth to train their model to predict the customized crown-filled depth. Their dataset contains 1500 training, 1570

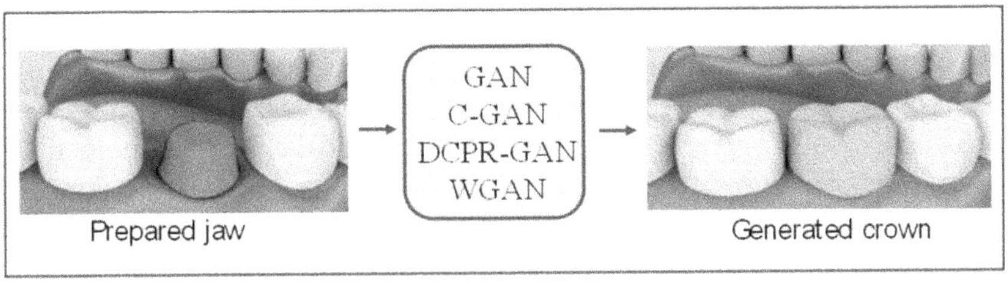

Figure 4.2. Using deep generative models to design crown.

validation, and 243 testing images. Each training sample included a scanned prepared jaw, a scanned opposing jaw, a gap distance map between the two jaws, and a crown that was manually designed. They used pix2pix algorithm, which is a type of generative adversarial network (GAN) model, to predict the 3D structure of crown. They achieved an IoU of 0.915 on their validation set with mean.

Similarly, Yuan *et al* benefited from GAN models to reconstruct the tooth occlusal surface [32]. The dataset was created by generating depth maps of 3D tooth models scanned with the optical intraoral scanner. The dataset contains 500 samples for training and 100 additional test samples. Each sample includes depth maps of the occlusal grooves and their corresponding original teeth. They trained their conditional GAN network in three stages: first, they trained the occlusal groove filter network and then froze the model. The generator model was then used to determine the occlusal groove filter loss, and finally, the generator model was used to determine the tooth crown. The peak signal-to-noise ratio (PSNR) with the highest value was reported to be 23.3044, while the root mean square error with the lowest value was 0.0697.

Tian *et al* developed a Wasserstein generative adversarial network (WGAN) with a specially designed loss measurement to generate a dental inlay surface with realistic crown details [33]. They acquired a database consisting of 830 dental samples. Each sample is a 3D dental IOS image obtained by a 3Shape dental scanner. These data were used later for the training and testing stages of the WGAN. They showed their approach outperformed the pix2pix method in generating the dental inlay surface. In another paper, Tian *et al* facilitated a dataset including 780 dental digital dental model samples, each containing an occlusal groove, an occlusal fingerprint, a preparation tooth, an opposing tooth, a target crown without the occlusal fingerprint, and a target crown with the occlusal fingerprint [34]. In their paper, they proposed a dental crown prosthesis restoration generative adversarial network (DCPR-GAN) which benefits from dental crown prosthesis restoration framework. Their framework consists of two stages which automatically generate the crown surface for a defective tooth. They achieved a root mean square between the generated occlusal surface and the target crown of less than 0.161 mm.

Based on the results of the above studies, it is possible to use a GAN model to predict the 3D structure of the crown and dental inlay surface with reasonable accuracy. However, generating a crown with eight to nine cusps is still a challenging problem that may not be solved by these generative approaches. The far more important part of crown design would be the mechanical load together with the prosthetic materials that can biomechanically relieve the stress from various forms and directions of forces [35, 36]. Thus, to give a usable AI design with crown or any other prostheses, a proper in silico evaluation such as a finite element method [37, 38] might be usable to testify the combination of the design and materials fit for the patient individually. Moreover, generative approaches typically require more data to train than regular CNN approaches that have been used in segmentation and object detection problems. As a result, having enough training samples will be a key point to use generative models.

4.3 AI in dental implant planning

Efficient planning for dental implant necessitates extensive experience in the field as well as expert knowledge. As a result, it is becoming more popular to consider the application of AI in this area. Herein, a study by Bayrakdar *et al* compared the performance of an AI-assisted system to that of manual dental implant planning [39]. They first performed all of the standard estimations in implant planning manually, then compared the results of manual assessment with AI prediction. A total of 75 CBCT images from patients were examined by oromaxillofacial radiologists. The jaws were separated and grouped based on different regions, then canals, sinuses, and fossae were detected, as well as missing teeth. InvivoDental 6.0 was used to measure bone height and thickness in missing regions. They used deep CNN trained in the Diagnocat platform to predict the canal detection and bone length or width computation in missing tooth regions. They found bone height measurements using a DL approach can be accurate as human experts, while they found a statistically significant difference between AI and manual measurements in bone thickness measurements. They had a 72.2% correct detection rate for canals, a 66.4% correct detection rate for sinuses/fossae, and a 95.3% correct detection rate for missing tooth regions. The findings indicated that AI can be useful in the planning of dental implants. Additionally, Görler and Akkoyun used a feed-forward artificial neural network (ANN) using the NeuroSolutions v6.02 software [40]. The ANN was trained using 120 panoramic CT images to predict the appropriate implant size.

Besides, resolving patients' implant problems is complicated if the dental implant device is unknown or if the patient visits a new dentist. As a result, a framework is needed to classify dental implant systems (DISs) based on minimal or small amounts of data without relying on the individual's expertise and knowledge. To boost the accuracy and speed of recognizing patient implants, AI is attracting the attention of researchers. Sukegawa *et al* assessed the effectiveness of five DL models for classifying DIS [41]. They collected 8859 panoramic x-ray images, between 2005 and 2019, which contained 11 implant systems. A basic CNN with three convolutional layers, VGG16 and VGG19 transfer-learning models, and finely tuned VGG16 and VGG19 were employed for the classification. The researchers evaluated the performance of models by recall, precision, accuracy, and *f*-measure. The highest performance results were from VGG16 fine-tuning, with a recall, precision,

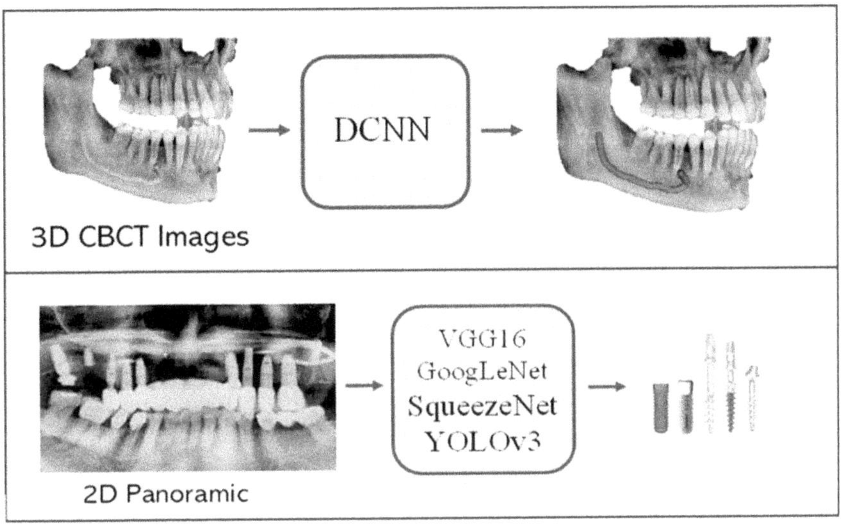

Figure 4.3. Deep learning approach for dental implant planning (top), classification of dental implant system (bottom).

accuracy, and *f*-measure of 0.907, 0.928, 0.935, and 0.916, respectively. Furthermore, DL models like SqueezeNet, GoogLeNet, ResNet-18, MobileNet-v2, YOLOv3, and ResNet-50 were used by different research groups for DIS classification [42–45] (figure 4.3).

Based on these studies, the AI system's results are found to be consistent with manual measurements in the maxilla molar/premolar and mandible premolar region. These findings provide hope for the AI platform usability in implant planning. By incorporating AI into implant planning, dentists will be able to provide better decision-making and will have a support mechanism in their implantology practice. The success of AI models in detecting sinus/mandibular canal and missing teeth, as well as the measurements they provide for implant planning, boosts this possibility. While the mandibular canal was successfully determined, it has been reported that the bone height could not be accurately determined in these regions using AI. To solve these issues, the implant diameter and thickness should be taken into account during the model's training phase. Also, models like GoogLeNet, SqueezeNet, and ResNet-18 can be used to perform DIS classification. However, one limitation of the aforementioned approaches is that the majority of them used predefined CNN structure models such as VGG16 and VGG19. That would be beneficial if more DL algorithms with different structures were required in the future to solve these problems. Furthermore, image quality and resolution provided by different equipment will vary; therefore, the performance of these models on images from different types of equipment will be a key issue. Developing a model that can detect implants without the need for manual image cropping, or one that can apply techniques to detect multiple implants at the same time, would be a more valuable direction for future research.

4.4 Predicting the lifespan of dental implants

In the early stages of implant design, analyzing aspects that affect dental implant lifetime and predicting failure is essential. A variety of factors influence the longevity of implants and reconstruction. Taking all these factors into account to predict the future state of implants will be a daunting task. Different methods are proposed like statistical and computational approaches for implant survival prediction. Based on the papers we reviewed, two general approaches have been used for dental implant lifespan prediction. A group of papers investigated the predictability of dental implant failure, while another group prioritized the factors affecting dental implant survival (figure 4.4).

Hashem *et al* investigated the longevity of dental restorations using Hebbian adversarial networks clustering with gradient boosting recurrent neural network (GBRNN) [46]. The data they used were collected from patients between 1993 and 2003 by reviewing patients' personal and dental information in a clinical setting, including both restored and normal patient records. The data were then used to conduct tests on restorative materials between 2003 and 2011, with 1714 cases identified having a problem from the dental material filling process. Finally, the GBRNN method predicted the longevity of dental restorations with an accuracy of 99.27%. Aliaga *et al* likewise used the same data to examine the longevity of dental restorations and the most appropriate restoration (amalgam and composite), as well as to monitor the progress of the dental restoration [47]. To perform the classification, the model was built using a combination of a Bayesian network (BN) and a multilayer perceptron NN.

Liu *et al* conducted a semi-comparison analysis with a few ML classifiers in order to develop a prediction model for early warning of dental implant failure [48]. Medical data from 681 patients with 1034 fixture implants were collected from electronic medical records, dental implant surgery records, prosthodontic treatment records, and automated x-ray interpretation. WEKA [49] was used to perform classification using decision trees (DT), support vector machines (SVMs), logistic regressions (LR), and classifier ensembles (i.e. Bagging and AdaBoost). The AUC of 0.741 was obtained by DT using bagging and AdaBoost techniques. Yamaguchi *et al* obtained 8640 2D images from stereolithography models scanned by an oral scanner [50]. Moreover, Ha *et al* studied different factors influencing the prognosis

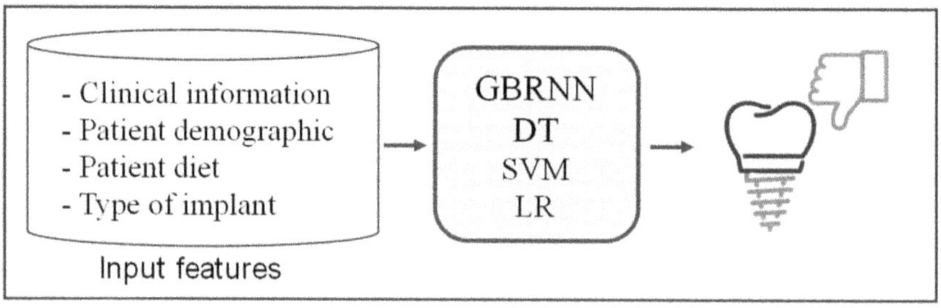

Figure 4.4. Lifespan prediction of the dental implant.

of dental implants [51]. They obtained the data through a 1-year systematic search of chart files at Seoul National University Bundang Hospital. In this period, 667 implants were placed in 198 patients following consultation with a prosthodontist, and a year later, the researchers evaluated the implant's position, characteristics, and biomechanical aspects related to the outcome. The data were analyzed using a DT model and an SVM, and the mesio-distal location was discovered to be the most important factor for the prognosis with an accuracy of 93%. These studies show that ML/DL approaches can be used to predict the failure of dental implants. However, in order to have robust models, it is necessary to use patient behavioral variables such as alcohol consumption and smoking in addition to clinical and oral situation variables to train the model [53]. Also, using features from different time points would be beneficial to train a more robust model.

4.5 AI to identify marginal bone loss prediction

Peri-implant bone tissue and marginal bone absorption around the implant influence the early stability and longevity of dental implants. In the first year of implementation, marginal bone loss (MBL) of less than 1.5–2.0 mm is considered an acceptable norm for implant performance. The MBL assessment using radiographs is a reliable method for examining implant success. However, there is still no reliable tool for predicting the incidence of MBL and the survival rate of implants.

Accordingly, Kim *et al* developed a DCNN to detect periodontal bone loss (PBL) in panoramic dental radiographs [52]. They collected 12 179 panoramic dental radiographs from the Korea University Anam Hospital. They used DentNet, which is based on DCNN and transfer learning for PBL detection. The proposed method detects PBL in all tooth styles and outperforms human experts with an *F*1-score of 0.75. Chang *et al* further proposed a hybrid system for the classification of PBL of each individual tooth from panoramic radiographs that combines DL and traditional CAD processing [53]. A total of 340 panoramic dental radiographs were acquired in 2018 at Seoul National University Dental Hospital. The researchers also performed data augmentation to increase the number of images for the DL architecture. They created a DL architecture based on R-CNN that includes two stages: identifying ROI and extracting features from the ROIs for classification. They achieved the Jaccard index, pixel accuracy, and dice coefficient values of 0.92, 0.93, and 0.88, respectively, for the detection of periodontal bone level (figure 4.5).

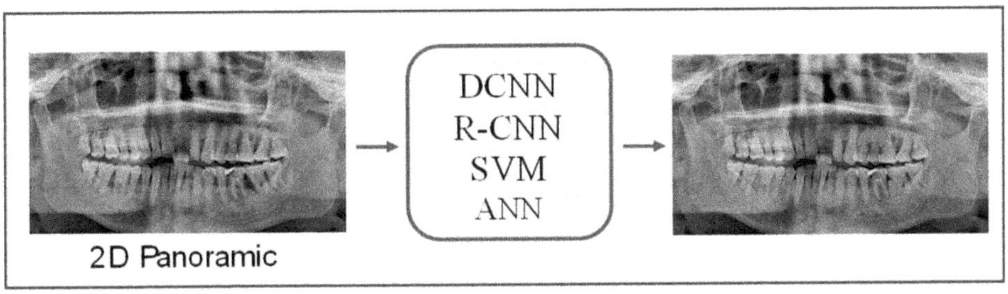

Figure 4.5. Using deep learning to predict MBL.

Similarly, Krois *et al* trained a CNN model with 1456 panoramic images and validated it with 353 images [54]. The mean classification accuracy, sensitivity, and specificity were 0.81 (0.02), 0.81 (0.04), and 0.81 (0.05), respectively, demonstrating outstanding efficiency compared to experts' identification of PBL in panoramic radiographs. Thanathornwong and Suebnukarn also used DL to identify periodontally affected teeth on panoramic radiographs [55]. Based on the ResNet architecture, they built a faster regional CNN. They gathered 100 panoramic radiographs and obtained the ground truth for the images by annotating the images with periodontal experts. They achieved relatively significant results with an average precision rate of 0.81, an average recall rate of 0.80, a sensitivity of 0.84, a specificity of 0.88, and an *f*-measure of 0.81. Lee *et al* developed a computer-assisted system to diagnose and predict periodontally compromised teeth (PCT) [56]. Three periodontists examined the images and categorized them to determine the PCT severity. The images were also resized and cropped. They adopted the VGG19 to preprocess the data to perform image augmentation. Deep CNN architecture was achieved the diagnostic accuracy for PCT of 81.0% for premolars and 76.7% for molars. Zhang *et al* investigated the use of ML for predicting the frequency of extreme MBL [57]. They included CBCT photos of 81 subjects, 41 of whom had significant MBL. To predict the MBL, SVM, ANN, LR, and random forest (RF) models were used. The SVM model achieved the best results, with an AUC of 0.967, a sensitivity of 91.67%, and an accuracy of 1.

Based on our review, radiograph images can be used to train DL models to predict MBL and PBL. Some studies used panoramic dental radiographs to train their models. Panoramic dental radiographs have a large field of view, resulting in low resolution for individual teeth. This makes it more difficult to detect local morphological changes of bone loss, and consequently, the model's overall sensitivity performance will be lower than expected. Additionally, the trained model for MBL and PBL prediction may not be accurate enough for all tooth types due to the lack of training data for a specific tooth. Thus, clinical validation is required to determine whether using panoramic images is possible to train a DL model to predict MBL and PBL.

4.6 AI for early diagnosis of oral cancer

Oral cancer is a subset of head and neck cancers, which are frequently regarded as a difficult disease with a complicated etiology [58]. This type of cancer is usually diagnosed in the late stages, which makes the treatment planning complicated when detected. Therefore, an automated approach for early diagnosis would be great [59]. Fu *et al* have investigated the use of DL in the early detection of oral cancer [60]. They employed DL CNN model to identify patients with oral cavity squamous cell carcinoma by processing their photographic images. They collected their data from 11 hospitals from 2006 to 2019. This dataset was used for training and external validation of the approach. They also collected an external dataset from six dentistry and oral surgery journals. An automated, cascading DL algorithm was used to execute the detection. Their validation showed significantly better results in

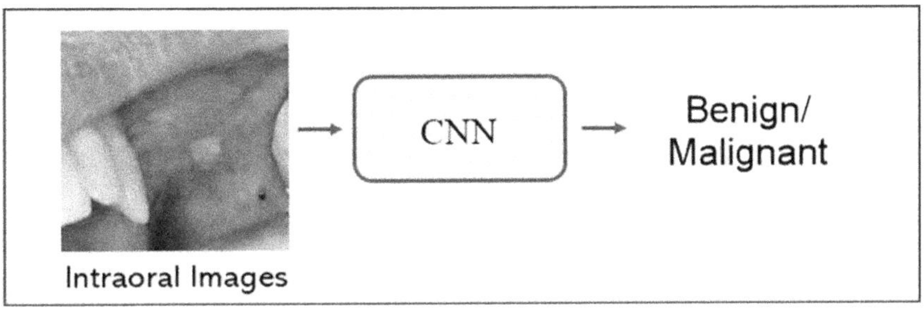

Figure 4.6. Using deep learning model to identify oral cancer lesions automatically.

comparison with seven other oral cancer specialists. They achieved an AUC of 0.980 and 0.935 for the clinical and validation datasets, respectively. This algorithm can serve as a trained assistant in the early detection of oral cancer, which is crucial in oral cancer treatment planning (figure 4.6).

Uthoff *et al* developed a deep CNN to detect cancerous and precancerous lesions using 170 autofluorescence images and white light images [61]. They developed a smartphone application to use their AI model, which makes their model more accessible to use. They compared their results with expertise's diagnosis, which showed the high capability of CNN in this field. They achieved an 85% sensitivity and 88.75% specificity. Also, hyperspectral imaging has been used to build CNN models for early diagnosis of oral cancer [62]. The model, after training, could classify the images as benign or malignant. The authors proposed a regression-based partitioned CNN learning algorithm for such complex images, which showed high classification quality in comparison with the traditional medical image classification algorithms. They reported an accuracy of 91.4%, a sensitivity of 94%, and a specificity of 91%.

AI will significantly alter studies on the early diagnosis of oral cancer, hence improving clinical practice in general. AI has been discovered to be promising in terms of improving the diagnostic procedure. Incorporation of AI with smartphone applications will help to provide a teledentistry-based platform for early diagnosis of oral cancers, which will be helpful in remote areas or poor countries.

4.7 AI in cariology and endodontics

In endodontics, AI can be applied in clinical applications like diagnosis, treatment, and disease prediction [63, 64]. AI models are intended to guide and support dentists to provide better clinical practice. Setzer *et al* developed a U-Net based CNN model to detect periapical lesions from CBCT images [65]. A lesion detection accuracy of 0.93 and a specificity of 0.88 were achieved using this model. Moreover, Hiraiwa *et al* adopted a pretrained CNN structure (AlexNet) to identify root morphologies using panoramic CBCT images [66]. The system evaluates the images to identify whether there is a single or multiple roots. They compared the system's performance with the identification of two radiologists and reported an accuracy of 86.9%.

Hung *et al* developed a DL system which identifies root caries using 15 factors related to personal, nutrition, lifestyle, and clinical factors [67]. Different ML models were employed to classify the data into absence and presence of root caries. Among these models, SVM showed the best performance, with an accuracy of 97.1%.

Also, AI models have been used for the prediction of the difficulty of endodontic cases. Mallishery *et al* [68] collected the data of 500 patients using the standard American Association of Endodontists endodontic case difficulty assessment form. Two endodontists have assessed the filled forms and extracted training features from them. SVM and the deep NN were trained using the extracted features. They reported an accuracy of 94.96%, which makes the importance of AI in this field clear. AI in endodontics could help with clinical applications, such as detecting periapical pathosis, detecting root fractures, determining the difficulty of endodontic cases, and predicting dental caries. It seems that AI could replace the conventional prediction methods and increase the speed of the procedure. It is still important for high-quality research to look at how AI works in terms of reliability, applicability, legal and ethical issues, and costs.

4.8 AI in orthodontics

Orthodontic treatments are typically lengthy, lasting an average of roughly 29 months. Also, choosing the best treatment plan in the field of orthodontics is often dependent on the practitioner's experience. The introduction of ML techniques can assist in saving time and energy and provide a better treatment plan in orthodontic treatment. Thanathornwong collected 15 orthodontic treatment variables from existing commonly used indexes (Index of Orthodontic Treatment Need (IOTN), Dental Aesthetic Index (DAI), and Index of Complexity, Outcome and Need (ICON)), which included missing teeth, overjet, overbite, anterior openbite, posterior openbite, diastema, anterior crossbite, posterior crossbite, anterior displacement, posterior displacement, supernumerary tooth, ectopic eruption, anterior-posterior molar relationship, upper lip to E-line, and lower lip to E-line [69]. They collected these features for around 1000 patients who were between 14 and 19 years old. Then, the BN learning algorithm was used on the training dataset to develop a model that assists the experts in orthodontic treatments. They evaluated their system by the evaluation set and compared the results with two human experts. The model showed a high degree of agreement with the two orthodontists.

Murata *et al* have developed a DL model for automated diagnostic imaging for orthodontic treatment [70]. The system includes a CNN and an RNN, which enables the system to classify the facial images of patients in a multi-label approach. The model helps to take all the facial features into account without increasing the operation requirements. They used the 352 frontal facial images of patients labeled by dentists and their students. However, regarding the low number of images and the training complexity of the system, it still needs improvement by acquiring more training images. So, it does not satisfy the practical applications yet, but it shows the possibility of using DL models to pace up the orthodontics planning process.

AI can also assist orthodontics in treatment timing. Kök *et al* employed AI techniques on cephalometric radiographs to detect cervical vertebrae stages (CVS) as a factor of growth and development of individuals [71]. They obtained radiographs from 300 individuals ranging in age from 8 to 17. They implemented seven different frequently used AI algorithms and eventually compared their performances. In this study, *k*-nearest neighbors (*k*-NN), naive Bayes, DT (Tree), ANNs, SVM, RF, and LR algorithms are used. They reported that the ANN had the highest accuracy in determining CVS, so it could be considered a suitable method for the initiation time of orthodontic treatment. Moreover, AI has shown advantages in evaluating the aesthetic outcome of orthodontics. Patcas *et al* collected 2164 pre- and post-treatment photographs from 146 patients [72]. They developed a model based on CNNs that consists of two major steps: face detection and then predicting the apparent age and facial attraction. They also took advantage of transfer learning to achieve higher accuracy in predictions. Their results showed the model helped improve facial attraction after orthodontic treatment.

4.9 Prosthesis color matching

The implant-based restoration treatment will only be satisfying if the dental implants and prostheses have a pleasing aesthetic appearance. As a result, color selection is critical in the construction of dental implants and maxillofacial prostheses. In most cases, shade matching is based on a set of decisions made by the dentist, the patient, and a technician. As the color selection is based solely on visual assessments made with the naked eye, it is indefinite and unappealing. Using AI and digital dentistry will not only speed up the process but will also result in more accurate shade matching.

Kim *et al* have developed a SVM digital shade matching device for dental color assessment [73]. They used an optical intraoral scanner to collect 3D color images of teeth. The 3D shade information was extracted and given a total of 35 color information sets. SVM was used to analyze the data to classify the color groups within each shade tab for the purpose of performing the color matching process. Using this approach, they achieved a match rate of more than 90%. Other classification algorithms, such as LR, RF, and *k*-NN, were also used to validate the results of the SVM. Additionally, as a manual shade matching algorithm, the Euclidean distance between representative colors of shade tabs in the database and the measured color was evaluated. The Euclidean distance was also used to compare representative colors between the AI-suggested and manual coloring (figure 4.7).

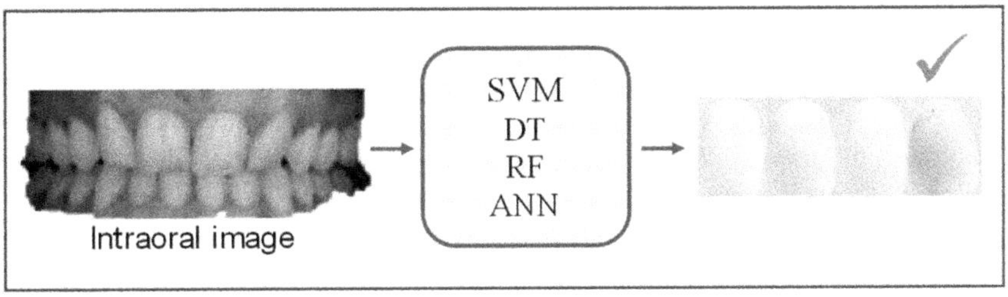

Figure 4.7. Automatic prosthesis color matching using machine learning models.

Besides, Chen *et al* suggested a shade matching method that included a fuzzy decision algorithm as the final stage [74]. They photographed each Vita 3D-Master shade tab using a digital camera. They provided several datasets, each of which contained 26 tagged images. They quantified each image's PSNR, structural similarity index, composite PSNR, and special international commission on illumination (S-CIELAB). Then, they used the fuzzy decision model to determine the optimal dental color for the teeth. They achieved a 99.78 percent accuracy rate. Justiawan *et al* performed a further comparative analysis between the color matching systems [75]. They set the VitaPan dental shade guide, which consists of 16 colors with standard real data parameters as the shade benchmark. Furthermore, they used a digital camera to capture various general dental photographs of patients and extracted the RGB and HSV. Following that, moment invariant was used to achieve the color function of the teeth. Finally, the *k*-NN, NN, and DT algorithms were used to define and classify these features into 16 different forms of dental shade. In the RGB characteristic, the best result obtained by the *k*-NN algorithm was 97.5%.

Color matching is also important in the case of maxillofacial prostheses because it has a direct impact on the patient's esthetical appearance. Mine *et al* suggested a coloration support system for maxillofacial prostheses construction to improve color matching [76]. They made 52 silicone elastomer samples of various colors by hand and used a spectrophotometer to calculate their CIE color space detail. They then used an ANN-based DL algorithm and an RF algorithm to predict the compounding quantities of four pigments. For the validation step, they compared the parameters of five participants' real skin colors with the silicone elastomer samples provided by the CIEDE2000 color comparison system. The color differences were 3.45 ± 0.87 (ANN) and 5.54 ± 1.41 (RF), indicating that the deep ANN approach performed better. According to these studies, ML/DL approaches can be used as an alternative to commercially available color matching systems for selecting the color of maxillofacial prostheses. However, the models we reviewed were designed primarily for use with a personal computer. These models can be extended to be used on mobile applications to make them more cost-effective and accessible to everyone in daily practices.

4.10 Predicting facial changes

Changes in facial appearance and soft tissues occur after maxillofacial surgery, maxillofacial prostheses, and full denture implementation. The post-facial appearance is critical to the patient's facial aesthetic and satisfaction. To obtain a satisfactory outcome, dentists and clinicians must predict the likely facial deformation, which is currently based on the dentist's experience and subjective opinion rather than an accurate prediction method.

Patcas *et al* aimed to improve facial appearance prediction in cleft patients after treatment [77]. They used a pretrained VGG16 to predict the facial attractiveness of cleft patients. They took frontal and left-sided photographs of each patient and divided them into two groups: those taken 0.5–2 years after treatment for cleft

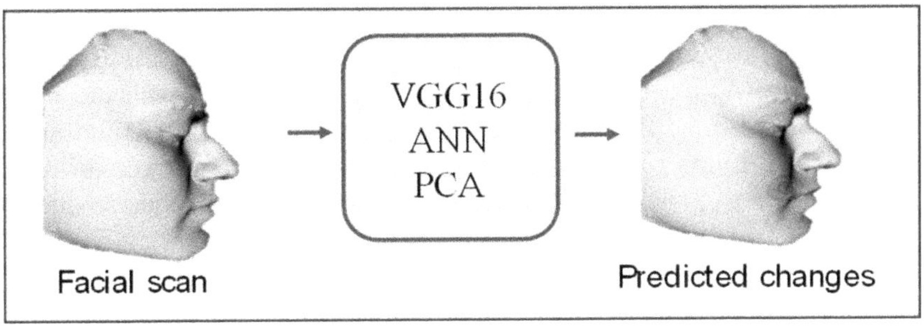

Figure 4.8. Facial change prediction using machine learning models.

patients and those taken 3–5 years after treatment for control patients. The VGG16 model identified the patients' faces in photographs first and then predicted their attractiveness. They also compared the model's results with three different scoring: layperson, orthodontists, and oral surgeons. Patcas *et al* used AI to study the effect of orthognathic treatment on facial attractiveness and age estimation [72]. They collected 2164 pre- and post-treatment photographs of 146 consecutive orthognathic surgery patients. All images contained the data about sex, age, malocclusion, and performed surgery. VGG16 architecture was employed to predict the attractiveness of the face and was trained on more than 0.5 million images from the public databases. For age estimation, the network was trained on APPA-REAL face images with age labels. Finally, the pretrained network was adjusted on the Chicago Face Dataset. The results indicated that most of the faces were more attractive after treatment and age estimations (figure 4.8).

Moreover, Yuan *et al* used a back-propagation NN to predict aesthetic facial deformation after complete denture insertion [78]. They collected facial scans from ten patients at the Peking University School of Stomatology's Department of Prosthodontics in Beijing, China. All patients underwent complete denture insertion. They extracted the external borderlines of the deformation areas and also measured the corresponding key features of the face. Their approach included developing a virtual prediction software module using a back-propagation NN and Laplacian deformation algorithm.

Also, Cheng *et al* proposed a method for predicting facial deformation following total denture implantation [79]. The data were obtained from the School of Stomatology, Peking University, containing 48 sets of facial models. All of the sets include both pre-treatment edentulous state and post-treatment dentigerous state. Face Scan 3D facial scanner, produced by 3D Shape, was used to collecting the facial models. Researchers applied principal component analysis (PCA) on the 3D point cloud data to reduce the feature dimension. The final model is an elastic deformation prediction model for complex skin tissue that is built using PCA output. Using this approach, the maximum deviation range between the prediction data and the facial model after treatment was 2.365 mm.

Attractiveness is often characterized as the ability to stimulate the observer's attention and desire, and as such, subjectivity is an intrinsic aspect of the definition.

Each person has his own reflection of its observation, whether experts or laypeople, and it would be hard to verify a person's judgment based on the conclusions of another. Similarly, AI-based metrics are a representation of a specific perspective that cannot be confirmed by comparison. As a result, DL-based findings cannot completely replace human judgment about attractiveness. However, using the DL approach will help to provide some rating for social attractiveness, which will be helpful to provide an independent assistant for attractiveness measurement.

4.11 Discussion and limitation

According to our findings, AI technology has had a significant impact on dentistry and oral health, and its role will grow in the near future. Dentists will be able to improve their decision-making and provide a better treatment plan with the help of ML and DL models. However, the potential errors in AI models should be considered when using them in clinical settings. Indeed, to date, no study has shown that AI has been put into real clinical practice. According to our review, AI models performed well in tooth and canal segmentation, teeth numbering, DIS classification, prosthesis color matching, and predicting dental implant lifespan. Some applications, such as crown design and facial deformation prediction, still require more robust models. Close collaboration among dentists, researchers, and engineers will aid in the development of more robust models for these applications. It will be beneficial to establish clinical trials in order to evaluate models and reduce the risk of AI errors for these applications.

DL models are usually data hungry, and having enough training data is necessary to build a robust model. Lack of enough training data may lead to the underfitting or overfitting the models. In some articles we reviewed, the author used a narrow number samples to train the models. They reported a good performance from their model, but it is important to consider that the reported accuracy is on the within-sample validation dataset, or they used an unseen independent validation dataset. Using within-sample validation on the small training dataset may not be enough to evaluate a model, as the model may overfit with the training dataset.

Furthermore, the quality of the input training data will have a significant impact on the model's performance. Even the most robust model will be unable to handle noisy and artifact-ridden images. As a result, the quality of the original images, as well as the quality of the image annotation, will have a significant impact on the model's final accuracy. As a result, clinicians must understand the data annotation procedure in order to provide high-quality training datasets. The majority of the articles we reviewed did not specify exactly how they performed data annotation. Providing data annotation details will aid in reproducing the results and better understanding about the preparing the data to feed into the model.

Furthermore, when developing AI models, generalizability is a critical factor. A generalized AI model can perform well on samples not included in the training/validation dataset. This can be used to train a model on samples from one clinic, which could then be used to predict data from other clinics. However, developing a fully generalized AI model for medical applications is a difficult task that remains unsolved in the research community. For generative models like GAN, generalizability will be a more important issue because these models are typically biased to generate new samples based only on the features they see in their training dataset. Despite some limitations in the AI models developed for these applications, we believe AI will assist dentists in providing better patient care in the fields of prosthodontics and implantology.

References

[1] Zhang C and Lu Y 2021 Study on artificial intelligence: the state of the art and future prospects *J. Ind. Inf. Integr.* **23** 100224

[2] Bohr A and Memarzadeh K 2020 The rise of artificial intelligence in healthcare applications *Artificial Intelligence in Healthcare* (Amsterdam: Elsevier) pp 25–60

[3] Yu K-H, Beam A L and Kohane I S 2018 Artificial intelligence in healthcare *Nat. Biomed. Eng.* **2** 719–31.

[4] Y-W C, Stanley K and Att W 2020 Artificial intelligence in dentistry: current applications and future perspectives *Quintessence Int.* **51** 248–57

[5] Zanjani F G, Moin D A, Verheij B, Claessen F, Cherici T and Tan T 2019 Deep learning approach to semantic segmentation in 3D point cloud intra-oral scans of teeth *Int. Conf. on Medical Imaging with Deep Learning* 102 (PMLR) pp 557–571

[6] Zanjani F G, Pourtaherian A, Zinger S, Moin D A, Claessen F, Cherici T, Parinussa S and de With P H 2021 Mask-MCNet: tooth instance segmentation in 3D point clouds of intra-oral scans *Neurocomputing* **45** 286–98

[7] Tian S, Dai N, Zhang B, Yuan F, Yu Q and Cheng X 2019 Automatic classification and segmentation of teeth on 3D dental model using hierarchical deep learning networks *IEEE Access* **7** 84817–28

[8] Zhang L, Zhao Y, Meng D, Cui Z, Gao C, Gao X, Lian C and Shen D 2021 TSGCNet: discriminative geometric feature learning with two-stream graph convolutional network for 3D dental model segmentation Proc. of the IEEE/CVF Conf. on Computer Vision and Pattern Recognition pp 6699–708

[9] Savoldi F, Yeung A W, Tanaka R, Mohammad Zadeh L S, Montalvao C and Bornstein M M *et al* 2021 Dry skulls and cone beam computed tomography (CBCT) for teaching orofacial bone anatomy to undergraduate dental students *Anat. Sci. Educ.* **14** 62–70

[10] Xu X, Liu C and Zheng Y 2018 3D tooth segmentation and labeling using deep convolutional neural networks *IEEE Trans. Visual Comput. Graphics* **25** 2336–48

[11] Cui Z, Li C and Wang W 2019 ToothNet: automatic tooth instance segmentation and identification from cone beam CT images *Proc. of the IEEE/CVF Conf. on Computer Vision and Pattern Recognition* pp 6368–77

[12] Ronneberger O, Fischer P and Brox T 2015 U-Net: convolutional networks for biomedical image segmentation *Int. Conf. on Medical Image Computing and Computer-Assisted Intervention* (Berlin: Springer) pp 234–41

[13] Lee S, Woo S, Yu J, Seo J, Lee J and Lee C 2020 Automated CNN-based tooth segmentation in cone-beam ct for dental implant planning *IEEE Access* **8** 50507–18.

[14] Lahoud P, EzEldeen M, Beznik T, Willems H, Leite A and Van Gerven A *et al* 2021 Artificial intelligence for fast and accurate 3D tooth segmentation on CBCT *J. Endod.* **47** P827–35

[15] Heckel F, Schwier M and Peitgen H O 2009 Object-oriented application development with MeVisLab and Python *Informatik 2009–Im Focus das Leben*

[16] Koch T L, Perslev M, Igel C and Brandt S S 2019 Accurate segmentation of dental panoramic radiographs with U-NETS *IEEE 16th Int. Symp. on Biomedical Imaging (ISBI)* (IEEE) pp 15–9

[17] Silva G, Oliveira L and Pithon M 2018 Automatic segmenting teeth in X-ray images: trends, a novel data set, benchmarking and future perspectives *Expert Syst. Appl.* **107** 15–31

[18] Jader G, Fontineli J, Ruiz M, Abdalla K, Pithon M and Oliveira L 2018 Deep instance segmentation of teeth in panoramic X-ray images *31st SIBGRAPI Conf. on Graphics, Patterns and Images* (IEEE) pp 400–7

[19] Zhao S, Luo Q and Liu C 2020 *Research Square Preprint* posted online 14 October 2020, accessed 10 May 2021 Automatic Tooth segmentation and classification in dental panoramic x-ray images https://doi.org/10.21203/rs.3.rs-89894/v1

[20] Leite A F, Van Gerven A, Willems H, Beznik T, Lahoud P and Gaêta-Araujo H *et al* 2021 Artificial intelligence-driven novel tool for tooth detection and segmentation on panoramic radiographs *Clin. Oral Invest.* **25** 2257–67

[21] Merdietio Boedi R, Banar N, De Tobel J, Bertels J, Vandermeulen D and Thevissen P W 2020 Effect of lower third molar segmentations on automated tooth development staging using a convolutional neural network *J. Forensic Sci.* **65** 481–6

[22] Huang G, Liu Z, van der Maaten L and Weinberger K Q 2017 Densely connected convolutional networks *Proc. of the IEEE Conf. on Computer Vision and Pattern Recognition* pp 4700–8

[23] Silva B, Pinheiro L, Oliveira L and Pithon M 2020 A study on tooth segmentation and numbering using end-to-end deep neural networks *33rd SIBGRAPI Conf. on Graphics, Patterns and Images (SIBGRAPI)* (IEEE) pp 164–71

[24] Zhao M, Xiong G, Shang X, Liu C, Shen Z and Wu H 2019 Nonlinear deformation prediction and compensation for 3D printing based on CAE neural networks *IEEE 15th Int. Conf. on Automation Science and Engineering (CASE)* (IEEE) pp 667–72

[25] Pan Y, Tsoi J K, Lam W Y and Pow E H 2021 Implant framework misfit: a systematic review on assessment methods and clinical complications *Clin. Implant Dent. Relat. Res.* **23** 244–58

[26] Pan Y, Tsoi J K H, Lam W Y, Zhao K and Pow E H 2021 Improving intraoral implant scanning with a novel auxiliary device: an in-vitro study *Clin. Oral Implants Res.* **32** 1466–73

[27] Dang T, Nguyen T T, McCall J, Elyan E and Moreno-García C F 2021 Two layer ensemble of deep learning models for medical image segmentation arXiv:2104.04809

[28] Chau R C W, Chong M, Thu K M, Chu N S P, Koohi-Moghadam M and Hsung R T-C *et al* 2022 Artificial intelligence-designed single molar dental prostheses: a protocol of prospective experimental study *PLoS One* **17** e0268535

[29] Chau R C W, Hsung R T C, McGrath C, Pow E H N and Lam W Y H 2023 Accuracy of artificial intelligence-designed single-molar dental prostheses: A feasibility study *J. Prosthetic Dentistry*

[30] Chen Y, Lee J K Y, Kwong G, Pow E H N and Tsoi J K H 2022 Morphology and fracture behavior of lithium disilicate dental crowns designed by human and knowledge-based AI *J. Mech. Behav. Biomed. Mater.* **131** 105256

[31] Hwang J-J, Azernikov S, Efros A A and Yu S X 2018 Learning beyond human expertise with generative models for dental restorations (arXiv preprint arXiv:1804.00064)

[32] Yuan F, Dai N, Tian S, Zhang B, Sun Y and Yu Q *et al* 2020 Personalized design technique for the dental occlusal surface based on conditional generative adversarial networks *Int. J. Numer. Methods Biomed. Eng.* **36** e3321
[33] Tian S, Wang M, Yuan F, Dai N, Sun Y and Xie W *et al* 2021 Efficient computer-aided design of dental inlay restoration: a deep adversarial framework *IEEE Trans. Med. Imaging* **40** 2415–27
[34] Tian S, Wang M, Dai N, Ma H, Li L and Fiorenza L *et al* 2022 DCPR-GAN: dental crown prosthesis restoration using two-stage generative adversarial networks *IEEE J. Biomed. Health Inf.* **26** 151–60
[35] Albelasy E, Hamama H H, Tsoi J K and Mahmoud S H 2021 Influence of material type, thickness and storage on fracture resistance of CAD/CAM occlusal veneers *J. Mech. Behav. Biomed. Mater.* **119** 104485
[36] Homaei E, Jin X-Z, Pow E H N, Matinlinna J P, Tsoi J K-H and Farhangdoost K 2018 Numerical fatigue analysis of premolars restored by CAD/CAM ceramic crowns *Dent. Mater.* **34** e149–57
[37] Maghami E, Homaei E, Farhangdoost K, Pow E H N, Matinlinna J P and Tsoi J K-H 2018 Effect of preparation design for all-ceramic restoration on maxillary premolar: a 3D finite element study *J. Prosthodont. Res.* **62** 436–2
[38] Genna F, Lopomo N F and Savoldi F 2021 Validation of a numerical model for the mechanical behavior of a continuous positive airway pressure mask *Comput. Meth. Biomech. Biomed. Eng.* **25** 1–11
[39] Bayrakdar S K, Orhan K, Bayrakdar I S, Bilgir E, Ezhov M and Gusarev M *et al* 2021 A deep learning approach for dental implant planning on cone-beam computed tomography images *BMC Med Imaging* **21** 86
[40] Görler O and Akkoyun S 2017 Artificial neural networks can be used as alternative method to estimate loss tooth root sizes for prediction of dental implants *Cumhuriyet Sci. J.* **38** 385–95
[41] Sukegawa S, Yoshii K, Hara T, Yamashita K, Nakano K and Yamamoto N *et al* 2020 Deep neural networks for dental implant system classification *Biomolecules* **10** 984
[42] Kim J-E, Nam N-E, Shim J-S, Jung Y-H, Cho B-H and Hwang J J 2020 Transfer learning via deep neural networks for implant fixture system classification using periapical radiographs *J. Clin. Med.* **9** 1117
[43] Lee J-H and Jeong S-N 2020 Efficacy of deep convolutional neural network algorithm for the identification and classification of dental implant systems, using panoramic and periapical radiographs: a pilot study *Medicine* **99** 26
[44] Hadj Saïd M, Le Roux M-K, Catherine J-H and Lan R 2020 Development of an artificial intelligence model to identify a dental implant from a radiograph *Int. J. Oral Maxillofac. Implants* **35** 6
[45] Takahashi T, Nozaki K, Gonda T, Mameno T and Ikebe K 2021 Deep learning-based detection of dental prostheses and restorations *Sci. Rep.* **11** 1–7
[46] Hashem M, Al-Kheraif A A and Wahba A A 2019 Examining the longevity of dental restoration using Hebbian adversarial networks clustering with gradient boosting recurrent neural network *Measurement* **141** 313–23
[47] Aliaga I J, Vera V, De Paz J F, García A E and Mohamad M S 2015 Modelling the longevity of dental restorations by means of a CBR system *BioMed Res. Int.* **2015** 540306

[48] Liu C-H, Lin C-J, Hu Y-H and You Z-H 2018 Predicting the failure of dental implants using supervised learning techniques *Appl. Sci.* **8** 698

[49] Hall M, Frank E, Holmes G, Pfahringer B, Reutemann P and Witten I H 2009 The WEKA data mining software: an update *ACM SIGKDD Explor. Newslett.* **11** 10–8

[50] Yamaguchi S, Lee C, Karaer O, Ban S, Mine A and Imazato S 2019 Predicting the debonding of CAD/CAM composite resin crowns with AI *J. Dent. Res.* **98** 1234–8

[51] Ha S-R, Park H S, Kim E-H, Kim H-K, Yang J-Y and Heo J *et al* 2018 A pilot study using machine learning methods about factors influencing prognosis of dental implants *J. Adv. Prosthodont.* **10** 395

[52] Kim J, Lee H-S, Song I-S and Jung K-H 2019 DeNTNet: deep neural transfer network for the detection of periodontal bone loss using panoramic dental radiographs *Sci. Rep.* **9** 1–9

[53] Chang H-J, Lee S-J, Yong T-H, Shin N-Y, Jang B-G and Kim J-E *et al* 2020 Deep learning hybrid method to automatically diagnose periodontal bone loss and stage periodontitis *Sci. Rep.* **10** 1–8

[54] Krois J, Ekert T, Meinhold L, Golla T, Kharbot B and Wittemeier A *et al* 2019 Deep learning for the radiographic detection of periodontal bone loss *Sci. Rep.* **9** 1–6

[55] Thanathornwong B and Suebnukarn S 2020 Automatic detection of periodontal compromised teeth in digital panoramic radiographs using faster regional convolutional neural networks *Imaging Sci. Dent.* **50** 169

[56] Lee J-H, D-H K, Jeong S-N and Choi S-H 2018 Diagnosis and prediction of periodontally compromised teeth using a deep learning-based convolutional neural network algorithm *J. Periodont Implant Sci.* **48** 114

[57] Zhang H, Shan J, Zhang P, Chen X and Jiang H 2020 Trabeculae microstructure parameters serve as effective predictors for marginal bone loss of dental implant in the mandible *Sci. Rep.* **10** 1–9

[58] World Health Organization 2020 *WHO Report on Cancer: Setting Priorities, Investing Wisely and Providing Care for All* (Geneva: WHO)

[59] Adeoye J, Koohi-Moghadam M, Lo A W I, Tsang R K-Y, Chow V L Y and Zheng L-W *et al* 2021 Deep learning predicts the malignant-transformation-free survival of oral potentially malignant disorders *Cancers* **13** 6054

[60] Fu Q, Chen Y, Li Z, Jing Q, Hu C and Liu H *et al* 2020 A deep learning algorithm for detection of oral cavity squamous cell carcinoma from photographic images: a retrospective study *EClinicalMedicine* **27** 100558

[61] Uthoff R D, Song B, Sunny S, Patrick S, Suresh A and Kolur T *et al* 2018 Point-of-care, smartphone-based, dual-modality, dual-view, oral cancer screening device with neural network classification for low-resource communities *PLoS One* **13** e0207493

[62] Jeyaraj P R and Samuel Nadar E R 2019 Computer-assisted medical image classification for early diagnosis of oral cancer employing deep learning algorithm *J. Cancer Res. Clin. Oncol.* **145** 829–37.

[63] Casalegno F, Newton T, Daher R, Abdelaziz M, Lodi-Rizzini A and Schürmann F *et al* 2019 Caries detection with near-infrared transillumination using deep learning *J. Dent. Res.* **98** 1227–33

[64] Fa S, Samek W and Krois J 2020 Artificial intelligence in dentistry: chances and challenges *J. Dent. Res.* **99** 769–4

[65] Setzer F C, Shi K J, Zhang Z, Yan H, Yoon H and Mupparapu M *et al* 2020 Artificial intelligence for the computer-aided detection of periapical lesions in cone-beam computed tomographic images *J. Endodontics* **46** 987–3.
[66] Hiraiwa T, Ariji Y, Fukuda M, Kise Y, Nakata K and Katsumata A *et al* 2019 A deep-learning artificial intelligence system for assessment of root morphology of the mandibular first molar on panoramic radiography *Dentomaxillofac. Radiol.* **48** 20180218
[67] Hung M, Voss M W, Rosales M N, Li W, Su W and Xu J *et al* 2019 Application of machine learning for diagnostic prediction of root caries *Gerodontology* **36** 395–404
[68] Mallishery S, Chhatpar P, Banga K, Shah T and Gupta P 2020 The precision of case difficulty and referral decisions: an innovative automated approach *Clin. Oral Invest.* **24** 1909–15.
[69] Thanathornwong B 2018 Bayesian-based decision support system for assessing the needs for orthodontic treatment *Healthcare Inf. Res.* **24** 22–8
[70] Murata S, Lee C, Tanikawa C and Date S 2017 Towards a fully automated diagnostic system for orthodontic treatment in dentistry *IEEE 13th International Conf. on E-science (E-Science)* (IEEE) pp 1–8
[71] Kök H, Acilar A M and İzgi M S 2019 Usage and comparison of artificial intelligence algorithms for determination of growth and development by cervical vertebrae stages in orthodontics *Prog. Orthod.* **20** 1–10.
[72] Patcas R, Bernini D A, Volokitin A, Agustsson E, Rothe R and Timofte R 2019 Applying artificial intelligence to assess the impact of orthognathic treatment on facial attractiveness and estimated age *Int. J. Oral Maxillof. Surg.* **48** 77–83
[73] Kim M, Kim B, Park B, Lee M, Won Y and Kim C-Y *et al* 2018 A digital shade-matching device for dental color determination using the support vector machine algorithm *Sensors* **18** 3051
[74] Chen S-L, Zhou H-S, Chen T-Y, Lee T-H, Chen C-A and Lin T-L *et al* 2020 Dental shade matching method based on hue, saturation, value color model with machine learning and fuzzy decision *Sens. Mater.* **32** 3185–207
[75] Justiawan D A W, Hadi R P, Nurhayati A P, Prayogo K, Sigit R and Arief Z 2019 Comparative analysis of color matching system for teeth recognition using color moment *Med. Devices (Auckl)* **12** 497
[76] Mine Y, Suzuki S, Eguchi T and Murayama T 2020 Applying deep artificial neural network approach to maxillofacial prostheses coloration *J. Prosthodont. Res.* **64** 296–300
[77] Patcas R, Timofte R, Volokitin A, Agustsson E, Eliades T and Eichenberger M *et al* 2019 Facial attractiveness of cleft patients: a direct comparison between artificial-intelligence-based scoring and conventional rater groups *Eur. J. Orthodont.* **41** 428–33.
[78] Yuan F, Cheng C, Dai N and Sun Y 2017 Prediction of aesthetic reconstruction effects in edentulous patients *Sci. Rep.* **7** 1–8
[79] Cheng C, Cheng X, Dai N, Tang T, Xu Z and Cai J 2019 Facial morphology prediction after complete denture restoration based on principal component analysis *J. Oral Biol. Craniofac. Res.* **9** 241–50

Chapter 5

Artificial intelligence applications in pathology

Ronald C K Chan, Curtis C K To, Nike Kwai Cheung Lau, Yeow Kuan Chong, Alfred L H Lee and Christopher K C Lai

Pathology is the study of diseases, and in the era of laboratory base medicine, pathologists have an important role in clinical care to identify and stage diseases, guide treatment, and manage laboratories of different disciplines. Pathology is a heavily data-driven speciality and at the same time deals with a wide disease spectrum. Different disciplines of pathology deal with vastly varying data types, incorporating the clinical information, to render a diagnosis. Tremendous work has been done to harness the power of artificial intelligence (AI) into different disciplines of clinical pathology in practice.

Similar to laboratory arrangements in clinical practice, this chapter is separated into three sections. Section 5.1 focuses on histopathology and cytology and the impact brought by advances in image analysis. Section 5.2 focuses on chemical pathology and the use of a gigantic volume of digitalized structured patient data. Section 5.3 focuses on clinical microbiology and its application in the management of infectious diseases.

5.1 Histopathology and cytopathology—new era in image analysis

5.1.1 What are histopathology and cytology?

Histopathology and cytology are branches of pathology that investigate human tissue and cells. The specimens are removed by clinicians through biopsies or surgeries. The removed tissue and cells are made into glass slides and then observed microscopically by pathologists and cytologists. Diagnoses can be made in the majority of specimens at this stage. Some specimens require histochemical stains and immunohistochemical stains to demonstrate the presence of certain biochemical molecules (such as elastic fiber, mucin, melanin, etc) and antigens. They can offer clues to tissue differentiation and target therapy responses. A tiny subset of cases would require molecular tests to look for mutations and translocations.

doi:10.1088/978-0-7503-4637-5ch5

5.1.2 Whole slide imaging as a new form of medical image

For the last century, histopathology and cytopathology have been built on the interpretation of tissue and cells mount on glass slides under microscopes. The unique format, high magnification, and huge tissue area have limited development of image analysis. In early 2000, advances in image acquisition techniques enabled Leica to make whole slide imaging (WSI) possible in 2004 [1]. To produce a WSI, a glass slide is scanned by a microscope with a motorized stage, patch by patch or line by line (see figure 5.1). The microscope must precisely scan through all slide areas at the correct focal length. Cytology specimens pose a greater challenge for auto-focus systems, as cytology specimens were whole mounted and cell clusters can be up to 10 μm in thickness, compared with formalin-fixed paraffin-embedded sections used in histology that are microtomed (thinly sliced) at 0.4 μm in thickness. The scanned images are scanned at 0.1–0.5 μm per pixel, and the entire slide area can be up to 200 000 × 100 000 pixels, a size far exceeding usual photography and even radiology images. If multiple layers have been scanned at different focal lengths to accommodate thick cytology specimens, a technique known as *z*-stack, the scanned files will be even larger.

5.1.2.1 Files and file types

All the acquired images are then compiled into a computer file that contains all images at various magnifications with headers containing information of the scan run. Unfortunately, scanner manufacturers, around a dozen at the time of writing, have not agreed on the file format and use various proprietary files formats. Most vendors provide software and sometimes cloud-based solutions, but large deployment sites with different machines usually will have difficulties in interoperability between different machines. Multiple projects (such as open microscopy environment (OME) and bio formats) have developed libraries and plugins to facilitate file input and output operation into non-vendor-specific pipelines. An array of software, both in proprietary and in open domains, have been developed for different uses.

Various vendor provided software	Aperio ImageScope, Zeiss ZEN, hamamatsu NDP.view2…
Image analysis	QuPath [2]/ImageJ (with bio formats plugin)
Image annotation	QuPath/ASAP (Automated Slide Analysis Platform) [3]
Image viewing and hosting	Pathomation PMA.studio
Libraries to extract data in programming environment	OpenSlide [4]/bioformats [5]

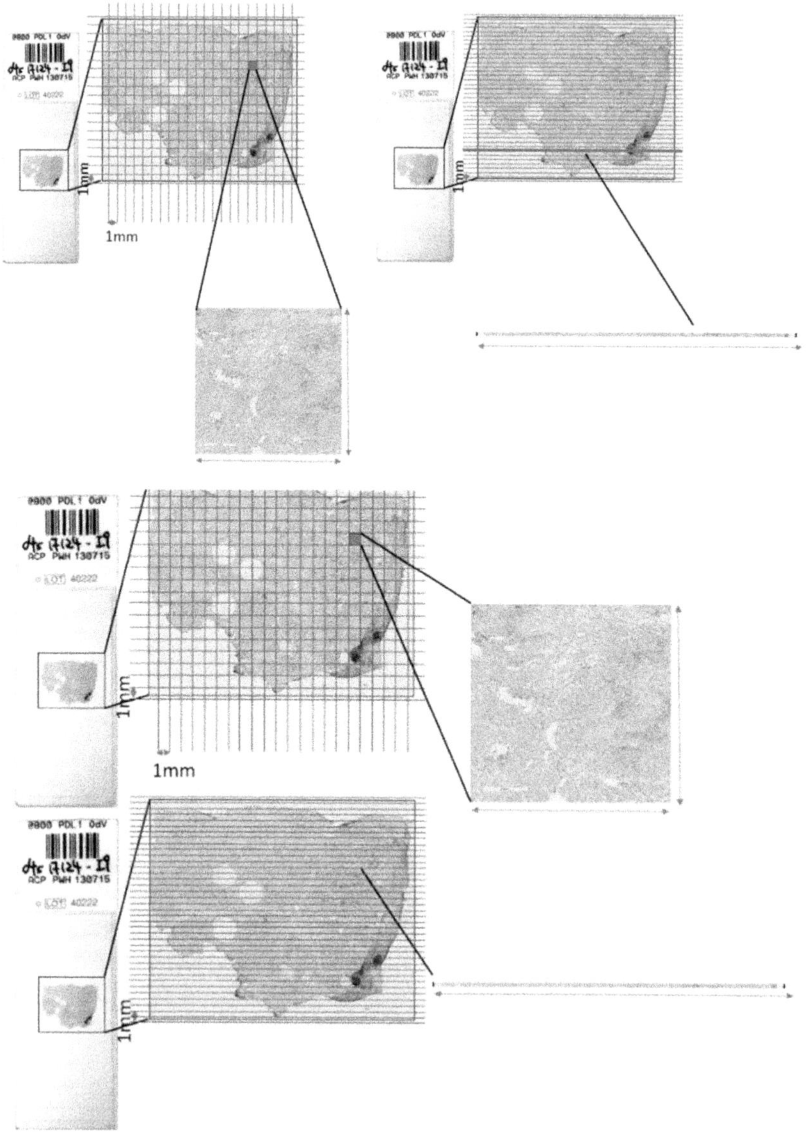

Figure 5.1. Tile scanning vs line scanning.

5.1.3 Common image processing techniques used in WSI analysis

Recent advancements in AI have been made possible with the prevalence of large-scale datasets and processing power, in particular parallel processing power enabled by graphics processing units (GPUs). The recent advancement in performance of AI in the field of medicine is an amazing feat and a testament of its flexibility. This section illustrates important considerations when planning to develop AI-based image analysis system on WSI images.

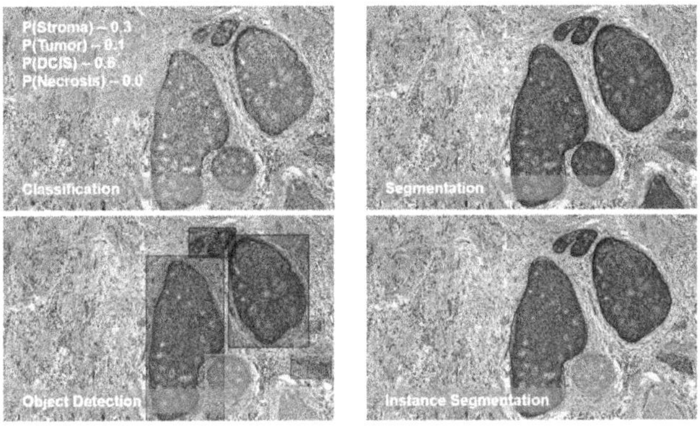

Figure 5.2. Visual representation of the different types of image analysis. (P(Stroma): Predicted probability of the image being the class Stroma). [126] John Wiley & Sons. © 2022 John Wiley & Sons Ltd.

5.1.3.1 Objective of image analysis in the context of pathology

There are several approaches for image analysis in pathology. The classical approach is to predict the label of an image, expressed in probability values of that image belonging to pre-defined classes. Another approach is to detect an object, roughly localizing meaningful objects within an image. For amorphous shapes, such as cancer area, segmentation, which outlines detection area at a pixel level, is a more precise approach than object detection. Finally, instance segmentation combines the best of the two and produces a high precision mask as well as instance count (figure 5.2).

5.1.3.2 Handcrafted features

Prior to the availability of powerful GPUs and modern deep learning architectures, machine learning algorithms could be trained to predict based on handcrafted cellular features known to be of importance. A classical dataset known as Breast Cancer Wisconsin (Diagnostic) Data Set [6] contained cell nuclear features such as radius, texture, concavity, etc, in a table of floating-point numbers. It contains 357 cases of benign and 212 cases of cancer cells. The original paper in 1992 reported a ten-fold cross-validation accuracy of 97% by multi-surface method-tree (MSMT) using just three nuclear features out of thirty. Hand-selecting and extracting useful features requires domain-specific knowledge. It is also a good deal of work to define, measure, and record the roundness or cavity of each cell under a microscope.

5.1.3.3 Alternatives to hand crafted features

It is difficult to design features for computer vision problems. For example, to teach a computer to identify whether a dog is in image, one might handcraft features such as number of legs, number of tails, etc. This approach works if the task is to distinguish pictures of humans versus pictures of dogs. However, these features are not useful once cat pictures are thrown into the mix. Deep learning models take an image as input and find the best filter/kernels to perform classification or segmentation tasks. The feature maps are generated automatically, so it is more flexible in

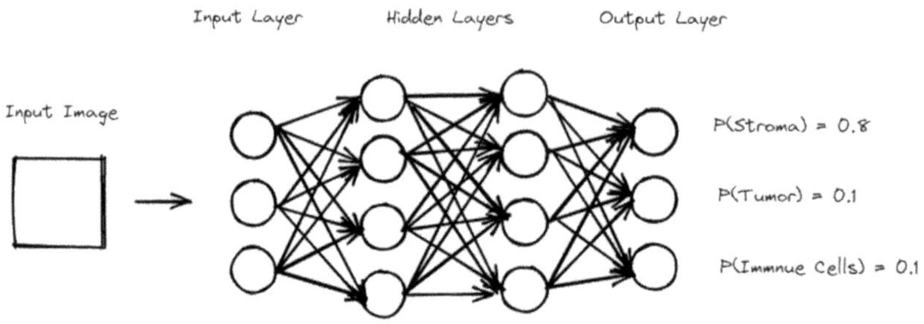

Figure 5.3. Simplified schematic diagram of a deep learning model.

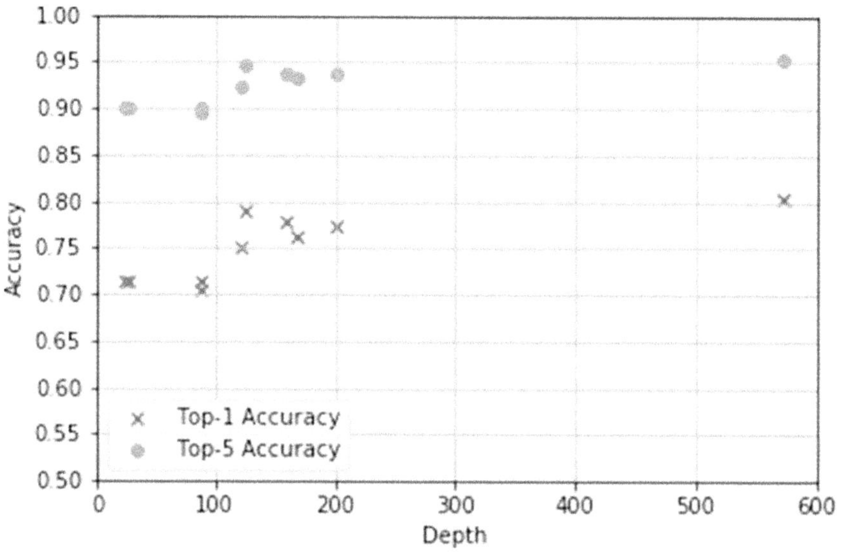

Figure 5.4. Accuracy in image classification using ImageNet data of different common architectures. Data from https://keras.io/api/applications/.

tackling different tasks. Various models architectures have been developed for different purposes using different input formats. A typical deep learning model consists of an input layer, multiple hidden layers, and an output layer (figure 5.3).

In general, model performance on training data can be improved by increasing the number of hidden layers, known as depth. However, the yield of further increasing depth is limited while increasing the risk of overfitting and requirements in computing resources. Modern model architectures contain dozens to more than a hundred layers (see figure 5.4). Readers are recommended to refer to 'Hands-On Machine Learning with Scikit-Learn and TensorFlow: Concepts, Tools, and Techniques to Build Intelligent Systems' [7] by Aurélien Géron for detailed discussion on how each architecture works.

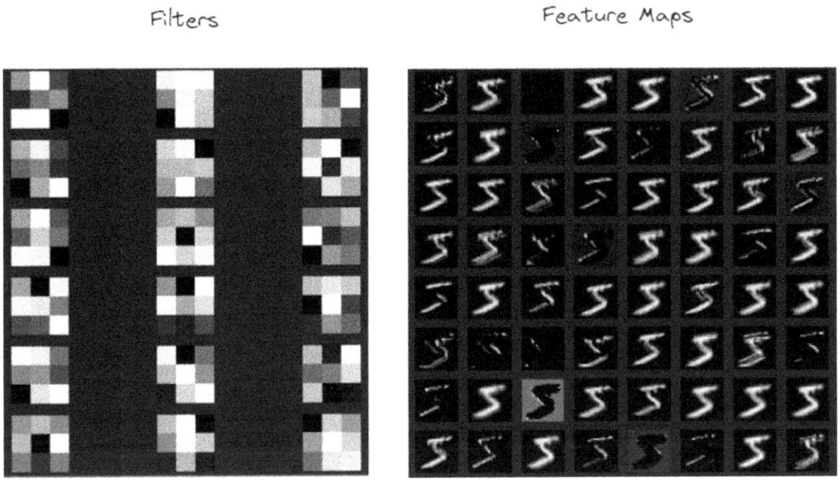

Figure 5.5. The filters extracted from hidden layers of the deep neural network are often difficult to understand.

Convolutional neural networks (CNNs) are a family of deep learning architectures for computer vision. CNNs makes use of convolution layers to extract low-level visual elements such as corners, straight lines, and edges. By stacking these convolutional layers, low-level visual elements are combined into high level elements. Based on the idea of CNN, a great of research efforts has been made on how best to stack different layers to achieve the best results. For typical classification tasks, VGG [8] and ResNet [9] are two examples of popular architectures. U-Net [10] could segment image and give a prediction to every pixel in an image. Faster region-based convolutional neural networks [11], mask region-based convolutional neural networks [12], and you only look once [13] are designed for object detection. Different models have their own specifications for training data.

Deep learning models are often referred to as 'black box', (almost) magically providing the prediction with no explainability. Examinations of the weights within the deep layers are seldom self-explanatory, particularly when the models are deep and complex. The lack of reasoning behind prediction significantly hinders its application in the medical field, as it is impossible to guard against obvious errors at a later stage. Doctors also have a hard time convincing patients to entrust their lives to a black box. Shapley value, gradient-weighted class activation mapping, and attention mapping are some of the more well known methodologies in explainable AI (figure 5.5).

5.1.3.4 Data preparation

Most CNN networks are not designed for pathology images. WSI is generally prohibitively large in size such that it is not feasible to directly feed the whole image into regular image analysis pipelines or into the memory of graphics cards. For example, the input size of Inception-ResNet v2 is 299 × 299 pixels. A common strategy is to divide and conquer, cutting or tessellating the whole slide images into tiles that are closer to model input sizes but are still visually distinguishable from a pathologist's point of view. In our experience, tile sizes of 125–250 μm [14] perform best when approaching a cancer detection problem. These can be good settings to start, adjusting and validating the settings by empirical data as needed.

The cut tiles are often paired with a label. The method of data labeling can be as simple as putting the tiles of class A into a folder named A, or it could be done with annotation software (e.g. QuPath and ASAP). Simple binary thresholding is often performed using a pre-determined value or Otsu's method [15] to remove the tiles from brightfield background. Image augmentations are often carried out by randomly flipping the images and altering the color, etc, such that dataset size is increased or as a means to balance a minority class.

5.1.3.5 Model training

Typically, a dataset is split into a training set and testing set, commonly at a 7:3 ratio. The training set is fed into the training loop to update the parameter of the model. The testing set is reserved for evaluating the true performance of the trained model. It is advised that the train–test split is performed at the case level since the training and testing images coming from the same WSI may have similar characteristics or even hidden bias. It is also crucial to make the best effort to encompass a wide, if not the entire, spectrum of morphology. Deep learning models have high degrees of freedom and can easily cause overfitting, in which case the model would have a high accuracy on training data but poor accuracy on unseen test data. Depending on the experiment design, one could elect to also conduct 'leave one out cross-validation' and '*K*-fold cross-validation'.

5.1.3.6 Model evaluation

In addition to the usual metrics such as accuracy, precision, recall, and *F*1-score, qualitative assessment is particularly important in this domain. Converting per tile prediction result into a heatmap is our institution's standard practice. Not only does it allow an overview on model performance, it also enables model evaluation on unannotated areas. It is a helpful method to identify model failure and bias. This information could indicate how the model would behave and, more importantly, what new data to collect for further model training (figure 5.6).

5.1.3.7 Up and coming

Data labeling is labor intensive and costly, particularly so when you need a pathologist to do it. A clean, high-quality dataset has become the bottleneck of the development of supervised learning models. While unsupervised models typically perform worse than their supervised counterparts, weakly supervised or semi-supervised models are emerging as an alternative with promising results [16]. Multimodal or sensor-fusion models, which could ingest images and textual and tabular data during inference, means clinical data can be combined with WSI data during inference. Generative adversarial networks, popularized by deep fakes, can generate super-resolution images. Transformer, a novel natural language processing architecture, has also demonstrated remarkable performance in computer vision

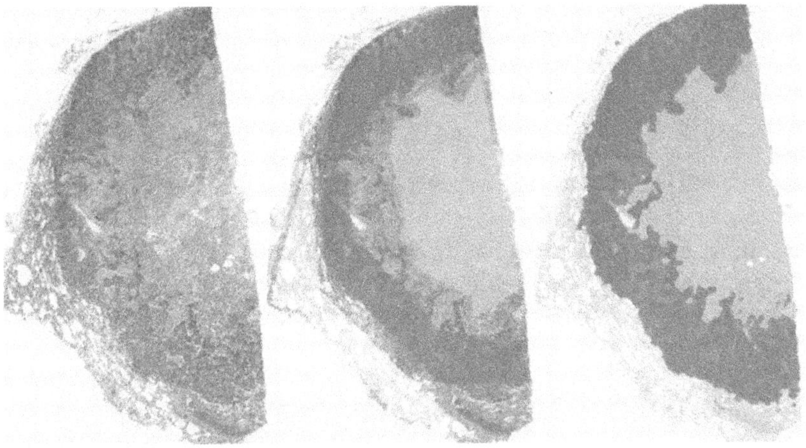

Figure 5.6. Cancer detection in lung WSI. Left: original WSI. Middle: with pathologist labels. Right: Model Prediction on both labeled and unlabeled regions. Red: tumor, green: necrosis, yellow: non-cancer lung tissue. Adapted from [14], Copyright (2022), with permission from Elsevier.

tasks . Connectivity and location of a tumor area can be represented in a computer graph and trained by graph neural networks. The AI industry is constantly getting more powerful GPUs, better cloud services, deep learning frameworks, and more experienced data scientists. The ever-growing ecosystem will be ever more capable in supporting advancements in the medical field.

5.1.4 Application in clinical pathology

There are countless attempts to develop image analysis systems for cancer (and pre-cancer) detection in both cytological and histology specimens. Specimens that benefited most are those with (1) high-volume specimens, such as common diseases that are nationally screened; (2) cancers that are not apparent to clinicians at the time of specimen collection; and (3) specimens that require tedious microscopic examination. Cancer detection tools are generally designed to be an assistive tool to look for suspicious areas, so high-risk cases can be triaged for earlier assessment by pathologists. Pathologists can also first look at areas flagged by the system to speed up the diagnosis.

5.1.4.1 Cytology

Cytology is the first area of pathology that has embraced AI with commercial success. Cytology specimens are inherently tedious to read, requiring microscopic examination at high power for a large slide area. Cytology specimens are also frequently first read by cytotechnologists to look for suspicious areas, then have diagnoses reviewed and endorsed by a pathologist.

Earliest attempts to detect abnormal cells in cervical smear took place in the early 1990s, so early that the US Food and Drug Administration (FDA) granted the pre-market approval [17] in a memorandum (typed by a typewriter!) in 1995. The product was named PAPNET and was developed by Neuromedical Systems Inc. It was approved for re-screening negative cases already reported by manual microscopic examinations. The system involved scanning the slides at a central facility and images analysis by a proprietary neural network, described as a 'non-algorithmic, connectionist system' in the FDA approval documents. The system chose 128 potentially abnormal areas, and they were subject to cytotechnologist review. The case would be completed if all 128 areas were negative. If any of these were positive, the entire case would be re-screened manually. Not surprisingly, PAPNET was able to increase the sensitivity of cervical smears by up to 30%. Despite being an excellent proof of concept, the high cost, limitation to re-screening, and trouble in mailing the slides prevented more widespread adoption and commercial success.

In the next 20 years, development in hardware and AI had evolved to allow on-site image capture and analysis. Vendors also realized the importance of AI use in initial screening instead of re-screening. ThinPrep Imaging System, approved by the FDA in 2003 [18], and various generations of AutoPap®Primary Screening System (later marketed as FocalPoint GS Imaging System), approved between 1998 and 2008 [19], gained reasonable market success. Multiple studies based on national screening programs have demonstrated an increase in productivity with these systems with comparable accuracy, particularly among routine cases [20–22].

Multiple recent studies have made use of deep learning (mostly some kind of CNN) to tackle the same problem and showed promising results. New generations of deep learning models must also have found their way into newer generations of commercial products. Large-scale studies with participation of multiple laboratories are lacking at the time of writing. However, it is safe to assume they will outperform earlier generations of products.

There are so many attempts to identify abnormal cells that practically all types of cytology specimens have been covered. However, none of them really took off. A detailed review covering different specimens has been covered by Landau and Pantanowitz [23] and is not further covered here.

5.1.4.2 Histology

Cancer detection in histological specimens was made possible only after the invention of the WSI system. Unlike with cytology specimens, cancer detection relies not only on a small area of a few cells but an overview of the entire tissue area. The first FDA-cleared cancer detection product, FullFocus by Paige.AI, Inc., only debuted in 2021 [24]. It was designed to detect cancer in prostate needle biopsy whole slide images and served as an assistive tool to pathologists. The system only accepted scans from the Philips IntelliSite Pathology Solution ultra-fast scanner. This system improved the average sensitivity from 74% to 90% with no change in specificity [25].

In the literature, researchers have attempted essentially every aspect of histological assessments, including cancer (and pre-cancer) detection [26, 27], subtyping [28], grading [29, 30], lymph node metastasis detection [31], mitotic counting [32, 33], and immune cell counting [34]. For non-neoplastic specimens, there were also attempts to segment glomeruli and classify nephropathies [35] [36], score liver injuries in biopsies [37], identify celiac disease in duodenal biopsies [38], and classify skin biopsies into diagnostic classes [39]. Most of the more recent studies have used some variations of deep learning architecture previously mentioned in section 5.1.3.

5.1.4.3 Molecular subtype predictions of cancers

For all examples mentioned, the computer model is essentially detecting features that the pathologist has been identifying under microscope. In the precision and molecular medicine era, pathologists often offer predictive and prognostic information by different molecular tests, something not apparent under the microscope. With the help of The Cancer Genome Atlas dataset comprising both histological images and genetic data, Kather *et al* [40] and Fu *et al* [41] reported the potential in AI to predict genomic events using only histological images. They have recognized morphological genetic associations both commonly known and unknown to pathologists. Actionable mutations and genetic events, such as EGFR mutation in non-small cell lung cancer, KRAS/NRAS mutation in colorectal cancers, and microsatellite instability status, are valuable targets for predictions. Multiple studies demonstrated the potential of AI in molecular subtyping and the ability to identify microsatellite instability. Using gastrointestinal cancer histological images, the reported classification performance (measured as area under receiver operating characteristic curve) was around 0.8. [42, 43] The prediction accuracy for EGFR mutation in non-small cell lung cancer [44] and KRAS/NRAS mutation in colorectal cancers have also been attempted with variable success [45]. All these attempts have yet to be validated in large-scale studies or receive any regulatory approval.

5.1.5 Limitations and concerns

There is no doubt that histopathology and cytology will soon be revolutionized by AI technologies. However, most of the pipelines described in the literature have not been validated for clinical uses, not to mention their robustness when the system is fed with WSI generated by different scanners and staining protocols. Although there is potential time-saving in slide interpretation, using this system would inevitably incur time and cost in slide digitization and file storage, particularly for laboratories not using WSI in routine diagnostics or not using the designated scanner. In the authors' opinion, the potential of going beyond academic interest will only take place when glass slide digitization becomes routine; then AI can serve as an efficient screening tool to assist pathologists. In the prediction of molecular classifications and eligibility of target therapy, it will be difficult for AI-based predictions to compete with molecular tests that offer almost perfect accuracy at a relatively low cost when compared with the steep target therapy cost.

5.2 Chemical pathology—treasures within high dimension structured data

5.2.1 What is chemical pathology?

Chemical pathology is the branch of pathology that provides biochemical and molecular investigations of blood and other body fluids for the screening, diagnosis, prognostication, treatment, and monitoring of diseases. The role of chemical pathology in clinical practice can be considered using the framework of total testing process [46], which starts from the pre-pre-analytical phase at the clinician, through the pre-analytical, analytical, and post-analytical phases in the laboratory, and then back to the clinician for the post-post-analytical phase in the clinical management of the patient [47] (table 5.1). In this process, a large volume of digitalized and structured patient result data (and their metadata) is produced at a high rate on a wide breadth and depth of biochemical parameters in many patients, longitudinally over time. These features of chemical pathology make it particularly well-suited to embrace the AI revolution.

5.2.2 Application of AI in general chemistry

At the core of chemical pathology service are the high-volume tests in general chemistry. The timely and accurate provision of these tests is maintained by the quality system in the laboratory. Given that pre-pre-analytical errors outside of the laboratory account for up to 68.2% of total identified errors in the total testing process [46], there is a need for the laboratory to detect such errors to prevent reporting of potentially misleading results, which may lead to inappropriate investigations and/or treatments and, hence, patient harm. AI has been applied to detect these pre-analytical errors which may be difficult to detect by humans or rule-based systems, with examples including spurious glucose results due to 'drip-arm' error during phlebotomy with a decision tree algorithm [48], misidentified specimens as 'wrong blood in tube' errors with a support vector machine [49] or a gradient-boosting-decision-tree model [50], and spurious hyperkalemia due to hemolysis in point-of-care testing using a multivariate logistic regression model [51]. After instrumental analysis, an efficient auto-verification system would be required for reporting of the analytical results. Instead of the commonly used rule-based verification, such as sign-out range, delta check, etc, auto-verification of laboratory results with AI could potentially improve quality of reporting and manpower efficiency [52, 53].

AI systems were developed for the interpretation of analytical data to reduce manual workload and improve turnaround time. Examples include support vector machine algorithms for automated review of gas chromatography–mass spectrometry data for urine toxicology [54] and neural network algorithms for classification of serum protein electrophoresis [55–58]. AI is also suitable for the interpretation of profile tests containing several related analyses to be interpreted as a pattern. Examples include plasma amino acid profiles [59] and tandem mass spectrometry–based newborn screening [60] for inherited metabolic diseases, urine steroid profile to differentiate adrenocortical carcinoma from adenoma [61], and plasma steroid profiling for diagnosis of primary aldosteronism [62].

Given the power of AI to learn from patient demographic and laboratory data to predict disease and outcome, this is a popular area of study for the application of AI. Many studies have been published on the prediction of acute kidney injury before overt clinical or biochemical abnormalities [63–65]. Other similar examples include

Table 5.1. Example of AI applications in the total testing process inside and outside of the laboratory.

Phases in total testing process	Location	Example of activities	Examples of AI applications
Pre-pre-analytical	Clinician	Clinician requesting test, sample collection and transport	• Prediction of gamma glutamyl transferase [102] or serum ferritin results [103]
Pre-analytical	Laboratory	Sample handling and preparation	• Detection of 'drip-arm' error [48] • Detection of 'wrong blood in tube' errors [49] [50] • Detection of spurious hyperkalemia due to hemolysis in point-of-care testing [51]
Analytical	Laboratory	Instrument operation, signal and data generation, quality control	• Automated review of gas chromatography–mass spectrometry data [54]
Post-analytical	Laboratory	Validation of analytical data, result transcription, interpretative reporting by pathologists	• Auto-verification of laboratory results specialists [52, 53] • Classification of serum protein electrophoresis [55–58]
Post-post-analytical	Clinician	Interpretation of results and action by clinician	• Interpretation of plasma amino acid profiles [59] • Differentiation of adrenocortical carcinoma from adenoma in urine steroid profile [61] • Diagnosis of primary aldosteronism with plasma steroid profile [62] • Reduction of false positive rates of inborn errors of metabolism by tandem-mass spectrometry-based newborn screening [60] • Prediction of acute kidney injury [63–65] • Prediction of diabetes mellitus [66] • Prediction of neonatal hyperbilirubinemia [67] • Prediction of cardiac amyloidosis [68] • Prediction of adverse outcome in febrile patients in the emergency room [69]

the prediction of diabetes mellitus [66], neonatal hyperbilirubinemia [67], cardiac amyloidosis [68], and adverse outcomes in febrile patients in the emergency room [69]. These studies showed that the additional clinical value of a lead-time window for early intervention can be extracted with AI on demographics and well-established biochemical tests.

5.2.3 AI in the diagnosis of metabolic diseases

Providing diagnostics for inherited metabolic diseases is a fundamental part of chemical pathology practice. While individually rare, these metabolic diseases are not uncommon, with an incidence of about 1 in 4122 in Hong Kong [70]. Availability of treatments for metabolic diseases has improved significantly over the past two decades, with enzyme or cofactor replacement, hematopoietic stem cell transplantation, gene therapy, stop codon readthrough, and so on [71]. Therefore, AI may have a role in making an early diagnosis and treatment before irreversible damage. The modern model for the diagnosis of metabolic diseases is supported by deep phenotyping, biochemical analysis, and genetic testing [72].

The application of AI in phenotyping and biochemical analyses, in contrast to its widespread application in the field of genetics, remain limited. An example of its use in phenotyping is the use of a deep CNN in identifying facial features for the diagnosis of more than 200 syndromes, based on 17 106 images of 10 953 subjects [73]. Generalizability, however, remains a key challenge. It is not difficult to appreciate the difficulty when the accuracy decreased from 80% to just 36.8% when testing patients with a different ethnic background [74].

The challenges in applying AI in the diagnosis of metabolic diseases stems from the individual rarity. It is not unusual for a metabolic disease to affect less than one person per million. Therefore, even a human specialist may have to start learning about a particular disorder based on initial observation of just one patient and to diagnose the second case. In the context of AI, this is called ‘one-shot learning’ and has been tried in other branches of medicine [75, 76], with variable degrees of success.

There is a strong case for supervised models when highly informative markers are available. For example, a method for automated interpretation of the human acidic metabolome was developed more than 20 years ago [77]. The approach by Collaborative Laboratory Integrated Reports (CLIR; previously Region 4 Stork/R4S) is much more sophisticated, providing pattern recognition of newborn screening data based on adjustment by multiple covariates, while reducing heterogeneity of data through normalization and removal of outliers [78]. An AI-based model has been developed from this dataset. The success of the CLIR project lies in the curation of a large dataset with a high degree of analytical homogeneity, namely, newborn screening by tandem mass spectrometry.

The diagnostic test panels for metabolic diseases (e.g. urine and plasma metabolomes), with a smaller test volume and much wider range of metabolites tested, is more difficult to standardize. In the past decade, improvements in the diagnostic capability of metabolic laboratories were enabled by the circulation of patient samples in quality assurance schemes such as the ERNDIM qualitative urine organic acid scheme [79], which overcome the differences in technical procedures and analytical results. It is suggested that a fully quantitative approach of metabolic tests would makes results more comparable across laboratories and therefore allow for the development of models that translate well across institutions.

5.2.4 AI in the field of genetics

The clinical application of next-generation sequencing (NGS) has revolutionized the landscape of all specialties in pathology, and with it comes the vast amount of generated data. With a median of almost 20 000 variants per exome sequenced [80], manual review and classification of every individual variant in a patient is impossible. The application of AI has impacted most significantly the classification of variants. Early developments of variant classification were based on conservation of sequence between species or structural modeling of protein following amino acid changes. AI models based on machine learning algorithms such as support vector machine, neural networks, and naïve Bayes classifiers such as PolyPhen-2 have since been developed to integrate variant features such as allele frequencies, functional characterizations, and clinical-pathological effects [81]. The inclusion of features has cumulated into the development of meta-predictions which integrate multiple prediction scores such as MetaLR, MetaSVM [82], and CADD [83]. In the past few years, efforts have focused on the avoidance of overfitting and accuracy of performance metrics for non-synonymous variants [84].

Variant classification of non-coding variants has followed a similar trend, with early methods focusing on small regions surrounding the splice site, with GeneSplicer covering 80 bases on either sides [85] and MaxEntScan covering 3 exonic bases and 6 or 20 intronic bases for splice acceptor and donor sites, respectively [86]. The scoring of splicing variants has benefited from the widespread availability of deep learning AI frameworks like TensorFlow, with models such as MMSplice and SpliceAI being developed since 2016. Whereas MMSplice took a relatively biologically oriented approach, with deep learning neural network models scoring 3′-intronic, splice acceptor, 5′-exonic, 3′-exonic, splice donor, and 5′-intronic sites, and predicting splicing efficiency and pathogenicity by combining these scores [87], SpliceAI took a different approach by feeding a very long pre-messenger ribonucleic acid (mRNA) transcript sequence (up to 10 kb) into a 32-layer deep learning neural network model, which provides the prediction of whether a splice acceptor or donor site exists on that base [88]. The clinical application of these predictors have been facilitated by variant annotation software such as ANNOVAR [89] and Variant Effect Predictor from Ensemble [90], with the former utilizing pre-calculated score tables and the latter using a combination of pre-calculated caches and real-time calculation in the forms of plugins.

Another area of genetics in which AI has worked its way into clinical laboratories is through its involvement in third-generation sequencing (TGS) platforms, in terms of both base calling and variant calling. The permeation of the technology can be seen with Guppy, the default basecalling tool for the Oxford Nanopore platform, being based on deep learning neural networks [91]. On the side of variant calling, DeepVariant is one of the first variant callers that utilized the power of deep learning [92], which has been expanded to process single-molecule real-time technology and nanopore sequencing data. In the Truth Challenge V2 hosted by the FDA, top performers on TGS platforms, including DeepVariant, were all based on deep learning neural networks [93].

5.2.5 Ending remarks

The above are only some brief mentions of examples in this rapidly developing field, as well as the greater context of clinical medicine and healthcare, and the reader is recommended to refer to more in-depth reviews [94–99]. The potential of AI applications to improve our current practice of chemical pathology to provide better care for our patients is enormous. However, there are still practical obstacles in the generalized application of AI in laboratory medicine, including the need for quality data, issues with underrepresented or novel conditions, interpretability of models, lack of standardization of assays, regulatory and data privacy requirements, and ethical issues.

One interesting development in AI applications is the recent advocacy of 'data-centric' AI proposed by one of the leading figures in AI, Dr Andrew Ng, compared to the traditional 'model-centric' approach [100]. This is based on the observation that improvement of the data quality is a more efficient approach than improvement of the model in terms of the overall performance of the machine learning. In our laboratory practice, for example, we may improve the signal-to-noise ratio of the data with meticulous sample preparation in our liquid chromatography–mass spectrometry analysis. However, in the routine clinical laboratory, it may be technically challenging or prohibitively costly to improve the quality of raw data. As a result, improvement of the model may still be a major direction of development for laboratory applications. For example, the improvement in basecalling accuracy in Oxford Nanopore long-read sequencing has a significant component due to the improvement in the neural network algorithm [91], in addition to the sequencing chemistry [101]. This highlights the importance of the communication and exchange between the domain experts in laboratory medicine (who improve the data), and the experts in computer science and AI (who improve the algorithms) to introduce AI to routine practice of clinical laboratories.

With the technical maturity of AI algorithms and advancement in computational power, we now should ponder how to incorporate AI in our practice, implement and manage such AI systems, and integrate them into the bigger hospital and healthcare systems. The above pilot projects have demonstrated the feasibility of AI transformation in chemical pathology and the need to equip ourselves with the appropriate level of AI knowledge to better manage the changes brought by AI to our practice.

5.3 Clinical microbiology—application in the management of infectious diseases

5.3.1 What is clinical microbiology?

Clinical microbiology is the scientific study of microorganisms in relation to human health and disease. Human pathogens are divided into bacteria, viruses, fungi, and parasites, with corresponding laboratory methods to detect them and elucidate their relevant characteristics. Prompt and accurate identification of pathogens plays a crucial role in infectious diseases management.

5.3.1.1 Traditional microbiology laboratory practice

Most techniques adopted by clinical microbiology laboratories until the 1990s relied heavily on the cultivation or direct visualization of microorganisms, or the antibody reactions to their antigens. Culture-independent technologies, particularly nucleic acid amplification tests (NAATs), transformed clinical microbiology practice starting at the turn of the millennium and became an essential tool in all clinical microbiology laboratories. Nonetheless, bacterial culture remained the main bulk of work in most clinical microbiology laboratories. To understand the impact of AI in microbiology, it is essential to understand the usual workflow for bacterial culture. This sample processing workflow of a bacterial culture is illustrated in figure 5.7.

This workflow in figure 5.7 can be applied to most clinical samples encountered in daily clinical practice, for instance, sputum culture, blood culture, urine culture, and stool culture. The time from specimen reception to reporting is commonly 2–5 working days. This timeframe is extended for slow-growing organisms, the prime example being *Mycobacterium tuberculosis*, the causative agent of tuberculosis, for which a minimum incubation of 6–8 weeks is required before a negative result is reported.

Diagnosis of fungal infections also heavily relies on cultivation methods. Growth of fungal organisms is slower than growth of bacteria. Yeasts typically take 2–3 days to form visible growth, and most medically important molds may take 1–2 weeks to sporulate sufficiently for identification. Non-culture-based diagnostics including fungal markers such as (1–3)-β-D glucan and galactomannan, and NAATs do not offer the same breadth and depth of clinical information compared with culture.

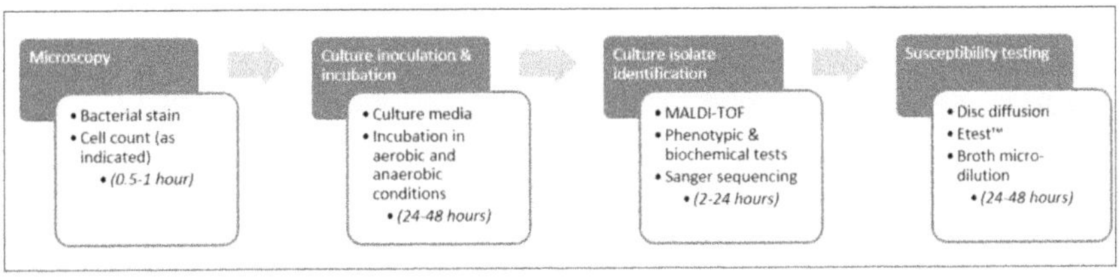

Figure 5.7. Typical sample processing workflow for bacterial culture. MALDI-TOF: matrix-assisted laser desorption/ionization-time of flight.

Viral infections can be diagnosed through direct detection of antigen, detection of antibody production through detection of serum serology, viral culture, direct visualization with electronic microscopy, or NAATs. The COVID-19 pandemic has seen the accelerated evolution of virology service away from traditional methods such as viral culture to NAATs, the latter being more sensitive, more specific, faster, and higher in throughput.

Diagnosis of parasitic infections in most microbiology laboratories is mainly through microscopy. Rapid antigen detection kits for detection of infection, for instance, falciparum malaria and visceral leishmaniasis, are exceptions rather than the rule in parasitology diagnostics. While NAAT and serological methods exist, they are not widely available in most laboratories. Owing to the paucity of parasitic infections in developed countries, these assays are also difficult to validate clinically.

5.3.1.2 Non-culture technologies in microbiology—matrix-assisted laser desorption/ionization-time of flight, Sanger sequencing, and NGS

Traditional methods of bacterial identification rely on phenotypic and biochemical tests on cultivated bacterial colonies. Classical phenotypic tests of catalase, coagulase, and oxidase tests performed directly on pure growth colonies are supplemented with an array of biochemical tests performed with in-house prepared bijou bottles or commercially available systems such as VITEK® 2 (bioMériaux), BD Phoenix™ (BD), or API® ID strips (bioMériaux). This approach is now largely superseded by matrix-assisted laser desorption/ionization-time of flight (MALDI-TOF), which analyzes the composition of ribosomal protein through mass spectrometry of prepared bacterial samples. MALDI-TOF is rapid, accurate, safe, and not operator-dependent, and its availability has made same-day species-level identification of most bacterial isolates possible.

Sanger sequencing is available in regional clinical microbiology laboratories and is usually used restricted for use for identification of difficult organisms (i.e. those organisms not readily identified by phenotypic and biochemical tests) or culture-negative samples from sterile sites such as heart valves. The targets of sequencing are typically 16S ribosomal RNA (rRNA) of bacterial organisms, and D2 region of rRNA gene, or the internal transcribed space region of fungal organisms.

NGS is another welcoming addition to the toolbox of clinical microbiologists. While a detailed discussion on technical aspects of NGS is beyond the scope of this section, it is worth noting that NGS has seen vast applications in epidemiological typing of organisms through whole-genome sequencing (WGS), polymicrobial pathogen detection, antimicrobial resistance determination, and microbiome studies. The availability of such a vast amount of genomic data also lends itself easily into the realms of AI.

5.3.2 Integration of AI in clinical microbiology

AI has seen multiple applications in various aspects of laboratory practice. AI is most useful for analyzing data-rich sources. The 'black box' diagnostics concept of MALDI-TOF makes it a natural next step for integration to AI [104]. Traditional phenotypic identification of microorganisms can easily be digitalized into data-rich images, a perfect match for AI. In fact, one application of AI in the clinical laboratory is in image interpretation, commonly known as 'computer vision' [105]. The vast amount of genomic data generated from sequencing, particularly NGS, is another area that symphonizes perfectly into machine learning processes. Finally, the existing total laboratory automation systems are already highly compatible with the integration of machine learning processes [106, 107]. In the following paragraphs, we will briefly discuss the applications of AI in microscopy, microorganism identification, and susceptibility testing.

5.3.3 Applications of AI in microscopy

Urine microscopy is an essential step before urine culture for the diagnosis of urinary tract infection (UTI). A positive urine culture only warrants treatment when the urine microscopy finding is suggestive of UTI in most clinical scenarios. Given the large number of urine specimens received every day, urine microscopy is a labor-intensive and operator-dependent process. Various machine learning methods have hence been proposed to automate the process of urine microscopy, with most of the recent models developed through neural networks [108–110]. Neural network models are accurate in classifying cells, casts, and crystals in urine microscopy, achieving a mean average precision of 86.9% in one study [108, 109]. Commercial platforms incorporating automated urine microscopy through AI are also available [110].

AI is also applied in parasite detection by microscopy. Diagnosis and speciation of *Plasmodium* spp., the causative agent of malaria, are classically done by light microscopy of thin and thick blood smears. Different AI algorithms applied to malaria diagnosis include *K*-means clustering, support vector machines, decision trees, and neural networks [111]. In field evaluations in resource-limited settings, the accuracy of digital image recognition was found to vary significantly across the site (sensitivity 52%–72%, specificity 75%–85%), with the main reason cited being the variability in volume of blood used for preparing smears. Higher accuracy was obtained with a higher volume of blood per smear [112]. Some models can be deployed on a cell phone, eliminating the need for a digital microscope for further analysis. This would further increase the affordability and flexibility of these algorithms in resource-limited settings [113].

5.3.4 Applications of AI in culture plate reading and microbial identification

Culture plate reading involves identifying significant bacterial or fungal colonies for further identification and processing from positive culture and discarding non-significant or negative culture. Colonial appearances vary by bacterial species, for example, the large beta-hemolytic zones of *Streptococcus pyogenes*, or chalky colonies of *Nocardia asteroides*. Computer vision has been employed in the interpretation of culture plates, either by screening out plates with no significant growth or by performing direct identification based on colonial morphology.

An approach of AI in culture plate classification is to sort culture plates into whether follow-up action is required for a particular specimen. In a multicenter evaluation study of the APAS™ image analysis system, a pre-defined algorithm classified blood agar and MacConkey agar culture plates into positive (follow-up action required), review (further review by microbiologist required), or negative (no further action required) based on camera images of plates, with a sensitivity of 99.0% and a specificity of 84.5%, respectively [114]. Variable performance was obtained in determining the morphotypes of bacterial colonies in the study. By eliminating the negative culture plates with AI, staff manpower could be diverted to other tasks.

Another approach was to classify bacterial colonies into bacterial species based on imaging. A commercially available example was the application of BD Kiestra™ Optis™ imaging software within a suite of total laboratory automation equipment [115]. In this study, urine specimens were inoculated on chromogenic agar and identified with automated imaging software. Images of culture plates obtained at a different time of incubation with different lighting were evaluated using a random forest model. The accuracy of identification in the study was high (98.3%–99.5%). However, it must be cautioned that the accuracy of such identification schemes is likely significantly lower with most other clinical specimens. Reasons for the potentially lower accuracy in other specimen sites include the wider variety of microbes with similar colony morphology in most other clinical specimens, the relative paucity of well-established chromogenic agar for other specimen sites, and the presence of slow-growing or fastidious organisms in some infections.

Machine learning methods are widely applied in microbiome studies using NGS. An example is the detection of gut microbiota alteration in patients with COVID-19. Using multivariate linear regression on metagenomic sequencing data, specific alterations in constituents of gut microbiota were identified [116].

5.3.5 Applications of AI in susceptibility testing

The time from visible bacterial growth to the availability of antimicrobial susceptibility test (AST) results can be shortened with the application of AI. By using computer vision to observe inhibition of bacterial growth in the pre-defined concentration of different antibiotics, Choi *et al* reduced the incubation time for susceptibility testing required from 24 to 6 h [117]. Categorical agreement was 91.11%, and the very major error rate was 1.45%. An alternative design with flow cytometry coupled with machine learning algorithms allowed same-day availability of susceptibility results for *Escherichia coli* and *Staphylococcus aureus* isolates, with a categorical agreement of 91% in these two species [118].

Stepping away from culture-based susceptibility testing, application of machine learning algorithms in MALDI-TOF has also been used to predict AST results with varying degrees of success [119]. Examples of antimicrobial resistance mechanisms that were identified through machine learning algorithms of MALDI-TOF include methicillin resistance in *S. aureus* [120], carbapenemase gene of *Bacteroides fragilis* [121], and carbapenem resistance in *Klebsiella pneumoniae* [122].

NGS has made possible WGS of bacterial isolates. The application of different machine learning algorithms has improved the prediction of AST based on WGS results. The application of XGBoost algorithm on WGS data of non-typhoidal *Salmonella* spp. allowed prediction of antimicrobial susceptibility with good accuracy (95%) [123]. In another study, logistic regression of WGS data also accurately predicted AST profile of clinical strains of Enterobacteriaceae with a 90.3% accuracy [124]. Taken together, these AST prediction models are superior to current molecular methods that detect the presence or absence of a limited set of resistance genes. These machine learning prediction–based WGS data would complement culture-based susceptibility methods, allowing for the precise prescription of appropriate antimicrobial therapy, leading to improved patient care [104].

5.3.6 Insights in future deployment

We are witnessing a period of rapid digitalization and transformation in the practice of clinical microbiology. Egli suggested several hurdles remained before the implementation of AI in daily practices: the standardization of data and code formats, interoperable information technology environment, infrastructure with sufficient storage and computational capacity, validated algorithms, and inputs from microbiologists and infectious diseases experts [125]. Finally, we believe AI is best in augmenting human effort; human intelligence will remain an integral and essential part of clinical microbiology laboratories.

References

[1] Leica Biosystems Imaging Inc. 2000 Fully automatic rapid microscope slide scanner. US; US6711283B1

[2] Bankhead P, Loughrey M, Fernández J, Dombrowski Y, McArt D and Dunne P *et al* 2017 QuPath: open source software for digital pathology image analysis *Sci. Rep.* **7** 1

[3] Litjens G 2018 ASAP – automated slide analysis platform (available at: https://computationalpathologygroup.github.io/ASAP/#about) (accessed 29 January 2022)

[4] Satyanarayanan M, Goode A, Gilbert B, Harkes J and Jukic D 2013 OpenSlide: a vendor-neutral software foundation for digital pathology *J. Pathol. Inf.* **4** 27

[5] Linkert M, Rueden C, Allan C, Burel J, Moore W and Patterson A *et al* 2010 Metadata matters: access to image data in the real world *J. Cell Biol.* **189** 777–82

[6] Street W, Wolberg W and Mangasarian O 1993 Nuclear feature extraction for breast tumor diagnosis *SPIE Proc.* **1905** 861–70

[7] Géron A 2017 *Hands-On Machine Learning with Scikit-Learn and TensorFlow: Concepts, Tools, and Techniques to Build Intelligent Systems* (Sebastopol, CA: O'Reilly Media)

[8] Simonyan K and Zisserman A 2014 Very deep convolutional networks for large-scale image recognition arXiv:1409.1556

[9] He K, Zhang X, Ren S and Sun J 2015 Deep residual learning for image recognition arXiv:1512.03385

[10] Ronneberger O, Fischer P and Brox T 2015 U-Net: convolutional networks for biomedical image segmentation arXiv:1505.04597

[11] Ren S, He K, Girshick R and Sun J 2016 Faster R-CNN: towards real-time object detection with region proposal networks arXiv:1506.01497

[12] He K, Gkioxari G, Dollar P and Girshick R 2017 Mask R-CNN *IEEE Int. Conf. on Computer Vision (ICCV)* (IEEE) pp 2980–8

[13] Redmon J, Divvala S, Girshick R and Farhadi A 2016 You only look once: unified, real-time object detection arXiv:1506.02640

[14] Lee A L S, To C C K, Lee A L H, Li J J X and Chan R C K 2022 Model architecture and tile size selection for convolutional neural network training for non-small cell lung cancer detection on whole slide images *Inf. Med. Unlocked* **28** 100850

[15] Otsu N 1979 A threshold selection method from gray-level histograms *IEEE Trans. Syst. Man Cybern.* **9** 62–6

[16] Campanella G, Hanna M, Geneslaw L, Miraflor A, Werneck Krauss Silva V and Busam K *et al* 2019 Clinical-grade computational pathology using weakly supervised deep learning on whole slide images *Nat. Med.* **25** 1301–9

[17] Department of Health and Human Services and Alpert S 1995 *Premarket Approval of Neuromedical Systems, Incorporated's PAPNET Testing System - Action* https://www.accessdata.fda.gov/cdrh_docs/pdf/p940029.pdf

[18] Department of Health and Human Services and Gutman S I 2003 *RE: P020002 ThinPrep® Imaging System* https://www.accessdata.fda.gov/cdrh_docs/pdf2/P020002a.pdf

[19] Department of Health and Human Services 2008 *Summary of Safety and Effectiveness Data* https://www.accessdata.fda.gov/cdrh_docs/pdf/p950009s008b.pdf

[20] Palmer T, Nicoll S, McKean M, Park A, Bishop D and Baker L *et al* 2012 Prospective parallel randomized trial of the MultiCyte™ ThinPrep® imaging system: the Scottish experience *Cytopathology* **24** 235–45

[21] Roberts J, Thurloe J, Bowditch R, Hyne S, Greenberg M and Clarke J *et al* 2007 A three-armed trial of the ThinPrep Imaging System *Diagn. Cytopathol.* **35** 96–102

[22] Kitchener H, Blanks R, Dunn G, Gunn L, Desai M and Albrow R *et al* 2011 Automation-assisted versus manual reading of cervical cytology (MAVARIC): a randomised controlled trial *Lancet Oncol.* **12** 56–64

[23] Landau M and Pantanowitz L 2019 Artificial intelligence in cytopathology: a review of the literature and overview of commercial landscape *J. Am. Soc. Cytopathol.* **8** 230–41

[24] Department of Health and Human Services and Philip R 2021 *De Novo Summary (DEN200080)*)https://www.accessdata.fda.gov/cdrh_docs/reviews/DEN200080.pdf

[25] Raciti P, Sue J, Ceballos R, Godrich R, Kunz J and Kapur S *et al* 2020 Novel artificial intelligence system increases the detection of prostate cancer in whole slide images of core needle biopsies *Mod. Pathol.* **33** 2058–66

[26] Araújo T, Aresta G, Castro E, Rouco J, Aguiar P and Eloy C *et al* 2017 Classification of breast cancer histology images using Convolutional Neural Networks *PLoS One* **12** e0177544

[27] Bejnordi B, Zuidhof G, Balkenhol M, Hermsen M, Bult P and van Ginneken B *et al* 2017 Context-aware stacked convolutional neural networks for classification of breast carcinomas in whole-slide histopathology images *J. Med. Imaging* **4** 1

[28] Gertych A, Swiderska-Chadaj Z, Ma Z, Ing N, Markiewicz T and Cierniak S *et al* 2019 Convolutional neural networks can accurately distinguish four histologic growth patterns of lung adenocarcinoma in digital slides *Sci. Rep.* **9** 1

[29] Awan R, Sirinukunwattana K, Epstein D, Jefferyes S, Qidwai U and Aftab Z *et al* 2017 Glandular morphometrics for objective grading of colorectal adenocarcinoma histology images *Sci. Rep.* **7** 1

[30] Ryu H, Jin M, Park J, Lee S, Cho J and Oh S *et al* 2019 Automated gleason scoring and tumor quantification in prostate core needle biopsy images using deep neural networks and its comparison with pathologist-based assessment *Cancers* **11** 1860

[31] Litjens G, Bandi P, Ehteshami Bejnordi B, Geessink O, Balkenhol M and Bult P *et al* 2018 1399 H&E-stained sentinel lymph node sections of breast cancer patients: the CAMELYON dataset *GigaScience* **7** 6

[32] Roux L, Racoceanu D, Loménie N, Kulikova M, Irshad H and Klossa J *et al* 2013 Mitosis detection in breast cancer histological images An ICPR 2012 contest *J. Pathol. Inf.* **4** 8

[33] Albarqouni S, Baur C, Achilles F, Belagiannis V, Demirci S and Navab N 2016 AggNet: deep learning from crowds for mitosis detection in breast cancer histology images *IEEE Trans. Med. Imaging* **35** 1313–21

[34] Aprupe L, Litjens G, Brinker T, van der Laak J and Grabe N 2019 Robust and accurate quantification of biomarkers of immune cells in lung cancer micro-environment using deep convolutional neural networks *PeerJ* **7** e6335

[35] Gallego J, Pedraza A, Lopez S, Steiner G, Gonzalez L and Laurinavicius A *et al* 2018 Glomerulus classification and detection based on convolutional neural networks *J. Imaging* **4** 20

[36] Ginley B, Lutnick B, Jen K, Fogo A, Jain S and Rosenberg A *et al* 2019 Computational segmentation and classification of diabetic glomerulosclerosis *J. Am. Soc. Nephrol.* **30** 1953–67

[37] Yu Y, Wang J, Ng C, Ma Y, Mo S and Fong E *et al* 2018 Deep learning enables automated scoring of liver fibrosis stages *Sci. Rep.* **8** 1

[38] Hassanpour S, Wei J, Wei J, Jackson C, Ren B and Suriawinata A 2019 Automated detection of celiac disease on duodenal biopsy slides: a deep learning approach *J. Pathol. Inf.* **10** 7

[39] Ianni J, Soans R, Sankarapandian S, Chamarthi R, Ayyagari D and Olsen T *et al* 2020 Tailored for real-world: a whole slide image classification system validated on uncurated multi-site data emulating the prospective pathology workload *Sci. Rep.* **10** 1

[40] Kather J, Heij L, Grabsch H, Loeffler C, Echle A and Muti H *et al* 2020 Pan-cancer image-based detection of clinically actionable genetic alterations *Nat. Cancer* **1** 789–99

[41] Fu Y, Jung A, Torne R, Gonzalez S, Vöhringer H and Shmatko A *et al* 2020 Pan-cancer computational histopathology reveals mutations, tumor composition and prognosis *Nat. Cancer* **1** 800–10

[42] Kather J, Pearson A, Halama N, Jäger D, Krause J and Loosen S *et al* 2019 Deep learning can predict microsatellite instability directly from histology in gastrointestinal cancer *Nat. Med.* **25** 1054–6

[43] Muti H, Heij L, Keller G, Kohlruss M, Langer R and Dislich B *et al* 2021 Development and validation of deep learning classifiers to detect Epstein-Barr virus and microsatellite instability status in gastric cancer: a retrospective multicentre cohort study *Lancet Digit. Health* **3** e654–64

[44] Coudray N, Ocampo P, Sakellaropoulos T, Narula N, Snuderl M and Fenyö D *et al* 2018 Classification and mutation prediction from non–small cell lung cancer histopathology images using deep learning *Nat. Med.* **24** 1559–67

[45] Bilal M, Raza S, Azam A, Graham S, Ilyas M and Cree I *et al* 2021 Development and validation of a weakly supervised deep learning framework to predict the status of molecular pathways and key mutations in colorectal cancer from routine histology images: a retrospective study *Lancet Digit. Health* **3** e763–72

[46] Plebani M 2010 The detection and prevention of errors in laboratory medicine *Ann. Clin. Biochem. Int. J. Lab. Med.* **47** 101–10

[47] Plebani M, Laposata M and Lundberg G D 2011 The brain-to-brain loop concept for laboratory testing 40 years after its introduction *Am. J. Clin. Pathol.* **136** 829–33

[48] Baron J M, Mermel C H, Lewandrowski K B and Dighe A S 2012 Detection of preanalytic laboratory testing errors using a statistically guided protocol *Am. J. Clin. Pathol.* **138** 406–13

[49] Rosenbaum M W and Baron J M 2018 Using machine learning-based multianalyte delta checks to detect wrong blood in tube errors *Am. J. Clin. Pathol.* **150** 555–66

[50] Mitani T, Doi S, Yokota S, Imai T and Ohe K 2020 Highly accurate and explainable detection of specimen mix-up using a machine learning model *Clin. Chem. Lab. Med.* **58** 375–83

[51] Benirschke R C and Gniadek T J 2020 Detection of falsely elevated point-of-care potassium results due to hemolysis using predictive analytics *Am. J. Clin. Pathol.* **154** 242–7

[52] Demirci F, Akan P, Kume T, Sisman A R, Erbayraktar Z and Sevinc S 2016 Artificial neural network approach in laboratory test reporting *Am. J. Clin. Pathol.* **146** 227–37

[53] Wang H, Wang H, Zhang J, Li X, Sun C and Zhang Y 2021 Using machine learning to develop an autoverification system in a clinical biochemistry laboratory *Clin. Chem. Lab. Med.* **59** 883–91

[54] Yu M, Bazydlo L A L, Bruns D E and Harrison J H 2019 Streamlining quality review of mass spectrometry data in the clinical laboratory by use of machine learning *Arch. Pathol. Lab. Med.* **143** 990–8

[55] Kratzer M A A, Ivandic B and Fateh-Moghadam A 1992 Neuronal network analysis of serum electrophoresis *J. Clin. Pathol.* **45** 612–5

[56] Altinier S, Sarti L, Varagnolo M, Zaninotto M, Maggini M and Plebani M 2008 An expert system for the classification of serum protein electrophoresis patterns *Clin. Chem. Lab. Med.* **46** 1458–63

[57] Ognibene A, Graziani M S, Caldini A, Terreni A, Righetti G and Varagnolo M C *et al* 2008 Computer-assisted detection of monoclonal components: results from the multicenter study for the evaluation of CASPER (Computer Assisted Serum Protein Electrophoresis Recognizer) algorithm *Clin. Chem. Lab. Med.* **46** 1183–8

[58] Chabrun F, Dieu X, Ferre M, Gaillard O, Mery A and Chao de la Barca J M *et al* 2021 Achieving expert-level interpretation of serum protein electrophoresis through deep learning driven by human reasoning *Clin. Chem.* **67** 1406–14

[59] Wilkes E H, Emmett E, Beltran L, Woodward G M and Carling R S 2020 A machine learning approach for the automated interpretation of plasma amino acid profiles *Clin. Chem.* **66** 1210–8

[60] Peng G, Tang Y, Cowan T M, Enns G M, Zhao H and Scharfe C 2020 Reducing false-positive results in newborn screening using machine learning *Int. J. Neonatal Screen* **6** 16

[61] Arlt W, Biehl M, Taylor A E, Hahner S, Libé R and Hughes B A *et al* 2011 Urine steroid metabolomics as a biomarker tool for detecting malignancy in adrenal tumors *J. Clin. Endocrinol. Metab.* **96** 3775–84

[62] Eisenhofer G, Durán C, Cannistraci C V, Peitzsch M, Williams T A and Riester A *et al* 2020 Use of steroid profiling combined with machine learning for identification and subtype classification in primary aldosteronism *JAMA Netw. Open* **3** e2016209

[63] Koyner J L, Carey K A, Edelson D P and Churpek M M 2018 The development of a machine learning inpatient acute kidney injury prediction model *Crit. Care Med.* **46** 1070–7

[64] Parreco J, Soe-Lin H, Parks J J, Byerly S, Chatoor M and Buicko J L *et al* 2019 Comparing machine learning algorithms for predicting acute kidney injury *Am. Surg.* **85** 725–9

[65] Tomašev N, Glorot X, Rae J W, Zielinski M, Askham H and Saraiva A *et al* 2019 A clinically applicable approach to continuous prediction of future acute kidney injury *Nature* **572** 116–9

[66] Lai H, Huang H, Keshavjee K, Guergachi A and Gao X 2019 Predictive models for diabetes mellitus using machine learning techniques *BMC Endocr. Disord.* **19** 101

[67] Daunhawer I, Kasser S, Koch G, Sieber L, Cakal H and Tütsch J *et al* 2019 Enhanced early prediction of clinically relevant neonatal hyperbilirubinemia with machine learning *Pediatr. Res.* **86** 122–7

[68] Agibetov A, Seirer B, Dachs T-M, Koschutnik M, Dalos D and Rettl R *et al* 2020 Machine learning enables prediction of cardiac amyloidosis by routine laboratory parameters: a proof-of-concept study *J. Clin. Med.* **9** 1334

[69] Lee S, Hong S, Cha W C and Kim K 2020 Predicting adverse outcomes for febrile patients in the emergency department using sparse laboratory data: development of a time adaptive model *JMIR Med. Inf.* **8** e16117

[70] Lee H C H, Mak C M, Lam C W, Yuen Y P, Chen A O K and Shek C C *et al* 2011 Analysis of inborn errors of metabolism: disease spectrum for expanded newborn screening in Hong Kong *Chin. Med. J. (Engl.)* **124** 983–9

[71] Vernon H J and Manoli I 2021 Milestones in treatments for inborn errors of metabolism: reflections on where chemistry and medicine meet *Am. J. Med. Genet.* A **185** 3350–8

[72] Kuseyri Hübschmann O, Horvath G, Cortès-Saladelafont E, Yıldız Y, Mastrangelo M and Pons R *et al* 2021 Insights into the expanding phenotypic spectrum of inherited disorders of biogenic amines *Nat. Commun.* **12** 5529

[73] Gurovich Y, Hanani Y, Bar O, Nadav G, Fleischer N and Gelbman D *et al* 2019 Identifying facial phenotypes of genetic disorders using deep learning *Nat. Med.* **25** 60–4

[74] Lumaka A, Cosemans N, Lulebo Mampasi A, Mubungu G, Mvuama N and Lubala T *et al* 2017 Facial dysmorphism is influenced by ethnic background of the patient and of the evaluator *Clin. Genet.* **92** 166–71

[75] Wang S, Cao S, Wei D, Wang R, Ma K and Wang L *et al* 2020 LT-Net: label transfer by learning reversible voxel-wise correspondence for one-shot medical image segmentation *2020 IEEE/CVF Conf Comput Vis Pattern Recognit* 9159 68

[76] Cai A, Hu W and Zheng J 2020 Few-shot learning for medical image classification *Artificial Neural Networks and Machine Learning – ICANN2020* (Switzerland: Springer) Lecture Notes in Computer Science pp 441–52

[77] Kimura M, Yamamoto T and Yamaguchi S 1999 Automated metabolic profiling and interpretation of GC/MS data for organic acidemia screening: a personal computer-based system *Tohoku J. Exp. Med.* **188** 317–34

[78] Sörensen L, von Döbeln U, Åhlman H, Ohlsson A, Engvall M and Naess K *et al* 2020 Expanded screening of one million Swedish babies with R4S and CLIR for post-analytical evaluation of data *Int. J. Neonatal Screen* **6** 42

[79] Peters V, Bonham J R, Hoffmann G F, Scott C and Langhans C-D 2016 Qualitative urinary organic acid analysis: 10 years of quality assurance *J. Inherit. Metab. Dis.* **39** 683–7

[80] Backman J D, Li A H, Marcketta A, Sun D, Mbatchou J and Kessler M D *et al* 2021 Exome sequencing and analysis of 454,787 UK Biobank participants *Nature* **599** 628–34
[81] Hicks S, Wheeler D A, Plon S E and Kimmel M 2011 Prediction of missense mutation functionality depends on both the algorithm and sequence alignment employed *Hum. Mutat.* **32** 661–8
[82] Dong C, Wei P, Jian X, Gibbs R, Boerwinkle E and Wang K *et al* 2015 Comparison and integration of deleteriousness prediction methods for nonsynonymous SNVs in whole exome sequencing studies *Hum. Mol. Genet.* **24** 2125–37
[83] Rentzsch P, Witten D, Cooper G M, Shendure J and Kircher M 2019 CADD: predicting the deleteriousness of variants throughout the human genome *Nucleic Acids Res.* **47** D886–94
[84] Grimm D G, Azencott C-A, Aicheler F, Gieraths U, MacArthur D G and Samocha K E *et al* 2015 The evaluation of tools used to predict the impact of missense variants is hindered by two types of circularity *Hum. Mutat.* **36** 513–23
[85] Pertea M, Lin X and Salzberg S L 2001 GeneSplicer: a new computational method for splice site prediction *Nucleic Acids Res.* **29** 1185–90
[86] Yeo G and Burge C B 2004 Maximum entropy modeling of short sequence motifs with applications to RNA splicing signals *J. Comput. Biol.* **11** 377–94
[87] Cheng J, Nguyen T Y D, Cygan K J, Çelik M H, Fairbrother W G and Avsec Ž *et al* 2019 MMSplice: modular modeling improves the predictions of genetic variant effects on splicing *Genome Biol.* **20** 48
[88] Jaganathan K, Kyriazopoulou Panagiotopoulou S, McRae J F, Darbandi S F, Knowles D and Li Y I *et al* 2019 Predicting splicing from primary sequence with deep learning *Cell* **176** 535–48.e24
[89] Wang K, Li M and Hakonarson H 2010 ANNOVAR: functional annotation of genetic variants from high-throughput sequencing data *Nucleic Acids Res.* **38** e164
[90] McLaren W, Gil L, Hunt S E, Riat H S, Ritchie G R S and Thormann A *et al* 2016 The ensembl variant effect predictor *Genome Biol* **17** 122
[91] Wick R R, Judd L M and Holt K E 2019 Performance of neural network basecalling tools for Oxford Nanopore sequencing *Genome Biol* **20** 129
[92] Poplin R, Chang P-C, Alexander D, Schwartz S, Colthurst T and Ku A *et al* 2018 A universal SNP and small-indel variant caller using deep neural networks *Nat. Biotechnol.* **36** 983–7
[93] PrecisionFDA Challenge 2022 Truth Challenge V2: calling variants from short and long reads in difficult-to-map regions. PrecisionFDA Challenge. Available at: https://precision.fda.gov/challenges/10/results
[94] Haymond S, Julian R K, Gill E L and Master S 2021 Biochemical and molecular basis of pediatric disease *Biochemical and Molecular Basis of Pediatric Disease* (Amsterdam: Elsevier) 37–70
[95] Cabitza F and Banfi G 2018 Machine learning in laboratory medicine: waiting for the flood? *Clin. Chem. Lab. Med.* **56** 516–24
[96] De Bruyne S, Speeckaert M M, Van Biesen W and Delanghe J 2021 Recent evolutions of machine learning applications in clinical laboratory medicine *Crit. Rev. Clin. Lab. Sci.* **58** 131–52
[97] Punchoo R, Bhoora S and Pillay N 2021 Applications of machine learning in the chemical pathology laboratory *J. Clin. Pathol.* **74** 435–42

[98] Herman D S, Rhoads D D, Schulz W L and Durant T J S 2021 Artificial intelligence and mapping a new direction in laboratory medicine: a review *Clin. Chem.* **67** 1466–82
[99] Haymond S and McCudden C 2021 Rise of the machines: artificial intelligence and the clinical laboratory *J. Appl. Lab. Med.* **6** 1640–54
[100] Ng A 2021 MLOps: from model-centric to data-centric AI. Deeplearning.Ai. Available at: https://deeplearning.ai/resources
[101] Sereika M, Kirkegaard R H, Karst S M, Michaelsen T Y, Sørensen E A and Wollenberg R D *et al* 2021 Oxford Nanopore R10.4 Long-read sequencing enables near-perfect bacterial genomes from pure cultures and metagenomes without short-read or reference polishing *Nat. Methods* **19** 823–6 (bioRxiv. 2021.10.27.466057)
[102] Lidbury B A, Richardson A M and Badrick T 2015 Assessment of machine-learning techniques on large pathology data sets to address assay redundancy in routine liver function test profiles *Diagnosis* **2** 41–51
[103] Luo Y, Szolovits P, Dighe A S and Baron J M 2016 Using machine learning to predict laboratory test results *Am. J. Clin. Pathol.* **145** 778–88
[104] Smith K, Wang H, Durant T, Mathison B, Sharp S and Kirby J *et al* 2020 Applications of artificial intelligence in clinical microbiology diagnostic testing *Clin. Microbiol. Newslett.* **42** 61–70
[105] Rhoads D 2020 Computer vision and artificial intelligence are emerging diagnostic tools for the clinical microbiologist *J. Clin. Microbiol.* **58** e00511-20
[106] Smith K, Kang A and Kirby J 2018 Automated interpretation of blood culture gram stains by use of a deep convolutional neural network *J. Clin. Microbiol.* **56** e01521-17
[107] Andreini P, Bonechi S, Bianchini M, Garzelli A and Mecocci A 2016 Automatic image classification for the urinoculture screening *Comput. Biol. Med.* **70** 12–22
[108] Suhail K and Brindha D 2021 A review on various methods for recognition of urine particles using digital microscopic images of urine sediments *Biomed. Signal Process. Control* **68** 102806
[109] Liang Y, Tang Z, Yan M and Liu J 2018 Object detection based on deep learning for urine sediment examination *Biocybern. Biomed. Eng.* **38** 661–70
[110] Yüksel H, Kiliç E, Ekinci A and Evliyaoğlu O 2013 Comparison of fully automated urine sediment analyzers H800-FUS100 and LabUMat-UriSed with manual microscopy *J. Clin. Lab. Anal.* **27** 312–6
[111] Poostchi M, Silamut K, Maude R, Jaeger S and Thoma G 2018 Image analysis and machine learning for detecting malaria *Trans. Res.* **194** 36–55
[112] Torres K, Bachman C, Delahunt C, Alarcon Baldeon J, Alava F and Gamboa Vilela D *et al* 2018 Automated microscopy for routine malaria diagnosis: a field comparison on Giemsa-stained blood films in Peru *Malar. J.* **17** 339
[113] Yu H, Yang F, Rajaraman S, Ersoy I, Moallem G and Poostchi M *et al* 2020 Malaria Screener: a smartphone application for automated malaria screening *BMC Infect. Dis.* **20** 825
[114] Glasson J, Hill R, Summerford M, Olden D, Papadopoulos F and Young S *et al* 2017 Multicenter evaluation of an image analysis device (APAS): comparison between digital image and traditional plate reading using urine cultures *Ann. Lab. Med.* **37** 499–504
[115] Croxatto A, Marcelpoil R, Orny C, Morel D, Prod'hom G and Greub G 2017 Towards automated detection, semi-quantification and identification of microbial growth in clinical bacteriology: a proof of concept *Biomed. J.* **40** 317–28

[116] Zuo T, Zhang F, Lui G, Yeoh Y, Li A and Zhan H *et al* 2020 Alterations in gut microbiota of patients with COVID-19 during time of hospitalization *Gastroenterology* **159** 944–55.e8
[117] Choi J, Jeong H, Lee G, Han S, Han S and Jin B *et al* 2017 Direct, rapid antimicrobial susceptibility test from positive blood cultures based on microscopic imaging analysis *Sci. Rep.* **7** 1148
[118] Inglis T, Paton T, Kopczyk M, Mulroney K and Carson C 2020 Same-day antimicrobial susceptibility test using acoustic-enhanced flow cytometry visualized with supervised machine learning *J. Med. Microbiol.* **69** 657–69
[119] Weis C, Jutzeler C and Borgwardt K 2020 Machine learning for microbial identification and antimicrobial susceptibility testing on MALDI-TOF mass spectra: a systematic review *Clin. Microbiol. Infect.* **26** 1310–7
[120] Tang K, Tang D, Wang Q and Li C 2021 MALDI-TOF MS platform combined with machine learning to establish a model for rapid identification of methicillin-resistant *Staphylococcus aureus J. Microbiol. Methods* **180** 106109
[121] Ho P, Yau C, Ho L, Chen J, Lai E and Lo S *et al* 2017 Rapid detection of cfiA metallo-β-lactamase-producing *Bacteroides fragilis* by the combination of MALDI-TOF MS and CarbaNP *J. Clin. Pathol.* **70** 868–73
[122] Huang T, Lee S, Lee C and Chang F 2020 Detection of carbapenem-resistant *Klebsiella pneumoniae* on the basis of matrix-assisted laser desorption ionization time-of-flight mass spectrometry by using supervised machine learning approach *PLoS One* **15** e0228459
[123] Nguyen M, Long S, McDermott P, Olsen R, Olson R and Stevens R *et al* 2019 Using machine learning to predict antimicrobial mics and associated genomic features for nontyphoidal *Salmonella J. Clin. Microbiol.* **57** e01260-18
[124] Pesesky M, Hussain T, Wallace M, Patel S, Andleeb S and Burnham C *et al* 2016 Evaluation of machine learning and rules-based approaches for predicting antimicrobial resistance profiles in gram-negative bacilli from whole genome sequence data *Front. Microbiol.* **7** 1887
[125] Egli A 2020 Digitalization, clinical microbiology and infectious diseases *Clin. Microbiol. Infect.* **26** 1289–90
[126] Chan R C *et al* 2023 Artificial intelligence in breast cancer histopathology *Histopathology* **82** 198–210

Chapter 6

Artificial intelligence–powered imaging-based diagnostic tools for ageing and longevity

Yan Yu and Varut Vardhanabhuti

6.1 Introduction—healthspan, lifespan, and longevity concept

Longevity is an emerging field related to ageing research that has blossomed over the past decade. Increasingly, it is being accepted that ageing can be characterised as a disease. A recent commentary in contemporaneous literature purports that ageing is a disease and has been recently added to the World Health Organization (WHO) classification [1]. Whilst debate may continue as to whether ageing should be classified as a disease or not, it is undisputed that ageing or the amalgamation of chronic illnesses, morbidity, and frailty remains a critical challenge in the pursuit of optimising human health. There is a notion that ageing is the precursor, and the instigator of various chronic illnesses from metabolic syndrome, to atherosclerotic heart disease, to cancers and neurodegenerative diseases. The field of longevity has emerged and has gained traction over recent years largely due to the premise that if we tackle ageing at the source and develop interventions targeting ageing mechanisms aiming at systemic rejuvenation rather than a single organ or system at a time, one can potentially prevent these chronic illnesses (see figure 6.1). This gives rise to the very real possibility that we can increase our healthspan, which is defined as the number of years that we can live healthily, relatively free of chronic illnesses.

First, for contextual framing, we need to examine the current states in which we live and our lifespan. Modern medicine has increased life expectancy significantly over the past 100 years, and the global life expectancy has more than doubled. A region like Hong Kong, for example, has one of the highest life expectancies in the World. Women live up to the age of 87.6 years on average, while men live up to the age of 81.9 years—about 6 years longer than their US counterparts. However, the increase in life expectancy has not necessarily been accompanied by an equivalent increase in *healthy* life expectancy. People are living longer, but many of those years are burdened with chronic diseases such as heart disease, diabetes, and

doi:10.1088/978-0-7503-4637-5ch6

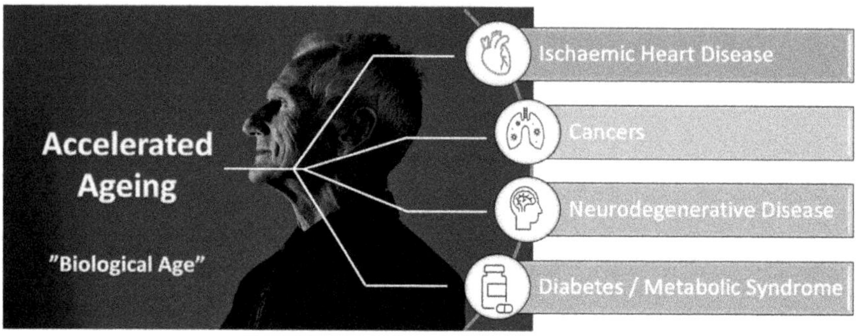

Figure 6.1. Conceptual framework for ageing as a disease and the source of various chronic illnesses including ischaemic heart disease, cancers, neurodegenerative disease, and metabolic syndrome.

even cancers. This is where it is important to understand the difference between lifespan and healthspan.

Lifespan is the total number of years we live, whereas **healthspan** is how many of those years we remain healthy and free from disease.

As we look into the future, researchers are also looking at the possibility of increasing lifespan, with particular emphasis on therapeutics to extend life, reverse the ageing process, or both, by tackling the building blocks or hallmarks of ageing that were recently defined [2]. Since the different steps of ageing is a combination of various molecular processes happening inside our bodies relating to our genes or physiological states as well as the interaction with exogenous agents and environmental factors, understanding the drivers of ageing processes is understandably complex. This is also the reason why recently researchers have leveraged the use of artificial intelligence to help to tackle such problems. When we talk about the broad research covering the ageing and longevity field, it can be initially split into two parts.

First is therapeutics, which is the development of drugs or the repackaging of existing drugs for the purpose of tackling the ageing disease process. Recent examples of this include the use of metformin in the Targeting Aging with Metformin trial, in which investigators are looking to see if the drug has an impact on lifespan extension. The trial plans to include 3000 non-diabetic subjects, aged 70–80 years and burdened with at least one chronic disease, in at least 14 health centres across the United States to evaluate the effects of metformin on its primary endpoint, which are composites of the incidence of age-related conditions such as myocardial infarction, congestive heart failure, stroke, cancer, dementia, and death.

The second focus is on the field of diagnostics. For the remaining part of this chapter, we will focus on the diagnostics aspects of ageing and longevity with particular emphasis on the use of machine learning and artificial intelligence.

6.2 Diagnostics aspects of ageing

The drug discovery and development fields are burgeoning with research on the possibilities of drugs that can be used to impact the process of ageing such as delaying the onset or even reversing the molecular processes that underlie ageing as a disease. To be able to intervene, we need a biomarker that can accurately establish and measure the process of ageing. This is a fundamental requirement because not only do we need to establish where an individual is in terms of their ageing process, but we also need to be able to monitor longitudinally whether an intervention is effective at delaying or reversing the process in question. To do this, we need to have an accurate and reproducible tool to be able to help us establish these processes.

In order to tell if we are living healthy lives, we need to be able to measure how we age accurately. One of the emerging concepts is something called 'biological age'. Various methods have been used to try and measure our biological age, notably including the assessment of telomere length, gene expression levels, and protein expression levels, with the most recent example that has gained prominence in the recent decade, is the assessment of epigenetics ageing by the use of DNA methylation. This was first developed by Steven Horvath and his team in 2013 [3]. This is a test based on DNA methylation data that was first applied to mice but has since been replicated in many organisms including humans to be able to predict the 'biological age' of the subject in question. The clocks were shown to have a high correlation with chronological age and intuitively are somewhat easy to understand for both patients and clinicians. For example,

> 'a chronologically 70-year-old individual with a biological age of 65 years has a similar risk of mortality and expected longevity as the average 65-year-old.'

In addition, it is hoped that substituting a more accurate 'biological age' for chronological age could improve the performance of existing risk prediction models.

The so-called first-generation clocks have focused on predicting biological age, based on chronological age (e.g. Horvath, Hannum *et al*, Weidner *et al*) [4, 5].

These clocks are based on DNA methylation, which is derived from a rich body of literature demonstrating that chronological age has a profound effect on genome-wide DNA methylation levels. It was discovered that several millions of so-called CpG dinucleotides in the human genome were seen to alter with age. The development of these was coupled with the advent of DNA methylation array technology that enabled the identification of specific CpG locations in the genome, which, in recent years, has also improved in terms of detection numbers as well as costs.

These so-called epigenetic clocks are typically built by regressing a transformed version of the chronological age on a set of CpGs using supervised machine learning methods. An example of this is the use of a penalised regression model such as Lasso or elastic net, which have been the basis of the Horvath clock. Subsequently, several age estimators have utilised similar methods, using different sets of CpGs and incorporating different sets of tissues and age spectra, with varying levels of accuracy. The advantage of the Horvath clock is that its correlation with chronological age has been demonstrated across multiple tissue types, with high accuracy seen even in children, and its strong correlation with gestational age, as well as homogeneity of its age estimates across the different tissue types [6]. It would also be notable to mention the Hannum's clock which was derived from the basis of 71 CpGs from DNA of blood, and subsequently also several distinct age estimators from other tissues [4].

The second-generation clocks that followed were developed to predict time to adverse events such as death. These are understandably broad and not specific to a particular disease process. They usually require a two-step model. An example is the PhenoAge [7], which was constructed by first generating a weighted average of clinical and blood-based parameters, of which values were then regressed on DNA methylations levels in the blood using a penalised regression model, resulting in the automatic selection of 513 CpG sites, effectively estimating the so-called phenotypic age, which outperformed the first-generation DNA epigenetics clocks in estimating or predicting mortality and many other diseases such as cardiovascular diseases and other measures of multimorbidity. Subsequently, another epigenetic ageing clock known as GrimAge [8] was also developed which combined physiological risk factors and stress factors such as plasma proteins and growth differentiation factors as well as smoking status into a composite biomarker of life span. It outperformed various other existing epigenetic clocks in terms of the prediction of time to death, time to coronary artery disease, and time to cancer as well as other related co-morbidities.

Some criticisms of the ageing clocks have been the lack of real-world repeatability and reproducibility. Specifically, studies have shown that test–retest reliability was not adequate, which may be due to the presence of technical noise in the methods [9]. It was shown that even in samples that were replicates (i.e. taken at the same time), technical noise produced deviations of up to 9 years for the prominent epigenetic clocks. This hugely limits the real-world utility. Investigators have come up with a solution using a computational approach to improve reliability using a machine learning method known as principal component analysis. The traditional epigenetic clock uses an elastic net regression to select a limited number of CpGs to represent a set of collinear CpGs while avoiding overfitting, but by doing so these models may retain technical noise from individual CpGs. Selecting numerous related CpGs could in theory improve reliability. It is hypothesised that PCA may be able to extract the covariance between multicollinear CpGs, including age-related covariance to gain a more accurate age estimation by using many CpGs for each principal component, could minimise the effect of noise from any single CpG.

To see this in a disease-specific cohort, researchers have utilised the combination of principal components analysis and regularised regression and applied it specifically at brain age to characterise epigenetic age in the context of Alzheimer's disease (AD), dubbed the 'PCBrainAge' [10]. It was demonstrated that acceleration of the PCBrainAge showed stronger associations with clinical AD dementia, pathologic AD, and APOE ε4 carrier status compared to prior epigenetic age predictors as well as maintaining reliability that has plagued prior ageing clocks.

6.3 The need for more specificity—organ or region-based ageing clocks

Biological age gives a person an idea of whether they are ageing appropriately. However, if a person is shown to have accelerated ageing, then unless we have a drug or an intervention that can tackle the ageing process as a whole (i.e. systemic rejuvenation), in order to increase lifespan, we do not yet know where to focus in order to improve or delay this process from the rapid deterioration. In this context, there is a need for more specificity. One emerging concept is to have organ-specific information such as organ-age whereby we can tackle these areas specifically for improvement. An approach to this was discussed in the prior section with application to 'brain age' using DNA methylation and principal component analysis and regularised regression. With the advancement in medical imaging, we do have existing data that shows that we can potentially derive useful organ-based ageing information. For this section, we will focus on medical imaging as tool for deriving age-related information.

6.3.1 Organ-based information

6.3.1.1 Chest x-ray biological age

Investigators utilised chest radiographs using a deep learning model based on convolution neural network (CNN) to train for 'chest x-ray biological age' (CXR-Age) using large datasets from the screening population with a long-term follow-up [11]. CNN-based CXR-Age was developed using more than 115 000 subjects using a chest x-ray image as input. The model then outputs an estimate of biological age. The datasets came from the large-scale population screening studies from the Prostate, Lung, Colorectal and Ovarian Cancer Screening Trial (PLCO) and the National Lung Screening Trial (NLST) in the United States. They then validated the performance of the so-called CXR-Age in two held-out testing sets. They demonstrated that CXR-Age outperformed standard chronological age, and a higher CXR-Age was associated with a higher risk of all-cause and cardiovascular-related mortalities compared with chronological age. This was assessed based on hazard ratios (HRs), and for the PLCO dataset, it was demonstrated that CXR-Age had HR: 2.26 (95% confidence interval [CI]: 2.24–2.29) versus chronological age HR: 1.77 (95% CI: 1.75–1.78) and was statistically significant ($p < 0.001$) for all-cause mortality. The cardiovascular mortality for the PLCO testing set was CXR-Age cause-specific HR: 2.45 per 5 years (95% CI: 2.34–2.56) versus chronological age HR: 1.82 per 5 years (95% CI: 1.74–1.90). In addition, they also demonstrated that adding CXR-Age to a multivariable model with risk factors, clinical findings, and chronological age resulted in modest but statistically significant improvements for both all-cause and cardiovascular mortality in PLCO and NLST datasets ($p < 0.001$ for all comparisons). Findings confirmed that information embedded in medical imaging may contain important age-related information that could potentially be used as a surrogate for biological ageing.

One additional interesting step that this study took was to derive activation areas based on gradient-weighted class activation mapping to highlight areas in the CXR that had the greatest contribution to the CXR-Age estimation. It was interesting to note that common activation areas were the mediastinum, aortic knob, and cardiac silhouette. These areas are known to become tortuous and dilate with age and conceivably could be important in terms of cardiovascular-related mortality.

6.3.1.2 Brain age

Several studies have examined using brain-specific imaging, more commonly magnetic resonance imaging (MRI) imaging data, to estimate brain-specific biological age, also termed 'brain age' [12–19]. We know that there are several imaging-specific findings that could be related to ageing, such as cerebral atrophy (generalised reduction in the brain volume), and signal alteration, such as white matter hyperintensities on MRI. MRI contains rich information in terms of structural information, functional information, and related vascular information, all of which could be important in approximating age. To this end, several investigators have examined using multi-modal information MRI data to try to improve brain age estimation. One investigator [12] combined structural MRI and angiography datasets from a large database of 2074 adults aged between 21 and 81 years. For this work, the investigators use a CNN-based approach, using three models, deriving the first model using structural MRI data based on T1W sequence (CNNT1) and the second model using the angiography (time of flight MRI sequence CNNTOF). The outputs from the CNN_{T1} and CNN_{TOF} models were combined and trained using a multiple linear regression model, using the two previously trained models as predictor variables and the chronological age as the target variable. Once trained, the linear regression model was concatenated with the previously trained CNN_{T1} and CNN_{TOF} models to form the $CNN_{Combined}$ model, which was used to predict the brain age of the test dataset. This resulted in the mean absolute error of 3.85 years comparing the predicted and chronological age. They also performed saliency maps to reveal areas that were important from the model. The predictive brain regions included the lateral sulcus, the fourth ventricle, and the amygdala, while the brain arteries contributing the most to the prediction included the basilar artery, the middle cerebral artery M2 segments, and the left posterior cerebral artery.

6.3.2 Region-based assessment for ageing

With the recent innovations in medical imaging segmentation, particularly with the success of 3D networks such as U-Net and nn-UNet, there has been interest in organ-specific segmentation. The organ or regions that are of particular interest in the field of ageing are fat, muscles, and bones.

6.3.2.1 Fat

Increasingly, researchers are realising that fat deposition needs to be assessed in terms of location. The usual area of fat is in the subcutaneous tissue, which is the fat that sits just under your skin. This is actually where most of your fat is stored. Some

Table 6.1. Percentage of body fat based on age, gender, and ethnicity [21].

Age and BMI	Women			Men		
	African American	Asian	White	African American	Asian	White
20–39 years						
BMI < 18.5	20	25	21	8	13	8
BMI ⩾ 25	32	35	33	20	23	21
BMI ⩾ 30	38	40	39	26	28	26
40–59 years						
BMI < 18.5	21	25	23	9	13	11
BMI ⩾ 25	34	36	35	22	24	23
BMI ⩾ 30	39	41	41	27	29	29
60–79 years						
BMI < 18.5	23	26	25	11	14	13
BMI ⩾ 25	35	36	38	23	24	25
BMI ⩾ 30	41	41	43	29	29	31

researchers have found this area of fat to be beneficial. Another location for fat is the so-called visceral fat that is located in the body cavity beneath the abdominal muscles, which is now emerging as a very important biomarker for metabolic syndromes. These are conditions like insulin resistance, type 2 diabetes, and fatty liver disease, for example. In general, visceral fat accounts for up to 20% of total fat in men and 5%–8% in women. There are some important changes with ageing that are noted with respect to visceral fat, which must be taken into account when assessing this in the context of how much an individual has with respect to gender and age. Both gonadal steroid and growth hormones secretion decline with age, which may explain the increase in visceral fat in males with ageing. Similarly, in postmenopausal women, the decline in oestrogen and age-associated decrease in growth hormones may account for the rapid increase in visceral fat.

Traditionally, we measure weight or body mass index (BMI) as a proxy for how much fat a body has, but this has now been shown to not be an accurate reflection of actual body fat. Slightly more sophisticated measures such as waist to height ratio have been shown to be more useful than weight or BMI but cannot differentiate subcutaneous fat from visceral fat, for example.

There are also certain scenarios where there will be discordant between BMI and total fat mass. Examples include bodybuilders, in whom BMI may be high but the amount of fat may be low, and in older adults or frail patients with sarcopenic obesity, in whom muscle mass is reduced but the amount of fat is high [20]. In some instances, it may also be important to assess fat percentage as the percentage of body fat varies with age, gender, and ethnicity (see table 6.1). For example, people of Asian ethnicity tend to have a higher percentage of body fat compared to their Black or White counterparts. In addition, at any given BMI, women have approximately 12% more body fat than men, and the percentage of body fat increases with age, even if total weight stays the same. The variation between different age, gender, and ethnicity has given rise to the need to monitor these parameters at an individual level, as we move from population-based diagnosis of obesity to more individualised therapy.

Researchers over the past decades have utilised various medical imaging techniques such as dual-energy x-ray absorptiometry (DEXA), CT, and MRI scans to assess the amount of fat we have in our body. DEXA being a relatively fast and cheap test has been demonstrated to be a good test for assessing fat in our body and can give an approximation of how much visceral fat we have in our body. The most accurate tests we have are computed tomography (CT) and MRI scans, which we can visualise and quantify precisely according to the precise location of this fat as seen on imaging. However, to delineate the whole fat volumes over several hundreds of CT or MRI slices in our body is labour intensive, and conventionally researchers have only utilised a 'single slice' assessment. Previous research has utilised a single slice with some success. For example, a study used a single cross-sectional image at the interspace between the L2/L3 and L4/L5 vertebrae and demonstrated that although CT-derived visceral fat estimations were predictive of diabetes, CT provided no important advantage over the simple metrics of waist circumference and waist/hip ratio [22]. These prior studies were limited by single slice assessment, mainly because to perform multi-slice, or full 3D volume, would be too labour intensive, but this has changed recently with the advent of automated segmentation using deep learning. In the future, it is anticipated that volumetric fat assessment could be made automatically on any CT or MRI scans and could accompany a radiology report and can be used as a biomarker or input into risk prediction models.

There are also fat depositions in other parts of our body or in our organs such as in the liver and around the heart. These are called 'ectopic fat' and can be measured by medical imaging techniques. With respect to the liver, this can be measured using various imaging modalities such as ultrasound elastography, CT, and MRI scan, with MRI scan using proton density fat fraction (PDFF) sequence being regarded as the gold standard. MRI that measures the PDFF has been proven to correlate well with magnetic resonance spectroscopy and histology-proven steatosis grade from contemporaneous liver biopsies [23, 24]. With the advent of deep learning automated quantification, these processes are expected to become more streamlined. Similarly, we have long known the importance of pericardial fat as one of the other sites for storage of so-called ectopic fat. Having more pericardial fat is associated with increased incidence of coronary heart disease and development of heart failure as well as systemic conditions including metabolic syndrome and non-alcoholic fatty liver disease [25–29]. More recently, investigators have also focused on a specific area known as the perivascular adipose tissue [30–32]. This is a very small area around the coronary vessels supplying the heart. Investigators [31] have adopted machine learning techniques, for example, using random forest classification technique with features derived from radiomic profile of the perivascular adipose tissue. They were able to demonstrate that there were able to discriminate cases from controls C-statistic 0.77 (95% CI: 0.62–0.93) in the external validation set.

Subsequently, they also tested the signature in 1575 consecutive eligible participants in the SCOTHEART trial, in which it significantly improved major adverse cardiac events prediction beyond traditional risk stratification. These included features that are already being used in traditional clinics such as clinical risk factors, coronary calcium score, coronary stenosis, and high-risk plaque features on coronary CT angiogram.

Traditionally, quantification of these various structures is time-consuming and labour intensive, but again, future utilisation of deep learning should help for more rapid adoption.

6.3.2.2 Muscle

There is increasing interest in muscle quantification, particularly with the acknowledgement that sarcopenia is an ageing-related entity. 'Sarcopenia' is defined by the decrease in muscle mass and loss of function of muscles which can be tested using several metrics. For example, muscle mass can be measured by an imaging modality such as DEXA and by using Appendicular Skeletal Muscle Index. Muscle function can be measured by loss of muscle strength, which can be estimated, for example, by handgrip strength, and/or bedside or clinic physical performance testing such as five-time chair stand, 6-m walk, or short physical performance battery with various cutoff thresholds for diagnosis. Recently, there has also been the use of imaging such as CT and MRI to be able to quantify the muscle volume as well as quantify the extent of fatty infiltration as a proxy for abnormal muscle composition thought to lead to the loss in muscle function [33, 34].

From the medical imaging perspective, the two most studied areas are the (1) paravertebral muscles (i.e. the psoas muscle), and (2) thigh muscles. The fat infiltration in the muscles can be detected on imaging, with the gold standard for assessment and quantification being MRI, with a specialised sequence of Dixon technique that allows for accurate separation of fat and water signal. Recently, several investigators, including our team at HKUMed, have developed a CNN-based segmentation model that can accurately segment various muscles in the thigh muscles as a whole volume, allowing for an accurate and reliable assessment of the fat infiltration [35]. These have advantages over traditional 'single slice' assessment because fatty infiltration can be sporadic and differentially involved in the early stage, and thus, a whole muscle volume assessment is highly desired. The innovation in deep learning is expected to make this process more automated and potentially will aid clinical adoption and utilisation. Not only will this aid diagnosis, but there is great hope that longitudinal tracking and monitoring at a patient level will help greatly in monitoring the impact of interventions.

6.3.2.3 Bones

The assessment of bone health on imaging is traditionally done based on quantification of bone mineral content, using DEXA scans. The amount of bone mineral density (BMD) a person has can be estimated and is based on measurements typically in specific areas, namely, the femur and the spine bones in the body. For example, the United States Preventive Services Task Force recommends that all women aged 65 years and older should have a BMD assessment [36]. DEXA is a robust clinical tool used for diagnosis, and indeed, the WHO criteria for the diagnosis of osteoporosis are based on reference data obtained by DEXA [37]. As a tool, DEXA has been extensively investigated for accuracy and robustness and is utilised routinely in clinics. For example, biomechanical studies have shown a strong correlation between mechanical strength and BMD measured by DEXA [38]. It offers excellent accuracy [39] and low radiation dose [40] and, in addition, has been validated in several randomised clinical trials that have shown a reduction in fracture risk with drug therapy based on BMD measured by DEXA [41]. Owing to the relatively robust and ease of use in bone density measurements, there have been few machine learning or deep learning approach performed with DEXA relating to BMD analyses. One study investigated the use of textural features on DEXA images and trained machine learning models to classify patients into whether they were normal or had osteoporosis or osteopenia, albeit with relatively modest performance (area under the curve values ranged from 0.50 to 0.78) and with a relatively small sample size (n = 147) [42]. Another study uses a deep learning approach comparing different deep learning–based CNN models and achieved an accuracy of up to 92.05% in classifying normal versus osteoporosis [43]. This was achieved by first running images through several image pre-processing steps (using denoising, image enhancement, and thresholding), data augmentation, and boosting of the minority class (using the SMOTE technique) before inputting them into the different CNN and hybrid models.

6.3.3 Physical activity and wearables devices

With increasing information being gathered including everyday activities such as physical activities, there is a huge potential for using this information based on commercially available wearable devices to enable machine learning and AI-based assessment. From a longevity perspective, exercise or being physically active is a very potent intervention that mitigates chronic diseases but also has a real impact on mortality reduction. For example, a previous study looking at older women has shown that there are incremental benefits of walking up to 7500 steps per day in terms of all-cause mortality [44]. In previous meta-epidemiological study [45], exercise has been shown to be as effective as drug interventions in the secondary prevention of coronary heart disease, rehabilitation after stroke, treatment of heart failure, and prevention of diabetes [46]. Exercise has been shown to outperform standard metformin treatment in preventing type 2 diabetes. In another study [47], just over 3000 persons at high risk of diabetes were randomised to three groups consisting of no intervention, metformin, or a lifestyle-modification programme with at least 150 min of physical activity per week. It was shown that lifestyle changes and treatment with metformin both reduced the incidence of diabetes in persons at high risk, with lifestyle intervention shown to be more effective than metformin.

With the advent of emerging technologies available to the everyday consumer such as smart watches and wearables used to track body metrics, there now lies enormous opportunities to utilise these data and gain more insights. For example, several investigators have utilised the UK Biobank study, which has a large amount of data from participants. Some investigators have used machine learning techniques to help categorise the type of activity. For example, Willets *et al* used balanced random forests with Markov confusion matrices to identify which one of four activity states (sleep, sedentary, walking, moderate intensity) an individual was in at any given time [48]. Given a large amount of data in >100 000 participants, an automated technique for sorting and categorising these data is highly desired. Investigators, therefore, have used AI-based methods to help with the automated process of categorising different activities.

6.4 Concluding remarks

Longevity and ageing have emerged from addressing those with chronic illness to the realms of preventative medicine in driving primary prevention to a new level, and with the advent of new technological tools as well as the emerging usage of machine learning and AI, there is now potential to solve one of life's most important questions. How exactly do we age, and what can we do to slow down or mitigate such effects? Before we have an actual real-world therapeutics strategy, we need to focus on measurable metrics that are available now, and this is the focus of the diagnostics area of ageing where we are just at the dawn of its utilisation. In the future, we hope that we can measure our health and optimise it in such ways that democratise individuals to be able to maintain their functional level to overall maintain their role as a productive member of society at large. Such technology comes with a deflationary force, such that the tools we develop in the future should become more affordable, and as a result, real health equity is in sight.

References

[1] Bischof E, Maier A B, Lee K F, Zhavoronkov A and Sinclair D 2022 Advanced pathological ageing should be represented in the ICD *Lancet Healthy Longev* **3** e12

[2] López-Otín C, Blasco M A, Partridge L, Serrano M and Kroemer G 2013 The hallmarks of aging *Cell* **153** 1194–217

[3] Horvath S 2013 DNA methylation age of human tissues and cell types *Genome Biol.* **14** 3156

[4] Hannum G, Guinney J, Zhao L, Zhang L, Hughes G and Sadda S *et al* 2013 Genome-wide methylation profiles reveal quantitative views of human aging rates *Mol. Cell* **49** 359–67

[5] Weidner C I, Lin Q, Koch C M, Eisele L, Beier F and Ziegler P *et al* 2014 Aging of blood can be tracked by DNA methylation changes at just three CpG sites *Genome Biol.* **15** R24

[6] Horvath S and Raj K 2018 DNA methylation-based biomarkers and the epigenetic clock theory of ageing *Nat. Rev. Genet.* **19** 371–84

[7] Levine M E, Lu A T, Quach A, Chen B H, Assimes T L and Bandinelli S *et al* 2018 An epigenetic biomarker of aging for lifespan and healthspan *Aging* **10** 573–91

[8] Lu A T, Quach A, Wilson J G, Reiner A P, Aviv A and Raj K *et al* 2019 DNA methylation GrimAge strongly predicts lifespan and healthspan *Aging* **11** 303–27

[9] Higgins-Chen A T, Thrush K L, Wang Y, Kuo P L, Wang M and Minteer C J *et al* 2021 A computational solution for bolstering reliability of epigenetic clocks: Implications for clinical trials and longitudinal tracking (accessed 7 January 2022) (available at: https://biorxiv.org/content/10.1101/2021.04.16.440205v1)

[10] Thrush K L, Bennett D A, Gaiteri C, Horvath S, Dyck C H and van, Higgins-Chen A T *et al* 2022 Aging the brain: multi-region methylation principal component based clock in the context of Alzheimer's disease *Aging* **14** 5641–68

[11] Raghu V K, Weiss J, Hoffmann U, Aerts H J W L and Lu M T 2021 Deep learning to estimate biological age from chest radiographs *JACC Cardiovasc. Imaging* **14** 2226–36

[12] Mouches P, Wilms M, Rajashekar D, Langner S and Forkert N D 2022 Multimodal biological brain age prediction using magnetic resonance imaging and angiography with the identification of predictive regions *Hum. Brain Mapp.* **43** 2554–66

[13] Stankevičiūtė K, Azevedo T, Campbell A, Bethlehem R and Liò P 2020 Population graph GNNs for brain age prediction (accessed 30 November 2021) (available at: https://biorxiv.org/content/10.1101/2020.06.26.172171v3)

[14] He S, Grant P E and Ou Y 2022 Global-local transformer for brain age estimation *IEEE Trans. Med. Imaging* **41** 213–24

[15] Cheng J, Liu Z, Guan H and Wu Z *et al* 2021 Brain age estimation from MRI using cascade networks with ranking loss *IEEE Trans. Med. Imaging* **40** 3400–12

[16] Brusini I, MacNicol E, Kim E, Smedby Ö, Wang C and Westman E *et al* 2022 MRI-derived brain age as a biomarker of ageing in rats: validation using a healthy lifestyle intervention *Neurobiol. Aging* **109** 204–15

[17] Basodi S, Raja R, Ray B and Gazula H *et al* 2022 Decentralized brain age estimation using MRI data *Neuroinformatics* **20** 981–90

[18] Lombardi A, Monaco A, Donvito G, Amoroso N, Bellotti R and Tangaro S 2021 Brain age prediction with morphological features using deep neural networks: results from predictive analytic competition 2019 *Front. Psychiatry* **11** 619629

[19] Du J, Pan Y, Jiang J, Lam B C P, Thalamuthu A and Chen R *et al* 2022 *White matter brain age as a biomarker of cerebrovascular burden in the ageing brain* MedRxiv Preprint https://doi.org/10.1101/2022.02.06.22270484 (posted online 7 February 2022)

[20] Prado C M M, Wells J C K, Smith S R, Stephan B C M and Siervo M 2012 Sarcopenic obesity: a critical appraisal of the current evidence *Clin. Nutr.* **31** 583–601

[21] Gallagher D, Heymsfield S B, Heo M, Jebb S A, Murgatroyd P R and Sakamoto Y 2000 Healthy percentage body fat ranges: an approach for developing guidelines based on body mass index *Am. J. Clin. Nutr.* **72** 694–701

[22] Bray G A, Jablonski K A, Fujimoto W Y, Barrett-Connor E, Haffner S and Hanson R L *et al* 2008 Relation of central adiposity and body mass index to the development of diabetes in the Diabetes Prevention Program *Am. J. Clin. Nutr.* **87** 1212–8

[23] Tang A, Tan J, Sun M, Hamilton G, Bydder M and Wolfson T *et al* 2013 Nonalcoholic fatty liver disease: MR imaging of liver proton density fat fraction to assess hepatic steatosis *Radiology* **267** 422–31

[24] Dulai P S, Sirlin C B and Loomba R 2016 MRI and MRE for non-invasive quantitative assessment of hepatic steatosis and fibrosis in NAFLD and NASH: Clinical trials to clinical practice *J. Hepatol.* **65** 1006–16

[25] Ding J, Hsu F C, Harris T B, Liu Y, Kritchevsky S B and Szklo M *et al* 2009 The association of pericardial fat with incident coronary heart disease: the Multi-Ethnic Study of Atherosclerosis (MESA) *Am. J. Clin. Nutr.* **90** 499–504

[26] Kenchaiah S, Ding J, Carr J J, Allison M A, Budoff M J and Tracy R P *et al* 2021 Pericardial fat and the risk of heart failure *J. Am. Coll. Cardiol.* **77** 2638–52

[27] Miao C, Chen S, Ding J, Liu K, Li D and Macedo R *et al* 2011 The association of pericardial fat with coronary artery plaque index at MR imaging: the Multi-Ethnic Study of Atherosclerosis (MESA) *Radiology* **261** 109–15

[28] Rosito G A, Massaro J M, Hoffmann U, Ruberg F L, Mahabadi A A and Vasan R S *et al* 2008 Pericardial fat, visceral abdominal fat, cardiovascular disease risk factors, and vascular calcification in a community-based sample: the Framingham Heart Study *Circulation* **117** 605–13

[29] Yun C H, Jhuang J-R and Tsou M-T 2022 Pericardial fat, thoracic peri-aortic adipose tissue, and systemic inflammatory marker in nonalcoholic fatty liver and abdominal obesity phenotype *Sci. Rep.* **12** 1958

[30] Oikonomou E K, Marwan M, Desai M Y, Mancio J, Alashi A and Hutt Centeno E *et al* 2018 Non-invasive detection of coronary inflammation using computed tomography and prediction of residual cardiovascular risk (the CRISP CT study): a post-hoc analysis of prospective outcome data *Lancet* **392** 929–39

[31] Oikonomou E K, Williams M C, Kotanidis C P, Desai M Y, Marwan M and Antonopoulos A S *et al* 2019 A novel machine learning-derived radiotranscriptomic signature of perivascular fat improves cardiac risk prediction using coronary CT angiography *Eur. Heart J.* **40** 3529–43

[32] Klüner L V, Oikonomou E K and Antoniades C 2021 Assessing cardiovascular risk by using the fat attenuation index in coronary CT angiography *Radiol. Cardiothorac. Imaging* **3** e200563

[33] Linge J, Ekstedt M and Leinhard O D 2020 Adverse muscle composition is linked to poor functional performance and metabolic comorbidities in NAFLD *JHEP Rep.* **3** 100197–7

[34] Linge J, Petersson M, Forsgren M F, Sanyal A J and Dahlqvist Leinhard O 2021 Adverse muscle composition predicts all-cause mortality in the UK Biobank imaging study *J. Cachexia Sarcopenia Muscle* **12** 1513–26

[35] Ding J, Cao P, Chang H C, Gao Y, Chan S H S and Vardhanabhuti V 2020 Deep learning-based thigh muscle segmentation for reproducible fat fraction quantification using fat-water decomposition MRI *Insights Imaging* **11** 128

[36] US Preventive Services Task ForceCurry S J, Krist A H, Owens D K, Barry M J and Caughey A B *et al* 2018 Screening for osteoporosis to prevent fractures: US Preventive Services Task Force recommendation statement *JAMA* **319** 2521–31

[37] Kanis J A 2007 *Assessment of Osteoporosis at the Primary Health-Care Level* (Geneva: World Health Organization Collaborating Centre for Metabolic Bone Diseases)

[38] Lotz J C, Cheal E J and Hayes W C 1991 Fracture prediction for the proximal femur using finite element models: Part I—Linear analysis *J. Biomech. Eng.* **113** 353–60

[39] Mazess R, Chesnut C H, McClung M and Genant H 1992 Enhanced precision with dual-energy X-ray absorptiometry *Calcif. Tissue Int.* **51** 14–7

[40] Njeh C F, Fuerst T, Hans D, Blake G M and Genant H K 1999 Radiation exposure in bone mineral density assessment *Appl. Radiat. Isot.* **50** 215–36

[41] Cranney A, Guyatt G, Griffith L, Wells G, Tugwell P and Rosen C *et al* 2002 Meta-analyses of therapies for postmenopausal osteoporosis. IX: summary of meta-analyses of therapies for postmenopausal osteoporosis *Endocr. Rev.* **23** 570–8

[42] Rastegar S, Vaziri M, Qasempour Y, Akhash M R, Abdalvand N and Shiri I *et al* 2020 Radiomics for classification of bone mineral loss: a machine learning study *Diagn. Interv. Imaging* **101** 599–610

[43] Varalakshmi P, Sathyamoorthy S, Darshan V, Ramanujan V and Rajasekar S J S 2022 Detection of osteoporosis with DEXA scan images using deep learning models *2022 Int. Conf. on Advances in Computing, Communication and Applied Informatics (ACCAI)* pp 1–6
[44] Lee I M, Shiroma E J, Kamada M, Bassett D R, Matthews C E and Buring J E 2019 Association of step volume and intensity with all-cause mortality in older women *JAMA Intern. Med.* **179** 1105–12
[45] Naci H and Ioannidis J P A 2013 Comparative effectiveness of exercise and drug interventions on mortality outcomes: metaepidemiological study *Brit. Med. J.* **347** f5577
[46] Lee C G, Heckman-Stoddard B, Dabelea D, Gadde K M, Ehrmann D and Ford L *et al* 2021 Effect of metformin and lifestyle interventions on mortality in the diabetes prevention program and diabetes prevention program outcomes study *Diabetes Care* **44** 2775–82
[47] Knowler W C, Barrett-Connor E, Fowler S E, Hamman R F, Lachin J M, Walker E A and Nathan D MDiabetes Prevention Program Research Group 2002 Reduction in the incidence of Type 2 diabetes with lifestyle intervention or metformin *N. Engl. J. Med.* **346** 393–403
[48] Willetts M, Hollowell S, Aslett L, Holmes C and Doherty A 2018 Statistical machine learning of sleep and physical activity phenotypes from sensor data in 96,220 UK Biobank participants *Sci. Rep.* **8** 7961

Chapter 7

Intra-operative image-guided interventional robotics—where are we now and where are we going?

Xiaomei Wang, Yingqi Li, Mengjie Wu, Yifeng Hao, Libaihe Tian, Zhuoliang He, Kwok Wai Samuel Au, Russell H Taylor, Iulian Iordachita, Jason Y K Chan, Joe King-Man Fan, Kenneth M C Cheung and Ka-Wai Kwok

7.1 Introduction

Surgical robots are designed with the intention of allowing remote operation and improvements in precision and steadiness [1]. Beginning around three decades ago with the earliest attempts in applications for orthopedic surgery [1] and neurosurgery [2], robotic systems have been developed to offer benefits to both patients and surgeons. For example, in laparoscopic prostatectomy, the assistance of medical robots has been proven to contribute to fewer intra-operative risks (e.g. blood loss), faster recovery (including shorter hospital stay), and lower reoperation rate [3]. Surgeons also benefit from the ergonomic design to shorten the learning curve, reduce physiological requirements (e.g. steadiness) [1], and relieve fatigue (e.g. reduce hand and wrist numbness) [4]. Minimally invasive surgery (MIS) has been performed on many parts of the human body, including but not limited to brain, heart, digestive tract, and spine. This chapter will introduce advanced medical imaging techniques from the view of assisting interventional surgeries (section 7.2), as well as representative robotic systems for various treatments (section 7.3), aiming to investigate some key techniques that are involved in their development (section 7.4) and discussing the current status, limitations, and future trends of intra-operative image-guided robotic platforms (section 7.5).

7.2 Medical imaging advances

Since their emergence in the 19th century, medical imaging modalities have played an important role in many clinical procedures, including pre-operative (pre-op)

doi:10.1088/978-0-7503-4637-5ch7

diagnosis and planning, intra-operative (intra-op) navigation, and post-operative (post-op) validation. The earliest application of medical imaging was radiography used in orthopedics pre-op diagnoses, where the surgeon could rely on x-ray images to pinpoint the affected anatomy [5]. However, the morphology of bones may change between the time of image acquisition and the actual operation, inducing inadvertent inaccuracies in operation. The problem prompted the development of real-time navigation systems using sequential fluoroscopic images. However, these images are usually distorted, and one-dimensional information would become lost due to the image projection. Different-perspective x-ray images were thus employed, which would be co-registered to a common coordinate established on the target structures, aiming to provide navigation for intra-op use [6].

Although possessing advantages of low cost and high speed, x-ray imaging still suffers from difficulties in standardizing the positioning and radiation dosage of the x-ray generator, which would affect imaging performance. Other advanced imaging modalities such as computed tomography (CT), magnetic resonance imaging (MRI), and ultrasound (US) imaging can offer three-dimensional (3D) views of anatomy, thus replacing the role of x-ray in intra-op guidance gradually. Not limited to pure use of the medical imaging, we can foresee the wider applications of robotic interventions will be considered in the future with these imaging modalities. The interventions will target not only bony structures but also soft tissues.

7.2.1 CT

CT is a non-invasive medical imaging technique using a series of x- or γ-rays to generate cross-sectional images of anatomy. The x-ray CT is the most common and is discussed in this section. CT can provide detailed images of bones, internal organs, soft tissues, and blood vessels. Additionally, a 360° view of the body's structure can be computerized through a series of cross-sectional slices. CT enables high spatial resolution, especially in high-density structures. It could provide angiograms and images of the skeleton/extremities, which is fast and even capable of intra-op guidance, thus having popularity in areas such as the diagnosis and therapy of head and neck cancers and lung intervention. However, the technique of CT involves exposure to ionizing radiation, which would put both the patient and physician at risk. Therefore, robotic systems designed for teleoperation under CT guidance have been developed more recently, which can mitigate the radiation exposure for physicians [7].

There have been developments in the technique of x-ray CT since its advent in 1979. The dynamic spatial reconstructor (DSR), a scanner capable of acquiring 240 slices with spacing of 1 mm in a time window of 0.01 s, was developed in 1979 at the Mayo Clinic [8]. DSR could show the heart, lungs, and blood flow precisely. The dual-source CT scanner was then developed to improve temporal resolution, and the multi-source CT made it accessible to rotate the focal spot freely [9]. Since the ionizing radiation of CT has a significant impact on cancer risk, researchers also focus on decreasing radiation dose [10]. There are several general strategies for reducing radiation dose while maintaining image quality. Lowering the x-ray tube current and voltage, both of which would affect the strength of the beam, is the most direct approach to reduce radiation dose and is appropriate for targets with small size or high contrast. Higher helical pitch, which is the ratio of table feed and collimated slice or beam width [11], could aid in reducing the exposure time. The individualization of scanning parameters further allows the optimization of dose, which is appropriate for patients of various body habitus. However, the reduction of radiation dose would bring image noise, which is inversely proportional to the square root of the radiation dose. Advanced image reconstruction algorithms such as iterative reconstruction could lower the requirement for high radiation dose [12].

One popular application of CT-guided robots is for positioning needles (or cannulas) to perform biopsies and therapies. In addition, robot-assisted spine surgery and orthopedics under CT have been developed recently. In a clinical report of pedicle screw insertion [13], it was proven that the robot-assisted approach improved the screw placement accuracy with decreased intra-op blood loss compared with freehand fluoroscopy-assisted insertion. Additionally, the research on the design of bedside- or patient-mounted robots (section 7.3.2) could boost the flexibility and reachable workspace of treatment tools. CT-guided robots are expected to simplify the surgical workflow and reduce radiation exposure for clinicians while improving patient outcomes.

7.2.2 MRI

MRI is a non-invasive and non-ionizing medical imaging modality that maps the internal body structure by employing a powerful magnetic field and radiofrequency (RF) waves to activate the atomic nuclei inside the body and analyzing electromagnetic (EM) signals emitted [14]. In addition to the absence of ionizing radiation, magnetic resonance (MR) has grown in popularity since its inception, thanks to its unique ability to capture 3D volumetric images with strong tissue contrast and arbitrary slice position in near-real-time [7]. Furthermore, MRI can offer precise monitoring of tissue temperature (i.e. MR thermometry), as well as morphological and functional information such as blood flow and tissue oxygenation [15, 16]. Despite its enormous potential, MRI-guided interventions are still in the early stages, facing significant challenges. The vast majority of commercially available MRI scanners rely on high-strength magnetic fields (1.5–3 T) for imaging, meaning that any EM interference induced by electric current would disrupt the magnetic field homogeneity in the MRI scanner and thus deteriorate image quality. Moreover, ferromagnetic materials cannot be used under MRI. Further challenges include the highly restricted workspace within scanners, where commonly used closed-bore scanners are small (600–700 mm). The workspace is further reduced by RF coils, such as a head/body coil, which are necessary for optimal image quality and RF heating risk reduction [17]. As a result, the space for operation and the dexterity of instruments are greatly limited. Another type of scanner architecture, open MRI scanners, avoid the closed 'doughnut' bore structure by using magnetic bottom and top coils and being open on all sides. Although it can expand the workspace to some extent, this comes at the cost of a magnetic field strength hardly higher than 0.5 T [18], thus inducing a low signal-to-noise ratio (SNR) and increased complexity in high-quality image reconstruction. Therefore, a closed MRI scanner is still the norm at present. The adoption of a robotics system is also problematic due to the confined available space [19]. Besides the restricted operating volume, more notably, the high-intensity magnetic fields preclude the use of metal materials (e.g. stainless steel) in a robotic system. Piezoelectric actuators are commonly employed as drives for MRI-adapted interventional robots, while fluid-driven actuators are also investigated. MR positional markers (section 7.4.1) are developed to achieve reliable real-time tracking and image registration without quality-degrading artifacts [20]. Due to limited available material choices and constrained space, designing versatile MRI-compatible systems is particularly complicated [7]. Developed robots are highly specialized in specific surgical procedures, integrated with customized actuation modules (section 7.4.2).

Most commercially available MRI scanners require complex and bulky electromagnets to generate high magnetic fields. Such scanners involve a high cost of installation, maintenance, and operation, resulting in scarce availability in low- and middle-income countries. The Swoop™ system from Hyperfine Inc. (USA) is a first-of-its-kind portable low-field MRI device which was cleared by the US Food and Drug Administration (FDA) in 2020 [21]. It is distinguished by its portable feature with a lightweight (630 kg) and compact size (140 cm high and 86 cm wide). This system uses a field strength of 0.064 T and consumes low AC power (<1200 W). Recent research conducted by Liu *et al* [22] also focuses on the cost-effective MRI scanner (figure 7.1). They utilize an ultra-low-field (0.055 T) scanner specially designed for brain disease diagnosis, which is powered by a standard AC power outlet. To eliminate the need for magnetic or RF shielding cages, a deep learning approach was applied for image reconstruction against EM interference. The four most universally adopted scan protocols for brain MRI, namely, T1W, T2W,

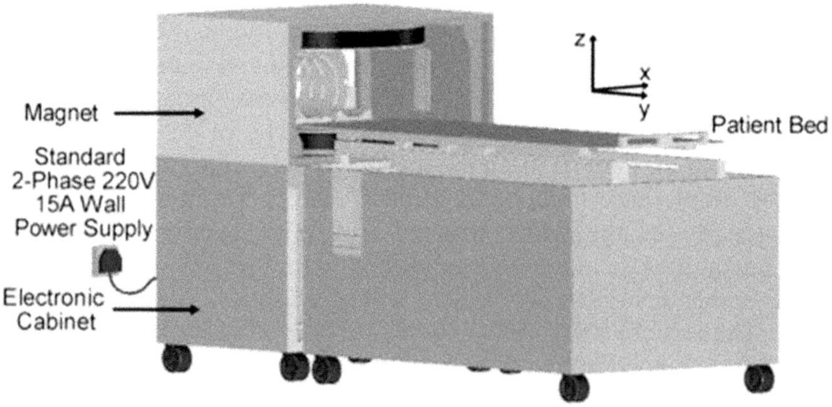

Figure 7.1. Example of the advanced MRI scanner prototype, 0.055 T ultra-low-field brain MRI system (reprinted by permission from Springer Nature Customer Servie Centre GmbH: Nature, Nature Communications [22], Copyright (2021)).

FLAIR, and DWI, have been implemented and validated on this device, and its feasibility of diagnosing brain tumors and strokes was successfully demonstrated.

7.2.3 Ultrasound

US, which utilizes high-frequency acoustic waves to reveal tissues, organs, blood, etc inside the body [23], has become a necessary medical imaging method for interventions and diagnoses. Unlike CT, x-ray, and MR imaging, US originates from mechanical energy rather than EM energy and does not cause ionizing radiation [24]. Although US images are relatively challenging to interpret, the lightness, portability, and affordability of US devices promote US as a flexible and cost-effective imaging solution [25]. As a result, US is widely used to show muscles, breasts, heart, vessels, eyes, thyroid, and the brain, with one of its most common usages being to monitor the growth of fetuses. Precise delineation of organs such as fetuses can be further offered by advanced 3D/4D US constructed from conventional 2D images [26]. Continued technical advances have boosted new imaging modes by leveraging the US contrast agents and harmonic signals produced by nonlinear wave propagation in tissues. These agents allow the visualization of micro-circulation vessels and even show the potential to improve US's sensitivity in liver lesion diagnosis to rival that of CT and MRI. The harmonic imaging approach particularly holds for obese patients and pelvic pathology owing to its improved SNR [27].

The advantages of US prompt its combined utilization with computer-controlled robots, which improves the execution efficiency, stability, and accuracy in interventional procedures and even enables autonomous operation. In urology, US is proposed to guide needles toward the direction of located lesions in prostate biopsy [28, 29] and brachytherapy [30, 31]. Meanwhile, some US-guided robots have been applied to needle-based breast biopsies, since real-time imaging can compensate for repositioning errors caused by physiological motion (e.g. breathing) and patient movement [32]. They have been proven to reduce targeting errors compared to manual positioning of biopsy needles [33, 34]. In addition to imaging, high-intensity focused ultrasound (HIFU) produced by customized transducer(s) can perform ablation therapy. Harmonic motion imaging for focused US has emerged as a new technique for concurrently conducting the HIFU ablation and imaging [35]. The detected oscillatory motion in the HIFU focal point was explored to image through a co-axially aligned transducer. It realized the continuous monitoring of ablation without mode switching between ablation and imaging, consequently decreasing the overheating risk during ablation.

7.3 State-of-the-art in surgical treatments

It was common to utilize modified industrial robots in surgeries before the emergence of special-purpose surgical robots. For instance, the industrial Programmable Universal Machine for Assembly (PUMA) robot was applied in neurosurgery [2]. In 1991, the world's first special-purpose surgical robot, PROBOT was developed for prostate resection [36], where the robot end-effector's movement was restricted in a pre-defined working envelope. In 1999, the first orthopedics robot, Acrobot, was invented for knee replacement surgeries, making orthopedics one of the first areas where robot applications were attempted. The motion of Acrobot's end-effector was limited to 3 degrees of freedom (DoFs), namely yaw, pitch, and translation, with small reach and angle range to decrease potential damage [37].

However, these first-generation surgical robots usually require frequent input of surgeons' control commands. Intra-op imaging guidance was not a routine in these initial surgical robots; *in situ* interventional navigation could not be carried out, either. Compared with surgeries for bones, those in soft tissue have higher requirements on imaging techniques due to the complex tissue deformations during operations. In terms of imaging on soft tissue and organs, CT is a quick choice for the chest and calcium deposit detection. MRI and US could provide ionizing radiation-free images, and the former excels in the spinal cord and brain due to its detailed visualization of structural abnormalities and tumors; the latter is commonly used in abdominopelvic diagnosis and cardiography (e.g. chamber-wall motion), as it can monitor the structure and movement of internal organs as well as blood flow. As for the cost, another factor that needs to be taken into account, it was reported that the mean charges of CT, US, and MRI were 1565, 410, and 2048 US dollars, respectively, for hospital diagnostic imaging procedures in Florida in 2002 [38]. Over the past two decades, surgical robots have been advanced gradually to combine with computer-controlled systems and imaging techniques, while intra-op image guidance has become the trend.

7.3.1 Stereotactic neurosurgery

Neurosurgery is regarded as one of the most challenging invasive operations because of the high precision requirement necessary to navigate delicate tissues and complex anatomical locations with individual variability [2, 39]. The risk of fatal complications (e.g. blood clots and seizures) is high in the brain with complicated blood vessel distribution and functional areas. There have been stereotactic platforms designed and validated for neurosurgery under MRI, such as the ClearPoint system (ClearPoint Neuro, USA), which could perform electrode placements and focal ablation with acceptable accuracy [40]. However, the workflow including frequent patient movement for imaging updates and manual operation on the instrument is still tedious. The application of robotics in neurosurgery is promising to provide stable and refined motion of instruments inside the cranial cavity, superior to humans particularly for intensive tasks that demand high precision [40, 41]. Robots can also contribute to reduce operating time and costs. The introduction of robot-assisted MIS also demonstrates considerable benefits for the patient's post-op recovery [42]. The rapid advancement of intra-op imaging has paved the way for the adoption of robotic platforms in neurosurgery [2].

The first application of robots in neurosurgery was in 1985 [2] when Kwoh and his colleagues successfully performed CT-guided biopsy cannulation by manipulating the PUMA 200 [2, 39]. Following this pioneering effort, other robots have

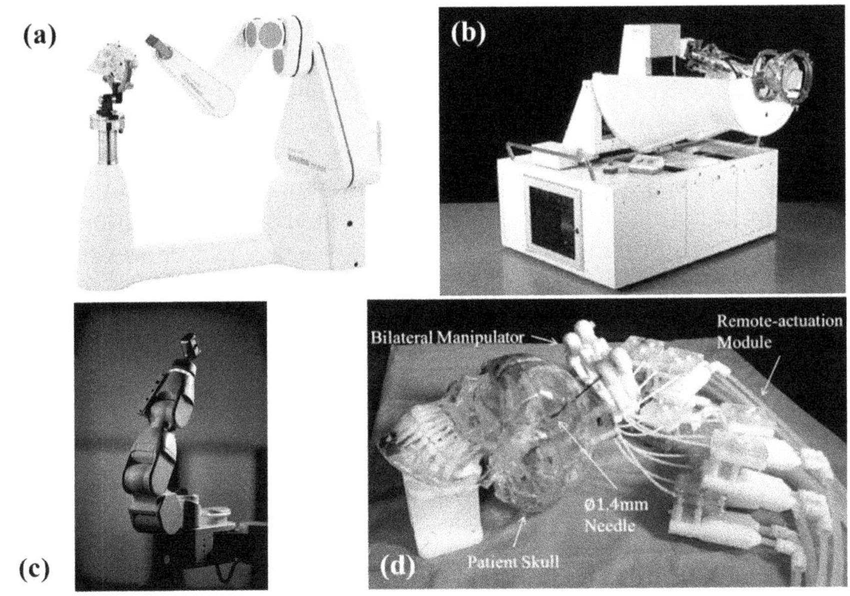

Figure 7.2. Commercial products and research prototypes of neurosurgery robotic platforms. (a) NeuroMate® stereotactic robot (Reprinted with permission of Renishaw. [43] ® Renishaw plc. All rights reserved.); (b) Minerva © system (reprinted by permission from Springer Nature Customer Service Centre GmbH: Nature, Neurosurgical Review, [44] , Copyright © 2014, Springer-Verlag Berlin Heidelberg.); (c) Mazor X Stealth Edition Spine Robot, image printed with permission of Medtronic and Mazor robotics.); (d) MRI-guided bilateral stereotactic neurosurgery platform (© 2018 IEEE. Reprinted, with permission, from [46]).

subsequently been proposed, e.g. the NeuroMate robot (Integrated Surgical Systems, USA) (figure 7.2(a)), which was approved by the FDA in 1999 as the first commercial robotic platform enabling stereotactic procedures such as deep brain stimulation (DBS) [44]. In these early robot-assisted neurosurgeries, surgeons pre-defined the path and motion of the robots relying on pre-op images. Even though this operation protocol simplified the positioning process, dynamic monitoring for instrument location or brain shifting was not available under this routine. The Minerva system was then devised as a dynamic CT-guiding system by which the surgeon could adjust the instrument trajectory in real-time (figure 7.2(b)). Incorporating a similar working process, SpineAssist, Mazor X Stealth Edition Spine Robot (Medtronic, USA) (figure 7.2(c)), and Cirq (Brainlab, Germany) have been widely used in spinal instrumentation. SpineAssist is the first share-control robot for spine surgery [47], which means that both the surgeon and the robot directly manipulate the surgical tool [48]. These systems are primarily dependent on the precise movements of the robot end-effector. Another kind of shared-control interface allows the surgeon to take the lead while the robot guarantees smooth motion. This retains surgeons' manipulation skills and manual dexterity. One of such dexterity-enhancing systems, the Steady Hand System (Johns Hopkins University, USA) [49], was designed to improve micro-surgery performance by filtering out tremors. Although the concept has shown potential for applications in neurosurgery, its current utilization is focused on retinal surgery [50]. One example of brain surgery robots employing shared control is the ROSA stereotactic robotic system (Zimmer Biomet, USA) [45], a system mainly used for depth electrode placement and intracranial biopsies.

Several teleoperated robotic systems have been developed for CT-guided stereotactic neurosurgeries, aiming at reducing harmful ionizing radiation exposed to clinicians. For example, NeuRobot (Shinshu University, Japan) incorporated a leader–follower operation mode to perform neurosurgical procedures such as tumor removal [51]. The teleoperation paradigm also provides a solution to interventional robots guided by MRI, where the surgeon's control command to the robot is given outside the scanning suite. NeuroArm (University of Calgary, Canada) is a commercial MR-conditional robot platform that allows teleoperation. Equipped with 3D force sensors, it can provide haptic feedback to the surgeon. Despite its success in neurosurgery in over 1000 cases [44], the pioneering surgical robot has drawbacks, most notably, its bulky size, high cost, and limited compatibility with only a specific MRI scanner. Researchers are constantly exploring solutions, attempting to optimize or even create new avenues in MRI-guided robotic neurosurgeries. Li *et al* (Worcester Polytechnic Institute, USA) [52] designed an MRI-guided table-mounted robot prototype for needle-based neural interventions (e.g. DBS), the mechanism of which referred to the kinematics of conventional manual stereotactic frames (e.g. Leksell frame). The robot enables 7-DoF operation driven by nonharmonic piezoelectric motors. Although its needle tip positioning accuracy achieved 1.37 ± 0.06 mm in a lab-based test, the imaging SNR reduction with robot running in the MRI bore reached 10.3% [53]. Guo *et al* (The University of Hong Kong, China) [46] proposed the first hydraulic-driven MRI-guided prototype of a bilateral intra-op robot for stereotactic neurosurgery. Mounted on the patient skull directly, the compact robot ($110.6 \times 206.8 \times 33.2$ mm) allows 8-DoF manipulation of the needle guide for DBS procedures (figure 7.2(d)) with a targeting accuracy of 1.73 mm, while the SNR loss with the robot in full motion was only within 3%.

7.3.2 Biopsy in prostate and breast

Biopsy is the main approach for cancer diagnosis, which involves the removal of tissue samples from the suspicious lesion for further pathological investigation [54]. Imaging modalities such as MRI, US, and CT are used to localize and pinpoint lesions prior to intervention and provide guidance through real-time imaging during operation. Traditional biopsies rely on manual needle insertion, posing a great challenge to the physician's perception and manipulation dexterity. Under these circumstances, robots hold great potential for more accurate biopsies, since it offers enhanced repeatability, rigidity, and precision by the use of stable mechanical manipulators.

Breast biopsy is routinely performed for pathological analysis if abnormal tissues are identified in breast mammography, US, or MRI. With breast cancer being one of the most commonly diagnosed cancers in women, breast biopsies are highly prevalent [56]. The breast is a deformable organ, making real-time imaging critical

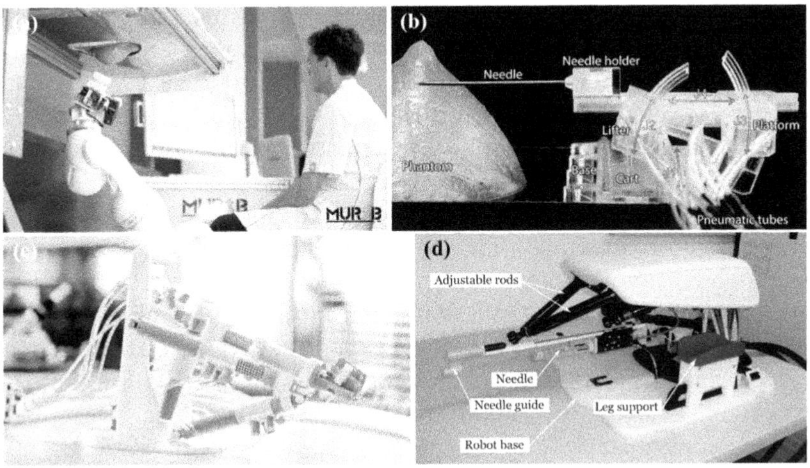

Figure 7.3. Robotic platforms for biopsy procedures. (a) MURAB project for US-guided breast biopsy with the pre-op MRI image (© 2020 IEEE. Reprinted, with permission, from [43], and the MURAB project.); (b) Stormram 4 MR-safe breast biopsy robotic system (Reprinted by permission from Springer Nature Customer Servie Centre GmbH: Medical Robotics, Annals of Biomedical Engineering [55], Copyight (2018)); (c) Soteria Medical MR-guided prostate biopsy platform (Image courtesy of Martijn Hoogenboom and Soteria Medical.); (d) MR-safe MIRIAM system for transperineal prostate biopsy (Image courtesy of Dr. Pedro Lopes Da Frota Moreira).

for its biopsy guidance. Biopsies for breast cancer are usually conducted under US guidance due to the ability to access all areas of the breast and axilla, alongside its adaptiveness to the deformable breast surface [57]. Such guidance also has the advantages of low-cost multi-directional sampling and patient comfort. However, the portable US manipulation also induces difficulties in robotization, including the alignment/coordination with the needle insertion instrument, particularly in guidance for such a soft organ. Both the US field of view and the needle will need to be tracked; thus, the US image can provide visualization of the needle. Compared to US, MRI has a higher sensitivity to abnormal tissues and can visualize tumors/lesions that are invisible under US. Combining pre-scanned MR images with real-time US guidance can provide more tissue details to guide the intervention.

In the MURAB system (figure 7.3(a)) [58], patient localization is performed with a stereo camera identifying projections or skin markers on the patient's body. With the position information, the robot combines the real-time volumetric US with pre-acquired MRI images to obtain the precise lesion location in robotic coordinate frame. Avoiding complex combination of several types of images, such as the deformable registration between different imaging modalities with diverse imaging sensitivity, MR-conditional robots can directly employ MRI as real-time feedback for the guidance of intervention. Navarro-Alarcon *et al* [59] developed an MR-safe biopsy robot which features a compact Cartesian mechanism with 3 DoFs of translation. It could perform needle insertion tasks from either the front or the side within an open bore scanner. Driven by a combination of piezoelectric and pneumatic actuators, it could achieve an accuracy of 1.5 mm in the insertion direction (z-axis) and 0.4 mm in the x–y stage. Stormram 4 [55] is a pneumatic-driven biopsy robot (figure 7.3(b)). Apart from the commercial needle, the robot itself is MR-safe. It is driven by four pneumatic stepper motors and its feasibility is demonstrated via a phantom study under MRI with an error of 1.29 ± 0.59 mm.

Prostate biopsy and needle therapy are among the most promising applications of robotic percutaneous methods. The gold standard for manual biopsy is fusion biopsy [60], which involves identifying suspicious lesions based on pre-op multiparametric MRI and targeting the lesion under intra-op US navigation. The biopsy outcome is heavily reliant on the surgeon's expertise, and the learning curve is long. Robotic assistance is introduced for procedure standardization and precision improvement. There are two main trends in robot-actuated prostate biopsies: (1) MR-fused biopsy, which fuses diagnostic MR images with *in situ* US navigation for needle targeting, and (2) in-bore solutions, i.e. MR-compatible robots.

Similar to breast biopsy, the in-bore solution avoids the cumbersome image registration process; however, the robot design needs to take into account issues such as the size of the MR bore and the material limitation. The remote-controlled manipulator system developed by Soteria Medical (The Netherlands) (figure 7.3(c)) [61] is a robotic device for needle guide positioning. It is constructed solely of plastic parts and tubing, aiming to perform fast and accurate in-bore MR-guided prostate biopsies. The system is driven by five pneumatic motors. In combination with dedicated intervention software for planning and remote control, the manipulator could move the needle to the target area under real-time MR imaging. The system is clinically used in over 25 different countries around Europe, USA, and Asia. Moreira *et al* [62] presented a parallel robot prototype capable of needle tracking and steering (figure 7.3(d)). This platform is driven by piezoelectric actuators and its dexterity was demonstrated by reaching targets hidden behind an obstacle.

Besides biopsy, needles or cannulas can assist various types of treatments, such as ablation, and even gene therapy, which developed rapidly in recent years. Gene therapy can be conducted to treat neurological disorders (e.g. central nervous system disorder) under intra-op MRI guidance. For example, the ClearPoint system (ClearPoint Neuro, USA) provides real-time visualization and trajectory planning for an MR-compatible infusion cannula named SmartFlow, which is steered by a skull-mounted rigid frame [63]. With visible cannula placement and infusate coverage, the intra-op adjustment can accomplish high targeting accuracy (<2 mm). Such a kind of drug delivery enables minimal incision and increased safety for the patient, as well as optimizes dose volume and infusion rates.

7.3.3 Abdominopelvic treatment

Common cancer types in abdominal or pelvic organs can usually be classified as (1) upper gastrointestinal (GI) cancers (e.g. liver, gall bladder/biliary tract, and pancreatic cancers), which are usually diagnosed by abdominal US and gastroscopies; (2) lower GI cancers usually by colonoscopies; (3) gynecologic cancers (e.g.

cervical and endometrial cancers) usually by transvaginal ultrasound and MRI; and (4) urological cancers by cystoscopies, abdominal CT, and MRI [64]. Their treatment approaches vary depending on the cancer position and grade. With the trend of MIS, several diagnostic imaging modalities have evolved as important alternatives to surgical/radiologic treatments. Endoscopic US guidance is a representative technique, which has been proven to have advantages over conventional surgical routines and percutaneous interventions in pseudocyst drainage and celiac plexus neurolysis [65]. Endoscopic US-guided liver biopsy has also been accepted as an effective choice to obtain liver tissue for both focal and parenchymal diseases [66]. Its improvement over fluoroscopy-guided transjugular routes is on the imaging quality for both the left and right hepatic lobes, thus facilitating more accurate access to focal liver lesions [67]. Currently such procedures are conducted manually, and the route toward the target is highly decided on the patient's risk profile, biopsy indications, and the endoscopist's experience [68].

Percutaneous approaches for both diagnosis and therapy of abdominopelvic disease (e.g. through biopsy, drainage, and tumor ablation) are usually performed by inserting a thin needle or probe through the skin to the target lesion. RF ablation for liver cancers is a typical application utilizing percutaneous approaches, particularly in treating remaining hepatocellular carcinoma after liver transplantation and resection [69]. Different from endoscopic US devices with inherent imaging guidance, additional imaging modalities are needed for visualization. Conventional workflows separate the guidance for needle insertion (e.g. using US or CT) and ablation assessment (e.g. using post-op CT or sonography), resulting in inaccurate monitoring for ablation margins (<1 cm) that may cause high recurrence or inadvertent organ damage [69]. Intra-op MRI-guided percutaneous systems thus have garnered attention, accredited to MRI's high soft-tissue imaging contrast and temperature monitoring resolution (<1 °C). Passive needle holders were developed and several of them have been commercialized, such as SeeStar (AprioMed, Sweden) and Simplify (NeoRad AS, Norway). For more autonomous manipulation, robot-assisted research prototypes have been investigated, with either table-, floor-, or patient-mounted mechanical designs. He *et al* [69] proposed a compact patient-mounted system allowing semi-autonomous needle orientation adjustment, i.e. coarse manual placement followed by fine automatic adjustment. The ablation management can also be enhanced by using intra-op MR thermometry.

Focused ultrasound (FUS), or specifically HIFU, provides an even less invasive option for therapies in the abdominal or pelvic cavity. The focused acoustic energy (from independently adjusted transducers) can result in micro-mechanical effects inside the patient body without requiring invasive access [70]. Although abdominal FUS/HIFU is still in the early stage, it has significant potential to ablate tumors in the prostate, uterus (e.g. uterine fibroids), and liver. As introduced, MRI has advantages in guiding and monitoring operations for soft tissues, including abdominal treatments. There have been commercial MRI-guided FUS platforms such as the Sonalleve MR-HIFU system (Philips, The Netherlands) and the ExAblate 2000 (Insightec, Israel). The focuses of the FUS system's advancement are related to the region-of-interest (RoI) expansion and acoustic-beam adjusting efficiency. The focal point is expected to have a workspace covering the RoI and be redundantly formed to circumvent skin burn induced by single ablation modes. Only by tuning the phases of the transducer array, the electronic adjustment range (<3.5 cm) of the focal spot may be insufficient to cover the target area. Therefore, platforms that enable additional mechanical focal spot adjustment have been gradually proposed. Dai *et al* [71] proposed a robotic platform that can provide 5-DoF mechanical adjustment for phase-array transducing. The compact robot can be placed in the water tank of an MRI operating table, which is built in the scanner specialized for US treatments. The robot workspace reaches about 100 mm × 100 mm × 35 mm without involving electronic focal-spot steering. It has the potential to conduct MR-guided FUS treatments for major abdominal or pelvic organs and to compensate for respiration-induced motion.

7.3.4 Cardiovascular catheterization

Endovascular intervention is an MIS option for cardiovascular diseases [72]. Using specially designed instruments such as catheters and guidewires, surgeons puncture the patient's skin surface to access blood vessels and, with intra-op imaging guidance, navigate through tortuous vascular branches to the lesion site [73]. Endovascular surgery shares all of MIS's advantages over open surgeries in terms of small incisions, shorter recovery time, minimal pain, and the possibility of local anesthesia rather than general anesthesia [74].

Because of its low cost and high temporal resolution, x-ray with iodine-based contrast agents has become the 'gold standard' technique for the diagnosis and treatment of coronary artery disease [79]. However, x-ray–guided interventions still suffer from significant drawbacks, including the use of ionizing radiation and the harm of iodine-based contrast agents to kidneys [80]. In an evaluation of a robotic-assisted coronary angioplasty system [81], it is reported that teleoperation can reduce radiation exposure to the operator by 97% compared to the operation conducted in the standard table position. Magellan™ (Johnson & Johnson, USA) is a commercial robotic platform designed for remote manipulation of a tendon-driven steerable catheter. However, its necessity for customized catheters leads to a high usage cost. CorPath GRX platform (Siemens, Germany) (figure 7.4(a)) was compatible with standard instruments, cleared by the FDA and certified with CE marking in 2011. In addition to tendon-driven approaches, which is the most-used steering method for off-the-shelf catheters, magnet driving is a newer actuation mode that tends to form sharper turning angles and thus gains access to more complex areas. One commercially available robotic platform that uses magnetic steering is the Niobe® system (Stereotaxis, USA) (figure 7.4(b)) [76]. It consists of two large permanent magnets, located on either side of the operation bed. Magnetic field changes will cause the movement of the catheter distal end where small magnets are embedded. Aeon Phocu (Aeon Scientific, Switzerland) (figure 7.4(c)) [77] is a CE-certified robotic platform for cardiac electrophysiological (EP) procedures, which also utilizes magnetic steering. Even though the radiation-related danger introduced by fluoroscopy to the surgeons is greatly reduced by teleoperation, it still poses a threat to patients.

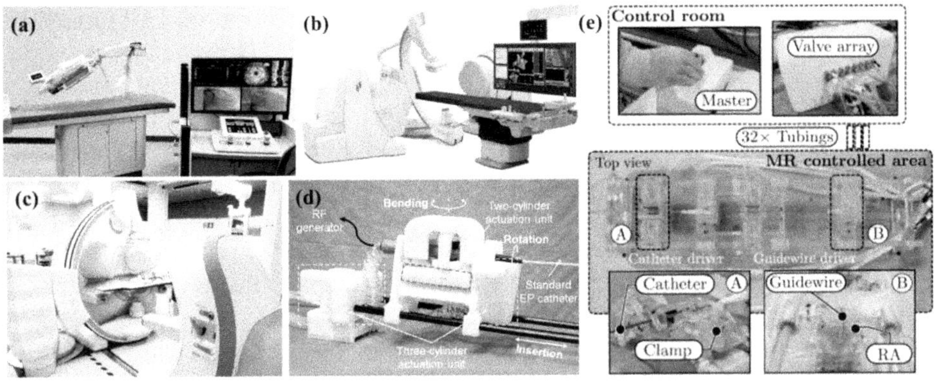

Figure 7.4. Robotic platforms for endovascular interventions. (a) CorPath GRX vascular robotic system ([75] John Wiley & Sons. © 2017 Wiley Periodicals, Inc.); (b) Niobe& magnetic navigation system ([76] John Wiley & Sons. Copyright © 2006, John Wiley and Sons.); (c) Aeon Phocus electromagnetic catheter steering system (© 2017 IEEE. Reprinted, with permissions, from [77]); (d) MR-safe intracardiac catheter manipulator; (e) MR-safe endovascular robotic platform (© 2020 IEEE. Reprinted, with permission, from [78]).

MRI is gaining increasing popularity as a non-ionizing alternative imaging modality for endovascular interventions, which can contribute to both navigation of the interventional procedure and temperature change monitoring of the ablation process [82]. Despite these strengths, MRI-guided endovascular interventions are still in the laboratory stage due to the intrinsic limitations of MRI scanning. The first robotic manipulator for MRI-guided cardiac EP intervention (figure 7.4(d)) was developed in 2018, with a compact size (780 × 105 × 210 mm) and a leader–follower hydraulic transmission actuator enabling teleoperation outside the MRI scanning room [83]. By plugging in a standard EP catheter, this platform was capable of catheter steering (−45° to 45°, 0.063°), rotation (−360° to 360°, 0.504°), coarse translation (0–200 mm, 0.115 mm), and fine translation (0–30 mm, 0.016 mm). Su *et al* [84] and Kundrat *et al* (figure 7.4(e)) [78] also employed the leader–follower fashion in their designs but used piezoelectric and pneumatic motors, respectively, for adaptation to the MR environment. Details of actuation mechanisms will be introduced in section 7.4.2. It is worth emphasizing that in MRI-guided cardiovascular intervention, real-time tracking of the surgical instruments, i.e. catheter, without sacrificing image quality is also a key concern. To address this issue, devices for localization and catheter shape sensing have been developed, which will be introduced in section 7.4.1.

7.4 Key advanced technologies

The localization of surgical tools and implants, particularly their intra-op positional tracking, is essential for precise and efficient treatments. Taking a commercial orthopedics platform, ROSA spine robot (Zimmer Biomet, USA) [85] as an example, light reflective spherical markers are used as the positional reference. Being attached on a fully automated robotic arm and the patient, the markers enable fast localization of the instrument and patient anatomy in the same coordinate frame. Alternatives can be found such as small wirelessly powered LED markers in the ExcelsiusGPS system (Globus Medical, USA) [86]. However, these optical markers are only available when implemented on rigid instruments outside the patient body, since the tracking relies on a direct and clear line of sight between cameras and markers [6]. Special localization approaches are required for interventional joint-linked or flexible instruments (e.g. catheters), as the instrument end-effector position cannot be calculated simply based on rigid transformation. Operations assisted by intra-op MRI also introduced requirements for sensor compatibility with high magnetic fields and limited space inside the scanner bore. Similar challenges in terms of compatibility also appeared in the actuator and mechanical design of robots, which should be sufficiently compact while maintaining a certain level of manipulation accuracy and workspace.

7.4.1 Localization and tracking of robots

Spatial positional tracking is crucial in robot navigation and automation. Stand-alone tracking devices can measure the location and orientation of objects (e.g. robot end-effector) in the 3D global coordinate space or provide the 3D rigid transformation in real-time. Various tracking approaches based on optics, EM, acoustics, and other principles have been applied in clinical surgical navigation. ***Optical*** tracking using an infrared camera has been widely applied in rigid instrument tracking scenarios such as in orthopedics. At least two optical cameras are fixed in the surgical environment. Both capture the active infrared LED or passive retroreflective markers that are rigidly attached on the instruments. At least three markers are required for deriving the 6D pose of each instrument. The pose estimation accuracy can be enhanced more at the core of measurement working volume than the edges, and an increased or redundant number of markers can result in improved accuracy, as reported in [87]. Representative commercial products like Polaris and Optotrak series (NDI, Canada) have been employed in neurosurgery, orthopedics, and others [88]. ***EM*** tracking markers/coils are not limited by the line-of-sight problem; however, they are commonly used in the tethering setting. The size of sensing marker unit can also be reduced significantly. However, they still need to be put in the measurement volume associated with the magnetic field generator. The tracking precision is susceptible to ferromagnetic sources, or EM motors nearby [89]. Although EM tracking enables technologies for both passive (wireless) and active (wired) markers, most interventional procedures utilized commercial active devices in view of the marker size. NDI (Canada), Ascension Technology Corp. (USA), and Polhemus Inc. (USA) have developed popular EM tracking platforms. Taking the NDI Aurora system as an example, it has been applied in interventional procedures such as cardiovascular surgery, abdominal interventions, as well as ear, nose, and throat surgery [88]. When applied in image-guided robotic interventions, all these optical- or EM-based tracking systems require alignment with the coordinates of robot kinematics and medical imaging. Such alignment may induce positional registration errors. Further challenges appeared in intra-op MRI-guided operations, where only specific position-tracking coils can be compatible and effective.

Shape/configuration sensing is increasingly in demand for interventional procedures. The use of continuum robots has been generalized in interventional devices, mainly because of their structural similarity with conventional manually operated instruments such as catheters [90]. There have been continuum robotic manipulators proposed for application in neurosurgery, otolaryngology, abdominal surgery, and particularly cardiovascular interventions, in the form of concentric tubes, fluid-driven (including hydraulic and pneumatic) and tendon-driven mechanisms [91, 92]. The configuration of continuum robots is in infinite DoFs theoretically, and there are no angle-encodable joints or rigid links available for kinematics calculation. Therefore, shape sensing for the continuum body inserted into the patient body will facilitate accurate and efficient end-effector control [93]. The EM tracking technique can be used in shape reconstruction if multiple markers are orderly attached to the manipulator. However, such approaches could only be applicable to cases that need simplified shape localization.

Fiber Bragg gratings (FBGs) have been accepted for uses of strain and curvature sensing in continuum surgical robotics. With sparse or continuous gratings inscribed inside a thin fiber, the sensor can reflect the axial strain changes along the fiber by the optical signal difference of the reflected spectrum. Besides biocompatibility and nontoxicity, their major advantages are the ability of long-distance transmission via fibers without inducing EM interference. These features make them compatible with the MRI environment without deteriorating the imaging quality and suitable for MRI-guided robots. Park *et al* [94] proposed to place three FBG fibers along grooves on a biopsy needle to measure the curvature, although each fiber was inscribed with only two FBG nodes. Such a triangular/triplet fiber configuration (120° interval) was then accepted as a common placement when using the combination of single-core fibers for 3D curvature estimation. The increased number of FBGs on each fiber can facilitate the improvement of accuracy [95, 96], since more locations can be considered in the reconstruction. FBGs have also been gradually extended for shape estimation of flexible manipulators, such as tendon-driven continuum robots [97] and endoscopes [98]. However, the use of multiple fibers met challenges in integration, particularly on the thin body like cardiovascular catheters. One solution is to use the multi-core fiber as a substitute. Each fiber (Ø 0.2mm) is inscribed by multiplc (e.g. seven) chains of continuous gratings and is interrogated quickly by the optical frequency domain reflectometry technique. A single multi-core FBG fiber enables the 3D curvature sensing of itself, appropriate to be integrated inside flexible manipulators with strict diameter limitations [99]. Dong *et al* [99] validated a method for tracking the cardiac catheter shape by combining a multi-core FBG fiber and positional tracking coils. Feasibility experiments were performed on a customized robot prototype with a commercial cardiac catheter [83], achieving a positional precision of 1.53 mm at the catheter tip and a path-following control accuracy of 0.62 mm. Current reconstruction models generally assume that strains on the continuum body can be totally reflected by FBGs integrated inside the manipulator [100], and FBGs only feedback deformation-induced strain changes without noises. This is because external-force–induced strain changes are difficult to identify and model. Although learning-based shape-sensing algorithms have been proposed employing FBG signals [101–103], improving the estimation accuracy under unstructured external forces is still a challenge.

Positional tracking in MRI coordinates is usually accomplished by MR-based tracking coil units, avoiding the registration between imaging and tracking coordinates [46]. These micro coils are often attached to devices (figure 7.5(a)), instrument end-effectors, or registration fiducial marks to either transmit RF signals or serve as receiver coils. They are typically made of conductive wire loops and peripheral electronic components such as capacitors [104]. The MR-based tracking coils are broadly subdivided into three types, i.e. passive [105–107], active [108–110], and semi-active tracking coils [111, 112]. The ***active*** types are connected to separate MR receiving channels by electrical cables. The MR system activates the small coils by RF pulse and then selectively acquires resonating signals around these coils [113]. It achieves higher temporal and spatial resolutions than the other two types [106, 110]. However, the heat issue involved by the long RF antenna could harm the

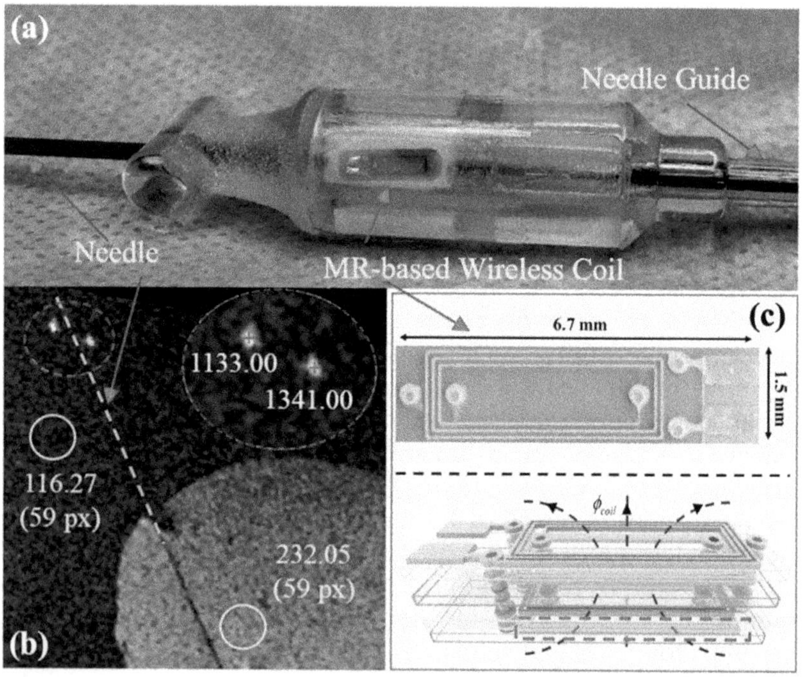

Figure 7.5. Integration and performance of passive tracking coils in MRI-guided needle insertion. (a) Needle guide with two tracking coils attached to the surface. One coil is visible on the front sidewall, and the other is on the back sidewall. (b) MR image of the brain phantom (in the coronal view) revealing the two tracking markers by the corresponding bright spots. The signal density at these bright spots (at the top-left) is much higher than that of the background and agar-gel phantom (© 2018 IEEE. Reprinted, with permission, from [46]). (c) Prototype and structure diagram of the four-layer coil [113] (© 2020 IEEE. Reprinted, with permission, from [78]).

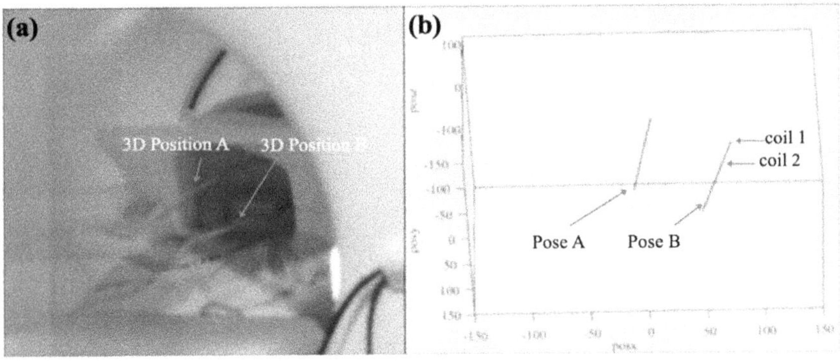

Figure 7.6. Real-time tracking demonstration using passive tracking coils. (a) Manipulation of a non-ferromagnetic rod attached with two tracking coils in the MR scanner. (b) Posture reconstruction and position tracking in the MRI coordinate.

patient, which remains a main concern of active tracking coils [114]. Unlike active coils, the ***passive*** type neither need to transmit RF nor require wired connections with the MR platform. It only amplifies the received MR signal to enhance the imaging contrast between itself and its immediate vicinity [115]. For example, in a phantom test [46] (figure 7.5(b)), two miniature coils attached to the needle guide amplify signal intensity around the marker locations by four times compared to the signal of background and agar-gel phantom. Its tiny and thin structure (figure 7.5(c)) simplifies the integration on both rigid and soft robots/instruments. Additionally, the wireless connection eliminates heating concerns. Such coils can also be used for real-time tracking applications. As in figure 7.6, the real-time 3D positions of two coils were obtained through the RTHawk (Heartvista, USA) interface, thus enabling pose tracking of a non-ferromagnetic rod in the MRI scanner. ***Semi-active*** coils enable passive visualization because they are not connected with the MR receiving channels, while being electrically activated by the MR sequences [116]. Herein, we categorize this hybrid tracking approach as semi-active. The semi-active coils possess the unique feature of being able to tune electrical characteristics, inducing coil resonance at or far from the Larmor frequency [117]. Although with the potential to achieve higher sensing robustness than the active and passive tracking coils, relevant studies are rarely reported due to the demand for complex hardware [118].

7.4.2 Surgical robot mounting and actuation mechanisms

Surgical robot mounting refers to the mechanical support of its actuation mechanisms, varied by the choice of imaging scanner, the required workspace of surgical manipulation, and the available footprint of operation theater. These factors directly determine how and where the robot should be based, either on the floor, bedside, ceiling, or patient. The SpineAssist (Mazor Robotics, Israel), mounted on the spine through a radiolucent frame, was the first robot system approved for spine surgery by the FDA. Stainless steel pins named Kirschner-wires, which were widely used in

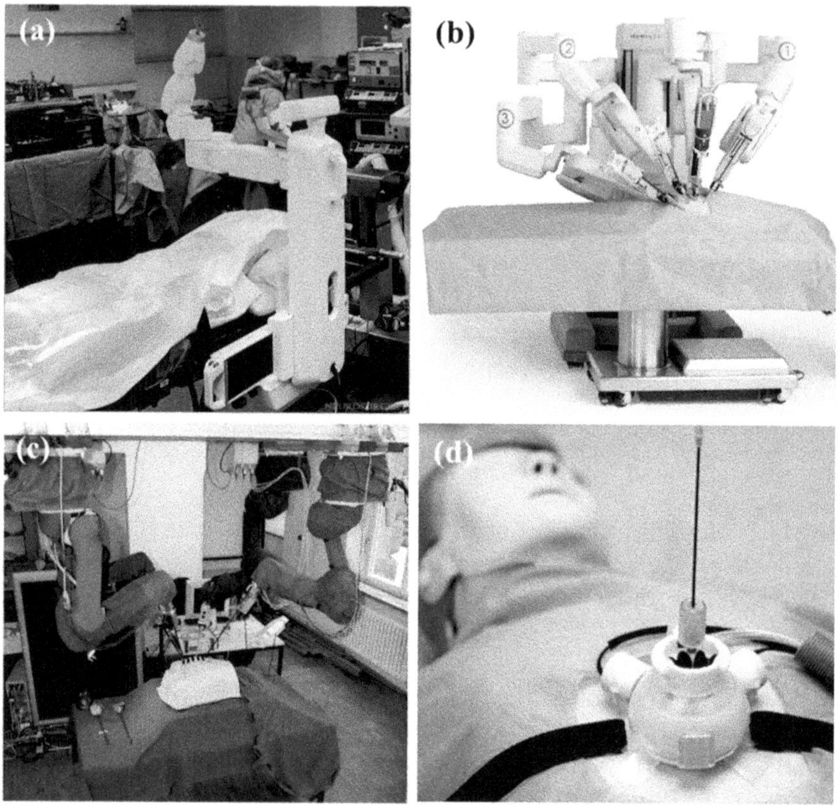

Figure 7.7. Mounting types of surgical robot systems and examples. (a) Mazor X Stealth Edition [47], bedside-mounted (reproduced from [120]); (b) da Vinci Surgical System, floor-mounted (Reprinted by permission from Springer Nature Customer Service Center GmbH: Springer Nature, Springer eBook [121], Copyright (2019)); (c) EndoPAR system, ceiling-mounted (© 2010 IEEE. Reprinted, with permission, from [122], cropped); (d) MR-compatible robot system [69], patient-mounted.

orthopedics surgeries, attached the frame to the patient. Ringel *et al* [119] conducted a controlled experiment of lumbar/sacral pedicle screw implantation, showing that the screw placement accuracy of this system was 85% and lower than the 93% in conventional freehand operation. This could be attributed to the dislocations of the Kirschner-wire. After the company was acquired by Medtronic, the latest version (released in 2019), Mazor X Stealth Edition (Medtronic, USA) (figure 7.7(a)), is integrated with Medtronic Stealth Navigation software and changed to bedside-mounting. A bone mount bridge, which is a rigid link extending from the bottom of the robotic arm, attaches the robot to the pins placed on posterior superior iliac spine (PSIS) or spinous process, enabling motion compensation for the patient's respiration and surgical manipulation.

Other commercial robotic systems targeting multi-arm manipulation for complex surgical operations are usually designed to be floor-mounted or mounted on mobile chassis due to their large setup, such as the da Vinci Surgical System (Intuitive

Surgical, USA) (figure 7.7(b)) [123]. Ceiling-mounted arrangements are designed to avoid the robotic system taking up large operation space, like the EndoPAR system [122], which consists of four robot arms mounted through an aluminum gantry (figure 7.7(c)). This mounting method saves floor space while retaining a large workspace and is mainly used in laparoscopic surgeries. However, there presents a requirement on the ceiling's loadbearing ability.

The patient's physiological motion during the operation may cause deviation in imaging registration. To tackle this problem, reference markers are usually used for motion tracking, hence, real-time motion compensation. For example, in the ROSA spine robotic system [85], markers were mounted on the spine and optically tracked to update the positional registration with the imaging. The ExcelsiusGPS system applied additional optical markers placed on the contralateral PSIS, and any location offsets greater than 1.0 mm would trigger the alert automatically [86]. Patient-mounting mechanism could be a promising solution for maintaining a relatively fixed position of the robot to the patient. It is also compatible with the narrow space in the CT/MRI scanner bore due to the compact system design. But the workspace could be limited at the same time; thus patient-mounted systems are usually used in percutaneous interventions like needle-based thermal therapy [124]. Small-sized robot design can even enable the cooperation of multiple robots. He *et al* [69] developed a compact MR-compatible needle robot (figure 7.7(d)) for treating large or multiple tumors, which allows percutaneous ablation to be performed at multiple locations simultaneously using several robots. However, the physiological motion of internal organs is usually independent to the skin and the robot. Inserting the needle during apnea phases or conducting motion compensation based on real-time MRI images [125] could further reduce the targeting deviation.

Actuation mechanisms are generally considered based on the performed tasks and required precision. EM motors are the most common actuators used in surgical robots [126]. The robot end-effectors usually rely on cables, gears, and pulleys to transfer the mechanical power of EM motors [127]. The cable tension, velocity, material, number of gears, and angles of cable wrapping around pulleys are the key parameters of EM actuation. With such actuations, a series of articulated robotic arms, such as KUKA LBR Med (KUKA Inc., Germany), have already been employed to assist surgical operations, allowing clinicians to carry out complex procedures with more flexibility and precision. However, the masses of mechanical links always generate much greater gravitational torques than dynamic torques [128]. Hence, control precision and safety become noteworthy concerns when motor power cannot withstand the arm weight and motion load [129]. To date, various solutions have been proposed to enable the robotic arm to serve in a 'gravity compensation' mode [129–132]. For instance, Montalvo *et al* [129] proposed a control method based on proportional derivative control with gravity compensation for low-cost robotic-arm systems. This method reduced the gravitational torques of manipulators by estimating the largest gravity torque. Hou *et al* [131] designed a parameter identification (PI) algorithm utilizing the least-squares theory and orthogonal triangle factorization to perform the PI. The torque generated by the

PI algorithm was transferred to the KUKA torque controller for gravity compensation. Lin *et al* [132] proposed a high-order polynomial model to measure the nonlinear disturbance forces applied to the master tool manipulator of da Vinci surgical robots. This method could sequentially identify both the disturbance and gravitational forces for each manipulator link, eliminating the uneven mass distribution on the manipulator. Furthermore, due to the incompatibility of EM actuation with high magnetic field, several other actuation approaches have been investigated to assist robotic surgeries under MRI, including Shinsei ultrasonic motors, Nanomotion ultrasonic motors [133], piezoelectric motors, and pneumatic and hydraulic actuators.

MR-conditional actuation is highly desired in MRI-guided robots, as a strong magnetic field is generated by the MRI scanner and the use of ferromagnetic materials is strictly prohibited in the scanning room. Pneumatic actuators fabricated with non-ferromagnetic materials, such as 3D printing materials like acrylonitrile butadiene styrene or other resin, can be inherently MR-safe. The first MR-compatible pneumatic stepper motor (figure 7.8(a)) was developed by Stoianovici *et al* [134]. The discrete rotary motion was generated from the sequential motion of three diaphragm cylinders. Chen *et al* [135] introduced a simplified pneumatic stepper motor similar to a two-stroke engine (figure 7.8(b)), which had a step angle of 3.6° and a maximum torque of 0.8 N·m. An MR-safe pneumatic stepper motor with high stepping frequency (320 Hz) and large torque (3.7 N·m) was developed by Groenhuis *et al* [136], and its stepping motion was generated using pistons and a rack/gear to produce either linear or rotary motion (figure 7.8(c)). However,

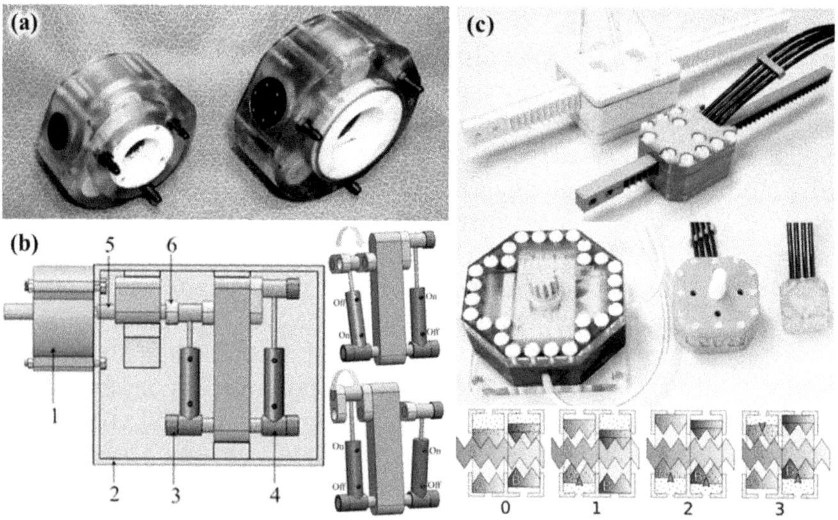

Figure 7.8. MR-conditional pneumatic actuators. (a) First MR-compatible pneumatic stepper motor (© 2007 IEEE. Reprinted, with permission, from [134]); (b) simplified pneumatic stepper motor (Adapted by permission from Springer Nature Customer Service Centre GmbH: Springer Nature, Annals Of Biomedical Engineering [135], Copyright (2014)); (c) linear and rotary MR-safe pneumatic stepper motors (© 2018 IEEE. Reprinted, with permission, from [136]).

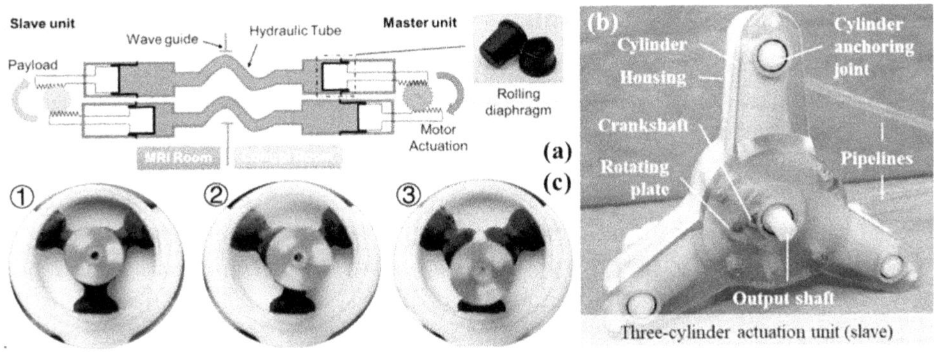

Figure 7.9. MR-conditional hydraulic actuators. (a) Leader–follower hydraulic actuator using rolling diaphragms (© 2018 IEEE. Reprinted, with permission, from [83]); (b) three-cylinder hydraulic motor (reproduced with permission from (© 2019 IEEE. Reprinted, with permission, from [139]); (c) hydraulic actuator that consists of three horizontal-mounted soft chambers (© 2020 IEEE. Reprinted, with permission, from [69]).

achieving precise control and maintaining high positional stability are still the major challenges of pneumatic actuation due to the nonlinear friction force and the high compressibility of air [137].

Hydraulic actuators can provide faster dynamic response and higher power density than pneumatic counterparts as incompressible liquid (e.g. water and oil) is used as the transmission medium. Lee *et al* [83] developed a leader–follower hydraulic system for MRI-guided intracardiac catheterization, in which the follower part located in the scanning room transferring hydraulic linear motion to rotation (figure 7.9(a)). The rolling diaphragms [138] that are used in pistons allowed efficient sliding with negligible friction. The torque under 0.1 MPa pressure was 1.47 N·m, and the dynamic response lag at 15 Hz frequency was 66 ms. The rolling diaphragm design was further implemented in a three-cylinder hydraulic motor (figure 7.9(b)) [139] for providing unlimited range of continuous bidirectional rotation, with the maximum output torque achieving 0.49 N·m. He *et al* [69] designed a hydraulic actuator (figure 7.9(c)) consisting of three horizontal-mounted soft chambers [140], to provide fine adjustment (accuracy within 0.9 mm) of the needle guide position for percutaneous ablation.

Nonmagnetic piezoelectric actuators could be more compact than fluid-driven actuators and could provide fast dynamic response without the issue of overshooting. The application can be found in the MRI-guided lumbar injection robot [141], with the linear guides and lead screws made of MR-conditional aluminum. The robot tip positioning accuracy reached 0.51 ± 0.27 mm in free space and 1.70 ± 0.21 mm in MRI-guided phantom study. When using piezoelectric actuation, the actuator and the cables must be covered with RF shielding to avoid artifacts caused in the imaging process, while the image SNR could still be reduced significantly during the robot motion due to the high-frequency EM signals [133, 142]. Su *et al* [143] developed a piezoelectric motor driver using linear amplifiers that could generate clean signals with precise waveform. However, high-performance drivers and control methods for piezoelectric actuators are still not commercially available yet.

7.5 Discussion and conclusion

Image-guided robotic interventions are a multidisciplinary research topic that requires combined efforts from surgeons, engineers, and radiologists to drive development. Increasing temporal and spatial resolution of images will be the research and commercialization focus for rapid and *in situ* guidance. We can foresee MRI, a radiation-free modality that provides high contrast soft-tissue imaging, will be widely adopted in intra-op image-guided interventions. MRI still meets challenges in popularization due to its high-cost construction/maintenance and bulky size. Under this condition, compact and portable MRI scanners become a direction for research and development. Regarding intra-op CT or positron emission tomography guidance, reduction of the radiation dose will be the priority, for which advances of artificial intelligences (AI) (e.g. generative adversarial network) enable low-dose image reconstruction and denoising. One reported [144] that 80% dose reduction can be accomplished with the use of AI-based algorithm or model, relative to the conventional filtered back projection used in the image reconstruction. Besides individual imaging modalities, multimodal fusion is also accepted as a promising direction to enhance surgical navigation, also through the augmented reality techniques for visual or even haptic guidance [145].

The design of MR-conditional mechanisms usually meets challenges of making robot structures or actuators compact and compatible with the strong magnetic field. Fluid-driven actuation becomes a popular option, but the trade-offs are usually imposed among the efficiency of mechanical transmission, the resolution of fluid-driven motion, and the overall size of actuators. Currently, the performances of fluid-driven actuators, in terms of output motion resolution and torque, are still not comparable to EM motors, while piezoelectric motors need further technical improvement to reduce the MR SNR degradation during actuating. Besides actuator size, robot structure should be sufficiently compact to operate in the space of scanning bore shared with the head/body coils. Patient-mounted designs are proposed with minimized robot size, and as a result, the DoFs and workspace may be sacrificed. Due to these limitations and high development costs, the existing robots for MRI-guided interventions are still procedure-specific, without a universal platform available. To empower the robot manipulation autonomy, further cooperation is required among fast imaging, positional tracking, and real-time control interfaces of MRI, which may have to be developed by a third-party company (e.g. RTHawk Heartvista, USA). This will lead to the trend for future software advances.

In addition to conventional surgical robots, nanorobots have emerged as a proof-of-concept technique in medical diagnosis and treatment. Nanorobots are generally smaller than a millimeter and made of biocompatible chemicals (e.g. iron molecules). After being injected into the human body, they are excreted or degraded by microbiological micro-ambiance [146]. Nanorobots have the potential to be applied in various treatments, such as blood clot defusing, drug delivery, gene delivery, or even pathogen isolation [147, 148]. Accurate delivery of the nanorobots requires precise actuation methods for control as well as detailed visual monitoring for navigation. Current actuation methods under investigation (e.g. magnetic, electric, and acoustic actuation) have been validated to drive nanorobot clusters but rarely refined to individuals. Although MRI [149], US [150], and x-ray [151] have been explored for the visual monitoring of nanorobot clusters, the tracking of ultra-small outliers is still challenging. When accessing highly eloquent areas of the patient brain, nanorobots have the potential to interfere with the patient's personality and character, which are collected and stored in the brain [152]. This raises significant ethical issues, complicating the regulatory approval (e.g. FDA, European Medicines Agency). Furthermore, nanorobots suffer from technical limitations related to biocompatibility and safety, which could elicit unwanted immunological responses and intrinsic inflammatory reactions. In the future, significant efforts will be concentrated on improving the fabrication, control intelligence, and the precision of real-time monitoring [147].

7.6 Disclosure statements

Russell Taylor and Johns Hopkins University (JHU) may be entitled to royalty payments related to technology discussed in this chapter, and Dr Taylor has received or may receive some portion of these royalties. Also, Dr Taylor is a paid consultant to and owns equity in Galen Robotics, Inc. These arrangements have been reviewed and approved by JHU in accordance with its conflict-of-interest policy.

Ka-Wai Kwok and The University of Hong Kong (HKU) may be entitled to royalty payments related to technology discussed in this book chapter, and Dr Kwok has received or may receive some portion of these royalties. Also, Dr Kwok is a co-founder and a paid director of Agilis Robotics, Ltd., and owns equity in Agilis Robotics, Ltd. These arrangements have been reviewed and approved by HKU in accordance with its conflict-of-interest policy.

References

[1] Simaan N, Yasin R M and Wang L 2018 Medical technologies and challenges of robot-assisted minimally invasive intervention and diagnostics *Annu. Rev. Control Robot. Auton. Syst.* **1** 465–90

[2] Kwoh Y S, Hou J, Jonckheere E A and Hayati S 1988 A robot with improved absolute positioning accuracy for CT guided stereotactic brain surgery *IEEE Trans. Biomed. Eng.* **35** 153–60

[3] Forsmark A *et al* 2018 Health economic analysis of open and robot-assisted laparoscopic surgery for prostate cancer within the prospective multicentre LAPPRO trial *Eur. Urol.* **74** 816–24

[4] Gofrit O N, Mikahail A A, Zorn K C, Zagaja G P, Steinberg G D and Shalhav A L 2008 Surgeons' perceptions and injuries during and after urologic laparoscopic surgery *Urology* **71** 404–7

[5] Peltier L F 1993 *Orthopedics: A History and Iconography* (San Francisco, CA: Norman Publishing)

[6] Zheng G and Nolte L P 2015 Computer-assisted orthopedic surgery: current state and future perspective *Front. Surg.* **2** 66

[7] Unger M, Berger J and Melzer A 2021 Robot-assisted image-guided interventions *Front. Robot. AI* **8** 221
[8] Robb R A, Hoffman E A, Sinak L J, Harris L D and Ritman E L 1983 High-speed three-dimensional x-ray computed tomography: The dynamic spatial reconstructor *Proc. IEEE* **71** 308–19
[9] Flohr T G *et al* 2006 First performance evaluation of a dual-source CT (DSCT) system *Eur. Radiol.* **16** 256–68
[10] Kubo T *et al* 2008 Radiation dose reduction in chest CT: a review *Am. J. Roentgenol.* **190** 335–43
[11] Silverman P M, Kalender W A and Hazle J D 2001 Common terminology for single and multislice helical CT *Am. J. Roentgenol.* **176** 1135–6
[12] Baumueller S *et al* 2012 Low-dose CT of the lung: potential value of iterative reconstructions *Eur. Radiol.* **22** 2597–606
[13] Feng S, Tian W, Sun Y, Liu Y and Wei Y 2019 Effect of robot-assisted surgery on lumbar pedicle screw internal fixation in patients with osteoporosis *World Neurosurg.* **125** e1057–62
[14] Wikipedia Magnetic resonance imaging. https://en.wikipedia.org/wiki/Magnetic_resonance_imaging (accessed 2022)
[15] Rogers T and Lederman R J 2015 Interventional CMR: clinical applications and future directions *Curr. Cardiol. Rep.* **17** 1–9
[16] Liu Z *et al* 2019 A two-stage approach for automated prostate lesion detection and classification with mask R-CNN and weakly supervised deep neural network *The Workshop on Artificial Intelligence in Radiation Therapy*
[17] Kwok W E 2022 Basic principles of and practical guide to clinical MRI radiofrequency coils *RadioGraphics* **42** 898–918
[18] Dale B M, Brown M A and Semelka R C 2015 *MRI: Basic Principles and Applications* (New York: Wiley)
[19] Fernández-Gutiérrez F *et al* 2015 Comparative ergonomic workflow and user experience analysis of MRI versus fluoroscopy-guided vascular interventions: an iliac angioplasty exemplar case study *Int. J. Comput. Assisted Radiol. Surg.* **10** 1639–50
[20] Kwok K-W *et al* 2014 Interfacing fast multi-phase cardiac image registration with MRI-based catheter tracking for MRI-guided electrophysiological ablative procedures *Circulation* **130** A18568
[21] Hyperfine Swoop portable MR imaging system https://hyperfine.io/products (accessed 16 February, 2023)
[22] Liu Y *et al* 2021 A low-cost and shielding-free ultra-low-field brain MRI scanner *Nat. Commun.* **12** 1–14
[23] FDA 2020 Ultrasound imaging https://fda.gov/radiation-emitting-products/medical-imaging/ultrasound-imaging (accessed 2022)
[24] Hides J and Nofsinger C C 2009 Musculoskeletal ultrasound clinical roundtable discussion *Athletic Train. Sports Health Care* **1** 104–5
[25] Heuvelings C C *et al* 2019 Chest ultrasound compared to chest X-ray for pediatric pulmonary tuberculosis *Pediatr. Pulmonol.* **54** 1914–20
[26] Palaniswamy S S and Subramanyam P 2018 Unusual sites of metastatic and benign i 131 uptake in patients with differentiated thyroid carcinoma *Indian J. Endocrinol. Metab.* **22** 740

[27] Merz E and Abramowicz J 2012 3D/4D ultrasound in prenatal diagnosis: is it time for routine use? *Clin. Obstet. Gynecol.* **55** 336–51

[28] Phee L *et al* 2006 Ultrasound guided robotic biopsy of the prostate *Int. J. Humanoid Rob.* **3** 463–83

[29] Bassan H, Hayes T, Patel R V and Moallem M 2007 A novel manipulator for 3D ultrasound guided percutaneous needle insertion *Proc. of the IEEE Int. Conf. on Robotics and Automation*

[30] Fichtinger G *et al* 2006 Robotically assisted prostate brachytherapy with transrectal ultrasound guidance—phantom experiments *Brachytherapy* **5** 14–26

[31] Hungr N, Baumann M, Long J-A and Troccaz J 2012 A 3-D ultrasound robotic prostate brachytherapy system with prostate motion tracking *IEEE Trans. Rob.* **28** 1382–97

[32] Boda-Heggemann J *et al* 2019 Ultrasound-based repositioning and real-time monitoring for abdominal SBRT in DIBH *Phys. Med.* **65** 46–52

[33] Phee L *et al* 2005 Ultrasound guided robotic system for transperineal biopsy of the prostate *Proc. of the IEEE International Conf. on Robotics and Automation* pp 1315–20

[34] Bax J *et al* 2011 A compact mechatronic system for 3D ultrasound guided prostate interventions *Med. Phys.* **38** 1055–69

[35] Grondin J, Payen T, Wang S and Konofagou E E 2015 Real-time monitoring of high intensity focused ultrasound (HIFU) ablation of *in vitro* canine livers using harmonic motion imaging for focused ultrasound (HMIFU) *J. Visual. Exp.* **105** e53050

[36] Harris S *et al* 1997 The Probot—an active robot for prostate resection *Proc. Inst. Mech. Eng. Part H J. Eng. Med.* **211** 317–25

[37] Jakopec M, Baena F R, Harris S J, Gomes P, Cobb J and Davies B L 2003 The hands-on orthopaedic robot' Acrobot': early clinical trials of total knee replacement surgery *IEEE Trans. Robot. Autom.* **19** 902–11

[38] Sistrom C L and McKay N L 2005 Costs, charges, and revenues for hospital diagnostic imaging procedures: differences by modality and hospital characteristics *J. Am. Coll. Radiol.* **2** 511–9

[39] McBeth P B, Louw D F, Rizun P R and Sutherland G R 2004 Robotics in neurosurgery *Am. J. Surg.* **188** 68–75

[40] Guo Z, Leong M C-W, Su H, Kwok K-W, Chan D T-M and Poon W-S 2020 Prospective techniques for magnetic resonance imaging–guided robot-assisted stereotactic neurosurgery *Handbook of Robotic and Image-Guided Surgery* (Amsterdam: Elsevier) pp 585–98

[41] Guo Z, Leong M C-W, Su H, Kwok K-W, Chan D T-M and Poon W-S 2018 Techniques for stereotactic neurosurgery: beyond the frame, toward the intraoperative magnetic resonance imaging–guided and robot-assisted approaches *World Neurosurg.* **116** 77–87

[42] Vitiello V, Kwok K-W and Yang G-Z 2012 Introduction to Robot-Assisted Minimally Invasive Surgery (MIS) *Medical Robotics* (Amsterdam: Elsevier) pp 1–P1

[43] Zanotto V *et al* 2011 A master-slave haptic system for neurosurgery *Appl. Bionics Biomech.* **8** 209–20

[44] Mattei T A, Rodriguez A H, Sambhara D and Mendel E 2014 Current state-of-the-art and future perspectives of robotic technology in neurosurgery *Neurosurg. Rev.* **37** 357–66

[45] Yamamoto T 2020 Recent advancement of technologies and the transition to new concepts in epilepsy surgery *Neurol. Med. Chir.* **60** 581–93

[46] Guo Z *et al* 2018 Compact design of a hydraulic driving robot for intraoperative MRI-guided bilateral stereotactic neurosurgery *IEEE Robot. Autom. Lett.* **3** 2515–22

[47] Huang M, Tetreault T A, Vaishnav A, York P J and Staub B N 2021 The current state of navigation in robotic spine surgery *Ann. Trans. Med.* **9** 86
[48] Payne C J, Vyas K, Bautista-Salinas D, Zhang D, Marcus H J and Yang G-Z 2021 Shared-control robots *Neurosurgical Robotics* ed H J Marcus and C J Payne (New York: Humana Neuromethods) 162 pp 63–79
[49] Taylor R *et al* 1999 A steady-hand robotic system for microsurgical augmentation *Int. J. Robot. Res.* **18** 1201–10
[50] Mitchell B *et al* 2007 Development and application of a new steady-hand manipulator for retinal surgery *Proc. of the IEEE Int. Conf. on Robotics and Automation (Piscataway, NJ)* (IEEE) pp 623–9
[51] Hongo K *et al* 2002 NeuRobot: telecontrolled micromanipulator system for minimally invasive microneurosurgery—preliminary results *Neurosurgery* **51** 985–8
[52] Li G *et al* 2015 Robotic system for MRI-guided stereotactic neurosurgery *IEEE Trans. Biomed. Eng.* **62** 1077–88
[53] Nycz C J *et al* 2017 Mechanical validation of an MRI compatible stereotactic neurosurgery robot in preparation for pre-clinical trials *IEEE/RSJ Int. Conf. on Intelligent Robots and Systems (IROS) (Piscataway, NJ)* (IEEE) pp 1677–84
[54] NHS 2021 Overview–Biopsy https://nhs.uk/conditions/biopsy (accessed 2022)
[55] Groenhuis V, Siepel F J, Veltman J, van Zandwijk J K and Stramigioli S 2018 Stormram 4: an MR safe robotic system for breast biopsy *Ann. Biomed. Eng.* **46** 1686–96
[56] WHO 2022 Breast cancer https://who.int/news-room/fact-sheets/detail/breast-cancer (accessed 2022)
[57] Helbich T, Matzek W and Fuchsjäger M 2004 Stereotactic and ultrasound-guided breast biopsy *Eur. Radiol.* **14** 383–93
[58] Welleweerd M K, Siepel F J, Groenhuis V, Veltman J and Stramigioli S 2020 Design of an end-effector for robot-assisted ultrasound-guided breast biopsies *Int. J. Comput. Assist. Radiol. Surg.* **15** 681–90
[59] Navarro-Alarcon D *et al* 2017 Developing a compact robotic needle driver for MRI-guided breast biopsy in tight environments *IEEE Robot. Autom. Lett.* **2** 1648–55
[60] Hansen N L *et al* 2017 Multicentre evaluation of targeted and systematic biopsies using magnetic resonance and ultrasound image-fusion guided transperineal prostate biopsy in patients with a previous negative biopsy *BJU Int.* **120** 631–8
[61] Bomers J, Bosboom D, Tigelaar G, Sabisch J, Fütterer J and Yakar D 2017 Feasibility of a 2nd generation MR-compatible manipulator for transrectal prostate biopsy guidance *Eur. Radiol.* **27** 1776–82
[62] Moreira P *et al* 2017 The Miriam robot: a novel robotic system for MR-guided needle insertion in the prostate *J. Med. Robot. Res.* **2** 1750006
[63] ClearPoint Neuro 2023 Biologics and drug delivery partners https://clearpointneuro.com/biologics-drug-delivery/ (accessed 16 February 2023)
[64] Jessen N H, Jensen H, Falborg A Z, Glerup H, Gronbaek H and Vedsted P 2021 Abdominal investigations in the year preceding a diagnosis of abdominal cancer: a register-based cohort study in Denmark *Cancer Epidemiol.* **72** 101926
[65] Fabbri C *et al* 2014 Endoscopic ultrasound-guided treatments: Are we getting evidence based-a systematic review *World J. Gastroenterol.* **20** 8424
[66] Shah A R, Al-Hanayneh M, Chowdhry M, Bilal M and Singh S 2019 Endoscopic ultrasound guided liver biopsy for parenchymal liver disease *World J. Hepatol.* **11** 335

[67] Saraireh H A, Bilal M and Singh S 2017 Role of endoscopic ultrasound in liver disease: where do we stand in 2017? *World J. Hepatol.* **9** 1013

[68] Johnson K D, Laoveeravat P, Yee E U, Perisetti A, Thandassery R B and Tharian B 2020 Endoscopic ultrasound guided liver biopsy: recent evidence *World J. Gastrointest. Endosc.* **12** 83

[69] He Z *et al* 2020 Design of a percutaneous MRI-guided needle robot with soft fluid-driven actuator *IEEE Robot. Autom. Lett.* **5** 2100–7

[70] Hsiao Y-H, Kuo S-J, Tsai H-D, Chou M-C and Yeh G-P 2016 Clinical application of high-intensity focused ultrasound in cancer therapy *J. Cancer* **7** 225

[71] Dai J *et al* 2021 A robotic platform to navigate MRI-guided focused ultrasound system *IEEE Robot. Autom. Lett.* **6** 5137–44

[72] Menaker S A, Shah S S, Snelling B M, Sur S, Starke R M and Peterson E C 2018 Current applications and future perspectives of robotics in cerebrovascular and endovascular neurosurgery *J. Neurointerv. Surg.* **10** 78–82

[73] Moscucci M 2020 *Grossman & Baim's Cardiac Catheterization, Angiography, and Intervention* (Ambler, PA: Lippincott Williams & Wilkins) 9th edn

[74] Saltzberg S S *et al* 2005 Is endovascular therapy the preferred treatment for all visceral artery aneurysms? *Ann. Vasc. Surg.* **19** 507–15

[75] Mahmud E, Pourdjabbar A, Ang L, Behnamfar O, Patel M P and Reeves R R 2017 Robotic technology in interventional cardiology: current status and future perspectives *Catheter. Cardiovasc. Interv.* **90** 956–62

[76] Armacost M P *et al* 2007 Accurate and reproducible target navigation with the Stereotaxis Niobe® magnetic navigation system *J. Cardiovasc. Electrophysiol.* **18** S26–31

[77] Chautems C, Tonazzini A, Floreano D and Nelson B J 2017 A variable stiffness catheter controlled with an external magnetic field *Proc. of the IEEE/RSJ Int. Conf. on Intelligent Robots and Systems (IROS) (Piscataway, NJ)* (IEEE) pp 181–6

[78] Kundrat D *et al* 2021 An MR-Safe endovascular robotic platform: design, control, and ex-vivo evaluation *IEEE Trans. Biomed. Eng.* **68** 3110–21

[79] Gruentzig A 1982 Results from coronary angioplasty and implications for the future *Am. Heart J.* **103** 779–83

[80] Vandenberghe W and Hoste E 2019 Contrast-associated acute kidney injury: does it really exist, and if so, what to do about it? *F1000Research* **8** 1–9

[81] Granada J F *et al* 2011 First-in-human evaluation of a novel robotic-assisted coronary angioplasty system *JACC: Cardiovasc. Interv.* **4** 460–5

[82] Fang G *et al* 2021 Soft robotic manipulator for intraoperative MRI-guided transoral laser microsurgery *Sci. Robot.* **6** eabg5575

[83] Lee K-H *et al* 2018 MR safe robotic manipulator for MRI-guided intracardiac catheterization *IEEE/ASME Trans. Mechatron.* **23** 586–95

[84] Su H, Li G, Rucker D C, Webster R J and Fischer G S 2016 A concentric tube continuum robot with piezoelectric actuation for MRI-guided closed-loop targeting *Ann. Biomed. Eng.* **44** 2863–73

[85] Lonjon N, Chan-Seng E, Costalat V, Bonnafoux B, Vassal M and Boetto J 2016 Robot-assisted spine surgery: feasibility study through a prospective case-matched analysis *Eur. Spine. J.* **25** 947–55

[86] Crawford N, Johnson N and Theodore N 2020 Ensuring navigation integrity using robotics in spine surgery *J. Robot. Surg.* **14** 177–83

[87] Elfring R, de la Fuente M and Radermacher K 2010 Assessment of optical localizer accuracy for computer aided surgery systems *Comput. Aided Surg.* **15** 1–12

[88] Sorriento A *et al* 2019 Optical and electromagnetic tracking systems for biomedical applications: a critical review on potentialities and limitations *IEEE Rev. Biomed. Eng.* **13** 212–32

[89] Poulin F and Amiot L-P 2002 Interference during the use of an electromagnetic tracking system under OR conditions *J. Biomech.* **35** 733–7

[90] Wang X *et al* 2018 Experimental validation of robot-assisted cardiovascular catheterization: model-based versus model-free control *Int. J. Comput. Assist. Radiol. Surg.* **13** 797–804

[91] Burgner-Kahrs J, Rucker D C and Choset H 2015 Continuum robots for medical applications: a survey *IEEE Trans. Rob.* **31** 1261–80

[92] Kwok K-W, Wurdemann H, Arezzo A, Menciassi A and Althoefer K 2022 Soft robot-assisted minimally invasive surgery and interventions: advances and outlook *Proc. IEEE* **110** 871–92

[93] Wang X, Li Y and Kwok K-W 2021 A survey for machine learning-based control of continuum robots *Front. Robot. AI* **8** 730330

[94] Park Y-L *et al* 2010 Real-time estimation of 3-D needle shape and deflection for MRI-guided interventions *IEEE/ASME Trans. Mechatron.* **15** 906–15

[95] Roesthuis R J, Kemp M, van den Dobbelsteen J J and Misra S 2013 Three-dimensional needle shape reconstruction using an array of fiber Bragg grating sensors *IEEE/ASME Trans. Mechatron.* **19** 1115–26

[96] van de Berg N J, Dankelman J and van den Dobbelsteen J J 2015 Design of an actively controlled steerable needle with tendon actuation and FBG-based shape sensing *Med. Eng. Phys.* **37** 617–22

[97] Roesthuis R J, Janssen S and Misra S 2013 On using an array of fiber Bragg grating sensors for closed-loop control of flexible minimally invasive surgical instruments *Proc. of the IEEE/RSJ Int. Conf. on Intelligent Robots and Systems* pp 2545–51

[98] Lunwei Z, Jinwu Q, Linyong S and Yanan Z 2004 FBG sensor devices for spatial shape detection of intelligent colonoscope *Proc. of the IEEE Int. Conf. on Robotics and Automation (ICRA'04)* pp 834–40

[99] Dong Z *et al* 2022 Shape tracking and feedback control of cardiac catheter using MRI-guided robotic platform—validation with pulmonary vein isolation simulator in MRI *IEEE Trans. Rob.* **38** 2781–98

[100] Shi C *et al* 2016 Shape sensing techniques for continuum robots in minimally invasive surgery: a survey *IEEE Trans. Biomed. Eng.* **64** 1665–78

[101] Wang X *et al* 2020 Eye-in-hand visual servoing enhanced with sparse strain measurement for soft continuum robots *IEEE Robot. Autom. Lett.* **5** 2161–8

[102] Lun T L T, Wang K, Ho J D, Lee K-H, Sze K Y and Kwok K-W 2019 Real-time surface shape sensing for soft and flexible structures using fiber Bragg gratings *IEEE Robot. Autom. Lett.* **4** 1454–61

[103] Wang K *et al* 2021 Large-scale surface shape sensing with learning-based computational mechanics *Adv. Intell. Syst.* **3** 2100089

[104] Wang T, Ciobanu L, Zhang X and Webb A 2008 Inductively coupled RF coil design for simultaneous microimaging of multiple samples *Concepts Magn. Reson. B: Magn. Reson. Eng. Educ. J.* **33** 236–43

[105] Seevinck P R, de Leeuw H, Bos C and Bakker C J 2011 Highly localized positive contrast of small paramagnetic objects using 3D center-out radial sampling with off-resonance reception *Magn. Reson. Med.* **65** 146–56

[106] Wang W 2015 Magnetic resonance–guided active catheter tracking *Magn. Reson. Imaging Clin.* **23** 579–89

[107] Dumoulin C L, Souza S and Darrow R 1993 Real-time position monitoring of invasive devices using magnetic resonance *Magn. Reson. Med.* **29** 411–5

[108] Dumoulin C L, Mallozzi R P, Darrow R D and Schmidt E J 2010 Phase-field dithering for active catheter tracking *Magn. Reson. Med.* **63** 1398–403

[109] Chen Y *et al* 2015 Design and fabrication of MR-tracked metallic stylet for gynecologic brachytherapy *IEEE/ASME Trans. Mechatron.* **21** 956–62

[110] Ooi M B, Aksoy M, Maclaren J, Watkins R D and Bammer R 2013 Prospective motion correction using inductively coupled wireless RF coils *Magn. Reson. Med.* **70** 639–47

[111] Galassi F, Brujic D, Rea M, Lambert N, Desouza N and Ristic M 2015 Fast and accurate localization of multiple RF markers for tracking in MRI-guided interventions *Magn. Reson. Mater. Phys., Biol. Med.* **28** 33–48

[112] Weiss S *et al* 2004 In vivo safe catheter visualization and slice tracking using an optically detunable resonant marker *Magn. Reson. Med.* **52** 860–8

[113] Cheung C-L, Ho J D-L, Vardhanabhuti V, Chang H-C and Kwok K-W 2020 Design and fabrication of wireless multilayer tracking marker for intraoperative MRI-guided interventions *IEEE/ASME Trans. Mechatron.* **25** 1016–25

[114] Bock M *et al* 2004 MR-guided intravascular procedures: real-time parameter control and automated slice positioning with active tracking coils *J. Magn. Reson. Imaging* **19** 580–9

[115] Rea M, McRobbie D, Elhawary H, Tse Z T H, Lampérth M and Young I 2008 System for 3-D real-time tracking of MRI-compatible devices by image processing *IEEE/ASME Trans. Mechatron.* **13** 379–82

[116] Eggers H, Weiss S, Boernert P and Boesiger P 2003 Image-based tracking of optically detunable parallel resonant circuits *Magn. Reson. Med.* **49** 1163–74

[117] Wong MSE E, Zhang Q, Duerk J and Lewin J 2000 MD, and M. Wendt PhD, An optical system for wireless detuning of parallel resonant circuits *J. Magn. Reson. Imaging* **12** 632–8

[118] Su H *et al* 2022 State of the art and future opportunities in MRI-guided robot-assisted surgery and interventions *Proc. IEEE* **110** 968–92

[119] Ringel F *et al* 2012 Accuracy of robot-assisted placement of lumbar and sacral pedicle screws: a prospective randomized comparison to conventional freehand screw implantation *Spine* **37** E496–501

[120] Kochanski R B, Lombardi J M, Laratta J L, Lehman R A and O'Toole J E 2019 Image-guided navigation and robotics in spine surgery *Neurosurgery* **84** 1179–89

[121] Douissard J, Hagen M E and Morel P 2019 The da Vinci surgical system *Bariatric Robotic Surgery* (Berlin: Springer) pp 13–27

[122] Staub C, Osa T, Knoll A and Bauernschmitt R 2010 Automation of tissue piercing using circular needles and vision guidance for computer aided laparoscopic surgery *Proc. of the IEEE Int. Conf. on Robotics and Automation* pp 4585–90

[123] DiMaio S, Hanuschik M and Kreaden U 2011 The da Vinci surgical system *Surgical Robotics* (Berlin: Springer) pp 199–217

[124] Bibi Farouk Z, Jiang S, Yang Z and Umar A 2022 A brief insight on magnetic resonance conditional neurosurgery robots *Ann. Biomed. Eng.* **50** 138–56

[125] Maurin B *et al* 2008 A patient-mounted robotic platform for CT-scan guided procedures *IEEE Trans. Biomed. Eng.* **55** 2417–25

[126] Stoianovici D 2005 Multi-imager compatible actuation principles in surgical robotics *Int. J. Med. Robot. Comput. Assist. Surg.* **1** 86–100

[127] Miyasaka M, Matheson J, Lewis A and Hannaford B 2015 Measurement of the cable-pulley coulomb and viscous friction for a cable-driven surgical robotic system *Proc. of the IEEE/RSJ International Conf. on Intelligent Robots and Systems (IROS)* pp 804–10

[128] Arakelian V 2016 Gravity compensation in robotics *Adv. Robot.* **30** 79–96

[129] Montalvo W, Escobar-Naranjo J, Garcia C A and Garcia M V 2020 Low-cost automation for gravity compensation of robotic arm *Appl. Sci.* **10** 3823

[130] Berthet-Rayne P *et al* 2018 The i2snake robotic platform for endoscopic surgery *Ann. Biomed. Eng.* **46** 1663–75

[131] Hou C, Zhao Y, Song G and Wang J 2018 Gravity compensation of KUKA LBR IIWA through fast robot interface *Proc. of the IEEE 8th Annual Int. Conf. on CYBER Technology in Automation, Control, and Intelligent Systems (CYBER)* pp 164–8

[132] Lin H, Hui C-W V, Wang Y, Deguet A, Kazanzides P and Au K S 2019 A reliable gravity compensation control strategy for dVRK robotic arms with nonlinear disturbance forces *IEEE Robot. Autom. Lett.* **4** 3892–9

[133] Fischer G S, Krieger A, Iordachita I, Csoma C, Whitcomb L L and Fichtinger G 2008 MRI compatibility of robot actuation techniques–a comparative study *Med. Image Comput. Comput. Assist Interv.* **11** 509–17

[134] Stoianovici D, Patriciu A, Petrisor D, Mazilu D and Kavoussi L 2007 A new type of motor: pneumatic step motor *IEEE/ASME Trans. Mechatron.* **12** 98–106

[135] Chen Y, Kwok K-W and Tse Z T H 2014 An MR-conditional high-torque pneumatic stepper motor for MRI-guided and robot-assisted intervention *Ann. Biomed. Eng.* **42** 1823–33

[136] Groenhuis V and Stramigioli S 2018 Rapid prototyping high-performance MR safe pneumatic stepper motors *IEEE/ASME Trans. Mechatron.* **23** 1843–53

[137] Yang B, Tan U-X, McMillan A B, Gullapalli R and Desai J P 2010 Design and control of a 1-DOF MRI-compatible pneumatically actuated robot with long transmission lines *IEEE/ASME Trans. Mechatron.* **16** 1040–8

[138] Whitney J P, Glisson M F, Brockmeyer E L and Hodgins J K 2014 A low-friction passive fluid transmission and fluid-tendon soft actuator *Proc. of the IEEE/RSJ International Conf. on Intelligent Robots and Systems* pp 2801–8

[139] Dong Z *et al* 2019 High-performance continuous hydraulic motor for MR safe robotic teleoperation *IEEE Robot. Autom. Lett.* **4** 1964–71

[140] Blumenschein L H and Mengüç Y 2019 Generalized delta mechanisms from soft actuators *Proc. of the 2019 2nd IEEE Int. Conf. on Soft Robotics (RoboSoft)* pp 249–56

[141] Li G *et al* 2020 Body-mounted robotic assistant for MRI-guided low back pain injection *Int. J. Comput. Assist. Radiol. Surg.* **15** 321–31

[142] Krieger A *et al* 2011 Development and evaluation of an actuated MRI-compatible robotic system for MRI-guided prostate intervention *IEEE/ASME Trans. Mechatron.* **18** 273–84

[143] Su H *et al* 2014 Piezoelectrically actuated robotic system for MRI-guided prostate percutaneous therapy *IEEE/ASME Trans. Mechatron.* **20** 1920–32

[144] Seah J, Brady Z, Ewert K and Law M 2021 Artificial intelligence in medical imaging: implications for patient radiation safety *Br. J. Radiol.* **94** 20210406

[145] Leibrandt K, Marcus H J, Kwok K-W and Yang G-Z 2014 Implicit active constraints for a compliant surgical manipulator *Proc. of the IEEE Int. Conf. on Robotics and Automation (ICRA) (Piscataway, NJ)* (IEEE) pp 276–83

[146] Jiang J, Yang L and Zhang L 2021 Closed-loop control of a Helmholtz coil system for accurate actuation of magnetic microrobot swarms *IEEE Robot. Autom. Lett.* **6** 827–34

[147] Dong Y, Wang L, Iacovacci V, Wang X, Zhang L and Nelson B 2022 Magnetic helical micro-/nanomachines: recent progress and perspective *Matter* **5** 77–109

[148] Al-Sharif M, Awen B and Molvi K 2010 Nanotechnology in cancer therapy: a review *J. Chem. Pharm. Res.* **2** 161–8

[149] Yan X *et al* 2017 Multifunctional biohybrid magnetite microrobots for imaging-guided therapy *Sci. Robot.* **2** eaaq1155

[150] Wang Q and Zhang L 2020 Ultrasound imaging and tracking of micro/nanorobots: From individual to collectives *IEEE Open J. Nanotechnol.* **1** 6–17

[151] Martel S *et al* 2009 MRI-based medical nanorobotic platform for the control of magnetic nanoparticles and flagellated bacteria for target interventions in human capillaries *Int. J. Robot. Res.* **28** 1169–82

[152] Capo L and Lafuente J 2022 Nanorobots in neurosurgery *Introduction to Robotics in Minimally Invasive Neurosurgery* (Berlin: Springer) pp 69–76

Chapter 8

Surgical applications in medical artificial intelligence

Jamie B J Chen and Jason Y K Chan

8.1 Introduction

8.1.1 What is artificial intelligence?

In 1955, John McCarthy defined artificial intelligence (AI) as 'the science and engineering of making intelligent machines' [1], which referred to the study of algorithms that empowered machines with the ability to realize self-learning, reason, and perform cognitive functions, solving problems that require human input [2, 3]. There are four characteristics that AI possesses according to the Defense Advanced Research Projects Agency, which include perceiving, reasoning, learning, and abstracting [4].

In the early stage of AI's development, these technologies have been universally implemented to solve advanced mathematical problems [1]. Nowadays, AI has gradually penetrated every corner of our daily life, such as autonomous driving and robot-guided systems, targeted advertising based on our shopping history, and intelligent housing systems. *AlphaZero*, an algorithmic program designed by Google subsidiary *DeepMind*, mastered moves and strategies for playing chess just after 4 h of learning, and unbelievably defeated the world champion, which put AI and its potential into the limelight.

8.1.2 The short but splendid history of AI in medicine

According to searching results of PubMed (a web-based search engine by the National Library of Medicine), the first published article or report with the idea of computer-assisted systems applied in medicine can be traced back to the 1950s. PubMed was also the main information source for those digital analyzers and established a solid foundation for future exploration and development of AI applications [5]. Then came the 'AI winter', due to reduced funding and interests. It was not until the innovation of collaborating systems, such as the *Stanford*

doi:10.1088/978-0-7503-4637-5ch8

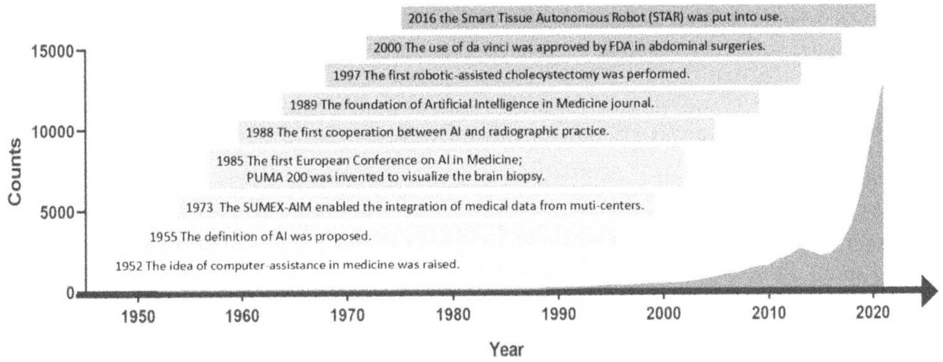

Figure 8.1. Great progresses and milestones of artificial intelligence in medicine during 1952–2022.

University Medical Experimental-Artificial Intelligence in Medicine (SUMEX-AIM) in 1973 that demonstrated the feasibility of applying AI to medicine. It built a time-shared intelligent communicating platform for clinicians and researchers in different areas and from various institutions to fulfill the collaboration, which brought the topic back to the spotlight. After that, the invention of neural network designs and the fifth generation of the computer in the 1980s greatly promoted the combination of medicine and computer science to a deeper level. The first European Conference on AI's clinical applications in 1985 and the foundation of *Artificial Intelligence in Medicine* journal in 1989 symbolized the step into a new era [6]. With the rapid development of medical knowledge and the increasing demands for the healthcare industry, the notion of the clinical transformation of AI in medicine was consequently jumpstarted [6] (figure 8.1).

8.2 AI subfields and their applications in clinical medicine

Since the objective of AI is to solve the problems with intelligent machines or computers, a constantly growing number of subfields were explored and enlarged to augment what AI could do to assist clinical work and medical research.

8.2.1 Machine learning

Machine learning (ML), as a principle subset of AI, is the computational algorithm that learns from experience and then improves its performance automatically [7]. One of the most common utilizations of ML in medicine is to predict outcomes from personal or exogenetic data produced in clinical processes, such as individual-patient profiles and epidemiological information [7]. The datasets would be separated into 'training sets' from which the machine can learn and analyze and 'testing sets' in which it can repeatedly adjust the weight of all data to improve its accuracy and deduce an ideal predictive model. If the algorithm is taught by direct programming, it can be called 'explicit learning', and the other that learns by observing and analyzing by itself can be termed 'implicit learning' [8]. The merit of ML is that it can frequently and instantly upgrade the information, integrate it, and provide a personalized treatment strategy, which surpasses the human's capability of speed and volume of data processing.

8.2.2 Deep learning and artificial neural network

Deep learning (DL), a more sophisticated algorithm in the field of ML, characterizes vast amounts of data without human guidance, driving the recent rise of AI to a large extent [9]. Refinement of the algorithm is attributed to automatically repeated training in an artificial neural network (ANN), a structure inspired by biological nervous systems and composed of an input layer, output layer, and numerous hidden layers between them, plentiful computational units similar to neurons. With well-developed mathematical operations and computational power, more autoencoders were created to realize different functions, such as elaborating complex relations between the input and output. Meanwhile, many algorithms were designed to simplify the calculation and skip some unnecessary procedures so that the AI could be more accessible to more devices [10, 11].

8.2.3 Natural language processing

By extracting useful information from massive free text and integrating it into structured documents, natural language processing (NLP) provides great help when doctors are working with electronic medical records (EMR) [10]. For instance, NLP could first connect with EMR systems, recognize the exact words by comparing them with medical dictionaries and associated acronyms, underline useful information, and provide doctors with appropriate diagnostic coding [10, 11]. The development of NLP and voice recognition technology gives a glimpse into its future purpose to distinguish the patient's complaints, decompose the record, and then integrate them into a unified structure, which is more time-saving and beneficial to standardize the medical record writing, ensure its quality, and make it more convenient to carry out more clinical studies. Additionally, the continuously updated EMR system can provide real-time predictions and statistic recommendations attributed to the huge amount of data collected.

8.2.4 Computer vision

Computer vision (CV) is the capability of a machine to recognize items in images, videos, or real scenes and then 'understand' or translate it into processible data [12]. It has been widely applied to complete image acquisition and interpretation in many departments' work, with the assistance of DL and the other latest algorithms. But there are also some bottlenecks to fulfill image recognition with videos, one of which was the failure in understanding and annotation of every time point during surgery. Current technologies enable the robotic systems to cope with more visual disturbances and keep track of operative instruments, providing better identification of the surgical step and real-time information of higher surgical value [12] (figure 8.2).

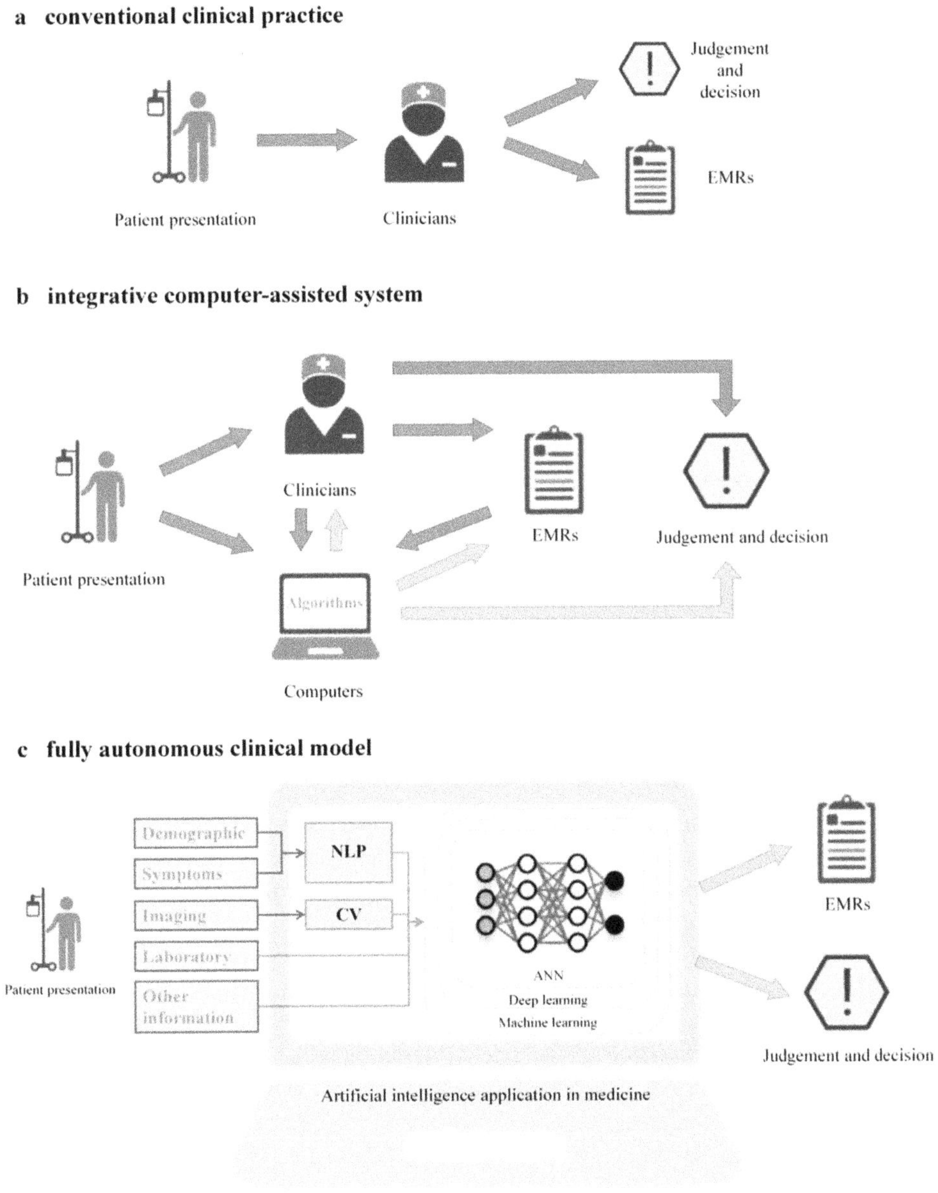

Figure 8.2. Three patterns of the clinical practice model.

8.3 AI in endoscopy

Endoscopy is thought to be amenable to AI applications because of its dependence on image-based diagnosis. Gastrointestinal endoscopy plays a major role in the diagnosis of many digestive diseases, in which AI is expected to potentially improve the quality and overcome current hurdles in diagnosis and management.

8.3.1 Alleviate the experience inequity of the endoscopists

In clinical work, repeated colonoscopies are necessary for diagnostic purposes, prior to surgical intervention and the follow-up of patients. The interpretation of the endoscopic findings varies with each observer, which reduces its reliability and objectivity. Work has been done on colonoscopy to realize standardization.

Narrow band imaging (NBI) is one of the preferred ways to detect early esophageal squamous cell carcinoma [13]. However, significant decreases in both sensitivity and specificity of using NBI were found in inexperienced endoscopists [14]. Therefore, it leaves a problem that the differing experience of endoscopists may lead to bias in disease incidence and patient outcomes, which with the introduction of AI techniques, computer-aided detection (CADe), and computer-aided diagnosis (CADx) are believed to have the potential for overcoming the lack of endoscopist experience.

8.3.2 Improve the detection and differentiation ability

Partly, the purposes of computer-aided systems are designed to elevate detection rates and differentiate early malignancies from the limited images collected during endoscopy. Different from humans, machines will not judge by the general appearance or overall pattern but elaborately measure parameters to reach a diagnosis, such as the color, shapes, texture, and the comparison with surrounding mucosa [15]. DL can extract lesion features from numerous pictures and integrate low-level findings into an abstract representation, which helps categorize and classify the images so that the machine can discover more and learn from the characteristic distribution of data collected for CADx accurately and within a short time. CADe aims to extend the scope that the polyps can be displayed and checked, and CADx is set to provide the precise diagnosis via an optical 'biopsy'. Compared to endoscopists, studies verified that the systems with CADe and CADx have a higher sensitivity and specificity, supported by randomized controlled trial (RCT) and real-time studies since 2019 [16].

In colonoscopies, adenoma detection rate (ADR), defined as the percentage of endoscopies performed by an operator in which more than one adenoma is detected. It is widely adopted as a quality metric and taken as an independent factor that predicts the risk of interval colorectal cancer and cancer mortality [17]. Several high-quality RCTs have demonstrated the CADe system augmented ADR, especially in diminutive adenoma detection [16].

8.3.3 How to further modify computer-assisted systems?

Many obstacles remain in endoscopic diagnosis. Gastric endoscopy, for instance, is always disturbed by 'noise', such as reflections, blurring, and foam, which makes it difficult for the endoscopist to distinguish, for example, erosive gastritis and ulcers from early gastric cancer (EGC) [18]. Since the endoscopic finding of EGC can be a subtle depression or elevation with faint redness compared to the surrounding mucosa, it is considerably hard to recognize the lesion, especially in low-quality images. According to previous studies, computer-assisted systems with DL and convolutional neural network models had an advantage on sensitivity over endoscopists when they were trained to filter out 'noise' by localization and segmentation, which significantly improved the detection rate [19].

Although the computer-assisted system seems promising for clinical application in the future, the improvement and modifications still depend on the endoscopist to some extent. Experienced endoscopists and standardized operations are beneficial to capture more high-quality images and a precise diagnosis. Therefore, the emphasis should be placed on how to assist the operator to perform better but not full automation. The reward and punishment mechanism was also introduced into DL models; once the output is correct or the captured photos are satisfying, it will receive positive feedback [19]. With 'experience' accumulation, it could remarkably reduce blind spots and detect more undistinguishable polyps. This kind of autonomous design was superior to the supervised model because it did not require any labeling by humans, which avoided the corresponding bias at the same time.

Another restriction of the system is the variation of the distance of the camera from the lesion. The computer first locates the lesion, completes the measurement of setting parameters, compares these findings with existing results in its database and finally gives its diagnosis. Therefore, attempts can be made to estimate the camera position, including: sensor-based localization and CV-based motion estimation [20]. The former means that the position of the camera is refined to the end and start of the colon, providing limited but accurate image information. The latter is considered to be more feasible and more likely to be put into the clinic because it doesn't require any additional equipment but at the expense of accuracy and image quality. In addition, another improvement can be made by expanding its database with more high-quality example images, especially of diseases in the early stage.

EndoBrain (Olympus, Tokyo, Japan) software is known as the first commercially available AI system carried in endoscopy *in vivo*, facilitating characterization of the colorectal tissue [21]. Currently, it is widely used to assist the differentiation between malignancies and benign diseases, which is expected to offer more information. The future of AI applications in the endoscopy is promising, and there are multiple potentials for its development.

8.4 AI in surgery for optimization

The earliest attempt of a surgeon turning to a machine for help to realize a better surgical performance can be traced back to the 1980s, when the Programmable Universal Manipulation Arm (PUMA) 200 was created to perform the trajectory of a brain needle biopsy and double the degrees of freedom (DOF) in the procedure when compared to a human's wrist [22].

Leonardo da Vinci's study of human anatomy and design of humanoid robots greatly enlightened future generations and gave rise to a surgical system named *da Vinci* (Intuitive Surgical Inc., CA). The system still functions as a 'master-slave' mode, in which the doctor sits behind a sophisticated console, remotely controlling the telemetry of the robot. Therefore, it is still faced with many hurdles that traditional open surgery possesses, mainly operator dependence without any autonomous robotic functions. In recent years, minimally invasive surgery has strengthened the concept of 'precision surgery' and personalized medical care [23], which calls for a new generation of robot-assisted surgery with a real sense of automation and intelligence.

Based on the problem in traditional endoscopic surgery, the visual and haptic sensors were implemented to receive the input and feedback from the body and tissue. Humans have never stopped exploring the feasibility of improving computer-assisted surgeries, and the well-known masterpieces include the *da Vinci*, the *TSolution-One* orthopedic robot providing guided acetabular reaming and assisted cup implantation in orthopedic operation [24], and the *Mazor X* platform integrating a three-dimensional (3D) camera with spatial tracking and a robotic arm to assist the spine surgery, which are considered to be partially autonomous with reduced human instructions.

8.4.1 Preoperative: comprehensive evaluation leads to the optimized strategies

A detailed preoperative evaluation based on clinical information from various aspects can effectively alleviate the risk of intraoperative accidents and postoperative complications. Firstly, AI algorithms can assist to decide whether the patients meet surgical indications, for example, a software created to triage abdominal pain and comprehensively evaluate some laboratory markers and ultrasonography, such as C-reactive protein, thrombocytes, leukocytes, and neutrophils, to elevate diagnostic accuracy of appendicitis and avoid unnecessary operations and surgical risks [25]. Moreover, the decision of surgery depends on many factors, especially when the patient has many treatment options. For instance, obese patients are advised to go on a diet at the beginning of weight loss therapy, and then their weight, blood glucose, food intake, physical activity, and many other indicators recorded on mobile facilities and their complaints, symptoms, family histories, and other information in their EMR can be integrated with the aid of AI, after which the surgeon can comprehensively evaluate whether they require surgical intervention [26].

As for detailed preoperative preparation, taking cataract surgery as an example, it is quite important to choose the correct intraocular lens (IOL) power that influences the refractive outcome of the patient. An AI-participating system modifies and improves the existing formula for selecting IOL from generation to generation by continuously updating the clinical data, especially postoperative outcomes, which takes full advantage of ANN. This AI-hybrid approach also provides the surgeons with the suggestion on the optimal time for surgery according to the progression of an epiretinal membrane [27].

8.4.2 Intraoperative: leaps and bounds in surgery

8.4.2.1 The navigation to the destination

One AI application in preoperative planning is to reconstruct the vital organs with the assistance of 3D printing. Currently, 3D printing is commonly used to remodel some vital organs, such as the liver and the kidney, since they present with a relatively constant shape and position with adjacent units. Its 3D visualization makes it superior to radiological images by providing the surgeons with more information about the anatomic structures so that they could determine the surgery extent, better avoid damage to the abdominal vessels, and reduce the risk of intraoperative complications [28]. An AI-assisted system overlaps the preoperative images on corresponding surgical findings and keeps real-time tracking. Moreover, advanced augmented reality devices are beneficial to visualize deeper structures by subtracting the images or rendering them transparent, which enables the surgeon to better perform the operation.

The introduction of robotic-assisted system also updates surgical navigation. As for pedicle screw instrumentation in spine surgery, the longer and wider screw should be inserted to pursue stronger fixation strength, but it also raises the stake of iatrogenic pedicle fracture and injury to surrounding neurovascular structures. Robotic navigation operative technique and the platform obtain the intraoperative scan and then provide navigation and real-time instrumentation planning to the robotic arm in a 'shared-control' mode with the surgeon, which allows for placement of screws with greater diameter and length, as well as high accuracy, comparing with a skin-based locating system [29]. This kind of intelligent device is under the joint control of the computer and the operator, taking advantage of great experience and high stability.

8.4.2.2 Pursuit for better performance

Physical improvement. On the basis of laparoscopy surgery, robotic surgeries are more flexible than laparoscopic surgeries since the instrument was equipped with more DOF, and they are not bothered by fatigue, ensuring steadiness. In previous studies, autonomous robotic surgery was put in limited applications, such as orthopedic surgery, because bones and other rigid anatomy are more predictable. In 2016, the Smart Tissue Autonomous Robot (STAR) was put into use, which surpassed humans in a series of *in vivo* operations [30]. STAR was mainly composed of a robot arm extended with an articulated laparoscopic suturing tool and 8 DOF. At the early stage of its application in surgical procedures, it was only utilized in simple planar suturing tasks. With the maturation of smart imaging technologies, STAR was equipped with near-infrared fluorescent imaging, 3D plenoptic vision, force sensing, and submillimeter positioning, which empowered it with a reconstruction accuracy of 1.14 mm and 3D visual tracking system. Integrating them with surgical tools, STAR presented a better performance in both *in vivo* and *ex vivo* suturing of the intestine, such as intestinal anastomosis, from the aspects of suture spacing, bite-size, completion time, lumen patency, leak pressure, and many other parameters. The researchers had full confidence in its outstanding performance in the *in vivo* experiments, while it has only been performed on the phantom tissues due to ethical reasons [31].

Intelligent assistance. One of the benefits that the global databases and 'big data' bring is creating an international surgical community, which enables the surgeons with poor experience to better complete the operation under the instruction of a continuously updating computer system and with the assistance of robots. Additionally, the intraoperative cooperation of CV and DL cultivates the dedicated man-machine combination. In surgeon-dominant operations, the assistance of AI could benefit patients. For example, when the microscope detects the hemorrhage during ophthalmic surgery, it will reflexively augment fluid-air exchange and consequently elevate intraocular pressure to alleviate the bleeding, and once it stops, the system will spontaneously cancel the intervention and leave the gas to be gradually absorbed.

Better outcome. Robotic surgery inherits the advantages of laparoscopic operations, including reduced intraoperative hemorrhage, alleviated postoperative pain, shorter hospital stay, and lower complication risks, which proved to improve the short-term prognosis. According to a cohort study recruiting patients with both benign and malignant liver tumors, the curative effectiveness of open, laparoscopic and robotic hepatectomy were compared, which found that the robot group had a shorter postoperative intensive care unit (ICU) stay and less frequent non-elective readmissions [32].

8.4.2.3 More objective decision-making

In the future, what the robotic platform can do is not just tremor filtration; it is expected to provide a globally connected data-harvesting surgical interface, which offers an intellectual suggestion based on biological, technical, and procedural data from its enormous database. On the basis of previous linear relationships or other simple mathematical models built on various surgical topics, with the help of ANN (overlapping and interweaving numerous layers with various nodes), AI algorithms demonstrate more sophisticated predictions and evaluations of the current status, which is also considered a driving force leading surgical workflow toward standardization and objectiveness. A complete preoperative assessment is definitely a great contributor to a successful operation, which not only includes laboratory tests and radiological examinations but also thoughtful provisions against the vicissitudes of all possible complications. Restricted by time, limited surgical experience, decision fatigue, omitted data, and other constraints, the intraoperative decisions by the surgical team are prone to errors, especially when physical stamina decreases and sleep deprivation happens. Moreover, the decision-making can also be influenced by the surgeon's heuristics or cognitive shortcuts, which probably induces bias and cognitive errors [33, 34]. For example, when the surgeon cannot determine whether to give up the abdominal exploration or stick to complete the cytoreductive surgery during the operation because the disease progresses too swiftly and violently after detailed preoperative evaluation. With an AI system, an alternative would be the comprehensive integration of all available information about the patient, connecting to vast databases to integrate other reported cases, assessing the capability and experience of this operator, and offering a suggestion for intervention within a short time. Although the final decision-maker is still the surgeon, the reference value and reliability of AI are believed to be well equipped to be applied in future clinical work.

8.4.3 Postoperative: prescient care and surgical education in the future

8.4.3.1 Prevent the complication and adverse events in advance

A comprehensive evaluation of preoperative information, such as EMR data, and intraoperative findings, including vital signs and procedures, greatly contributes to avoidance and real-time prediction of postoperative adverse events.

Camera manipulation, an indicator of robotic surgical expertise and a predictor of surgical performance, including the position and adjustment frequency, influences operative time. A DL model revealed the potential relationship between view exposure and surgical performance of radical prostatectomy, anticipating Foley catheter duration, and consequently proposed the removal time, which simply demonstrated the predictive values of AI algorithm on the postoperative complications from person to person [35].

The prediction by an AI algorithm is not a linear regression but a tree design with multiple levels, which displays strong predictive values in several common postoperative complications. The preoperative prediction aims to help to make a decision, identifying which patients could benefit from an intervention and which patients may take infructuous risks. The postoperative anticipation doesn't have to bother with whether or not the negative outcome will outweigh the positive benefits but more to remind the medical staff to anticipate complications with high probability and reassess the indication for transferring the patient out of ICU [36, 37].

8.4.3.2 Empower surgical education through accessibility

For medical students and young surgeons, the chance to be an assistant in surgery is quite precious; what they can learn from traditional open surgery is limited by the exposure, which can to a degree be overcome by the laparoscopic and robotic surgical views. The development of novel technologies and devices also pushes surgical education into a new era in which the onus of appropriate instruction is by seasoned tutors and AI as well. Cutting-edge technologies have their own niches, in providing surgical education. For instance, CV provides images for collection, ANN dynamically recognizes the phase of surgery from these images, and virutal reality systems reconstruct these data back into 3D images, for the trainee surgeons to have a preview before they enter the operating room, harvesting immersive experience from the processes that then allow the virtual practice of surgery.

Furthermore, an AI-assisted system can provide a more objective evaluation of the operator's performance rather than previous means of assessment, which depend on subjective surgeon evaluations: instrument movement, blood loss, camera manipulation, and other surgical skill performances that are captured by recorded surgical videos. An AI algorithm will then automatically analyze and classify them into the expert and novice groups by recognizing different but representative features of their operations. Beyond grading surgical skills, personalized training schemes can be drawn up to improve the specific skills, such as suturing and knotting, according to every trainee's capability respectively [38]. Meanwhile, the AI model can also refine itself and give more exact feedback with the accumulation of repeated practices of skills and evaluations.

8.5 Future of AI in surgery: Integration of images, surgeons, and robots for autonomous robotic surgery

8.5.1 Start with the operation room

Tele-surgery was proposed several decades ago, with researchers continually exploring conducting tele-surgery under extreme conditions, such as in the space station. Since 2019, the pandemic of COVID-19 has had an immense impact to the medical staff who are forced to face an unprecedentedly high risk of infection, which brought back the implementation of distant robotic surgery to the fore [39].

A smart operating room is one critical component when conducting tele-surgery and robotic surgery. In the same way as its learning model in surgical performance, it gets the utmost out of CV, DL, and other intelligent algorithms to learn and then imitate the daily workflow of a surgical team as well as the setting of the operation room; eventually, it is expected to allow autonomous procedures. As for the construction of a smart operating room, it composes medical equipment and facilities, including HD technology (the latest imaging quality with 8K ultra-high definition [40]), mechanical arms, control center, video/image hubs, and especially intelligent elements, including digital communication and navigation functions integrated with the electronic system [41]. Several medical equipment and systems are set on the mechanical arm suspended from the ceiling, eliminating the connections and floor installations, minimizing their footprint.

We are on the verge of a technical revolution. One day, the patient will be transported by automatic vehicles into the operation room, and then medical history and patient information will be collected by computer-assisted systems. Under anesthesia, the vital signs of patients are shown on an integrated screen so that the anesthetist can be reminded by AI algorithms and give a quick response before adverse events happen. The indoor conditions are steadily maintained by the system, under which the optimized surgical environments are perfected with the assistance of the algorithm. According to intraoperative procedures and patient features, complications are anticipated after the patient is transferred to ICU.

8.5.2 The valley of death between the trials and clinical work

8.5.2.1 Information bias

In terms of the disparity, AI application also seems to be a 'double-edged sword'. On the one hand, the algorithm learns from the data. Therefore, when it is trained by data with bias, the results it produces are biased, especially when the patient cannot be represented by training data. On the other hand, with vast databases and the algorithm's ability to upgrade the latest worldwide achievements, it can spontaneously improve itself and offer real-time suggestions referring to multi-center experience. Currently, AI application in clinical work is still limited, since the information disparity has not been overcome so far.

Another obstacle is that patients in the area or countries with low income have no access to robotic-assisted surgeries. Poor basic infrastructures, different education levels, drug stockpiles, and many other factors lead to different clinical decisions varying between these regions and other places, which further creates the heterogeneity of these cases and causes the loss of reference value.

To produce models that can be integrated with the electronic medical record in any setting, data is required to be standardized, which also creates difficulties during the permeation of AI algorithms globally in different hospital systems. Some frameworks are designed to capture key information from the history described by patients, assemble them into EMR, and then input them into the cloud flow, which ensures standardization and communication but still needs refinement.

Many factors hinder progress in the development of AI in surgery, such as nonstandard information collection, different features of population, and other pivotal socioeconomic elements influencing the outcome. However, with the enlargement of datasets and self-improvement by ML, this should be an addressable problem.

8.5.2.2 'Black box' conundrum

The establishment of a DL model begins with tremendous input, weighs different kinds of data with various portions, consequently and continually adjusts itself, and finally offers a result and an existing model. The basis of AI depends on a large sample size, but the pattern in which AI-assisted systems detect and deduce the conclusion is hard to ascertain. The phenomenon where AI cannot exactly interpret how it values the components but still presents an excellent result is called the 'black box' conundrum [42].

Diligent clinicians and informed patients wonder why the algorithm makes a certain recommendation. To earn their trust, some versions of AI models can display their interpretation mechanisms illustrating how and why predictions were made. For instance, attention mechanisms can reveal and even visualize the specific period in which the data has been processing, from the inputs to their distribution to data points and finally to the output, which enables each model to be visualized with disproportionate contributions and various phenotypic clusters [33]. Another method to understand the model is to conduct prospective studies or randomized clinical trials. Although external validation doesn't explain the underlying mechanism as well, the enhanced efficiency of a synthesized model brings confidence to the users [43].

8.5.2.3 The system of accountability

What follows the flourishment of AI application in health care is the issue of responsibility. Regulatory authorities, such as the US Food and Drug Administration (FDA), previously covered the duty for regulating and approving the use of certain medical devices. However, the FDA declared that certain types of software were no longer under its jurisdiction, which made the accountability much more difficult [44]. It also enforces these authorities to solve the accountability problems due to the maturation of AI technology. Although the joint custodianship of both surgeon and robot breaks the traditional 'master-slave' mode, there is still a long way to go to achieve autonomous robotic surgery to enter clinical practice. The first barrier is the evaluation of whether the algorithm is qualified to be put into real use. The robot learns from 'big data', but it may randomly choose a solution to the situation that it has never been trained in, which is not safe in clinical practice. Therefore, performance standards are necessary to ensure patient safety when it meets with unprecedented events.

When the robot surgery starts, a new question arises on when to cease. Some studies purported that costly miscalculations can be made if AI learns the pattern in the wrong way [45]. As a result, some researchers insist that, before we place great hopes on AI and make every effort to promote its clinical implementation, we should formulate legal and ethical rules in case AI does not evolve the way we would like it to. Then how do we enable a robot to realize its sense of responsibility? For example, the researchers designed a 'reward and punishment' mechanism in the ANN module, just like positive and negative feedback regulation in the neural system, to impose on AI a kind of 'memory' to increase the frequency of doing things right and reduce the probability of making mistakes [46].

The previous literature seems to exaggerate the efficiency of AI due to publication bias, which means the studies with significant findings are more likely to be submitted or published. In other words, numerous failures behind a successful model will not be reported to the public. Besides the setting of more strict standards, 'stress tests' can also play a role in the qualification, in which not only real data but also man-made wrong data can be input into the model to observe the accuracy of output and the capability of intelligent systems to detect these errors. Therefore, to guarantee the patients' rights, before clinical use, the AI algorithm with self-correction should be challenged by repeated testing from multiple vantage points, such as trial-and-error methods in the single-center and external validation, and the practice should start with a small-scale prospective study, which maximizes the objectivity and reference values of that model, to proactively reduce the risk that the patients will face.

8.5.2.4 More than thinking and moving

In this way, AI is just like an intern, who is facing the transition from theory to practice, receiving an explosive amount of information, learning to work in an ethical and logical way in different majors and fields, often making mistakes but sometimes giving surprisingly satisfactory answers. Surgeons and scientists work as guardians, teaching the AI how to solve problems, assign tasks, and correct its mistakes. So can interns eventually become guardians?

Logistic robots have been used to carry surgical instruments and other items in the operating room. Similarly, they are also widely used in restaurants, where they embody their advantages, as they require less time to refresh, have more maximum load, and considerably reduce errors caused by memory biases, such as sending or ordering the wrong food. However, when you go for a meal alone, robot waiters will not intend to make a doll bear to accompany you to ease your loneliness without an artificial setting. Robots are equipped with many abilities, including figuring out the real demand from conversations—NLP, drawing conclusions or raising suggestions based on big data—DL and ANN, and having image recognition and refined physical movement—CV and elaborate structure. However, in these human-related industries, one of the merits in which humans outperform robots is the emotional output. Trust is a critical element in the relationship between doctors and patients, which may be influenced by the reputation of the hospital, the title of the surgeon, the preferences of patients and their families, and most importantly, face-to-face interaction. A study found that the sense of trust would increase when people were committed, which also existed between humans and robots, but only in humanoid ones. Nevertheless, when computers were used instead, trust significantly decreased, which could be fatal to the doctor-patient relationship [47]. Although we are still in the stage of semi-automation, and many patients seem to prefer the intervention with advanced technology, such as AI and *da Vinci* surgery, they may turn to be deeply skeptical when they are informed that AI takes charge of decision-making. This is also the valley of death between theory and practice.

8.6 Conclusion

In the past decades, the incorporation of AI has led to the transformation of traditional medicine into a new stage. To meet the requirements in scientific research and clinical work, the subfields of AI were ameliorated separately and integrated comprehensively. In terms of technical levels, it makes up for limited knowledge reserve and augments the sensitivity and angles of joints. However, it still obeys to 'master-slave' mode due to some existing flaws, such as a lack of tactile feedback. More studies should be encouraged to explore its vast potential, but strict regulations on AI application should also be enacted to ensure patients' safety and wellbeing. With the improvement with each passing day, it is believed that the final realization of autonomous operation in the near future will bring hugely beneficial changes to clinical workflow.

In the past 70 years, increasing studies about AI applications in medicine have been published in the PubMed database. The x-axis indicates the publishing year of studies, and the y-axis presents the total number of the literature on the topic of medical AI algorithms in that year. Milestones in the development of computer-assisted systems are described in time sequence. An obvious increase in related studies can be seen since 2000; in that year the use of a representative surgical device was approved to be utilized in clinical work.

Different models with or without AI assistance are illustrated. (a) In conventional practice, the judgment and EMR are mainly completed by clinicians. (b) With the partial intervention of intelligent systems, doctors and computers shoulder the work together. Under the supervision of clinicians and with their modification, the AI systems continuously improve their performance; at the same time, the doctors benefit from it by saving time and making decisions based on 'big data'. (c) In the future, the fully autonomous computer system will probably be put into use. NLP and CV will collect various information from the patients and translate it into computer language. These data will consequently be processed by the algorithms to fulfill DL and go through numerous layers and nodes in an ANN and finally output precise prediction, valuable decisions, standardized EMRs, etc.

References

[1] Hamet P and Tremblay J 2017 Artificial intelligence in medicine *Metabolism* **69S** S36–40

[2] Bellman R E 1978 *An Introduction to Artificial Intelligence: Can Computers Think?* (San Francisco, CA: Boyd & Fraser Publishing Company)

[3] Topol E 2019 *Deep Medicine: How Artificial Intelligence Can Make Healthcare Human Again* 1st edn (New York: Basic Books)

[4] Sun B, Wood G and Miyashita S 2021 Milestones for autonomous *in vivo* microrobots in medical applications *Surgery* **169** 755–8

[5] Kaul V, Enslin S and Gross S A 2020 History of artificial intelligence in medicine *Gastrointest. Endosc.* **92** 807–12

[6] Maza G and Sharma A 2020 Past, present, and future of robotic surgery *Otolaryngol. Clin. N. Am.* **53** 935–41

[7] Beam A L and Kohane I S 2018 Big data and machine learning in health care *JAMA* **319** 1317–8

[8] Panesar S, Cagle Y, Chander D, Morey J, Fernandez-Miranda J and Kliot M 2019 Artificial intelligence and the future of surgical robotics *Ann. Surg.* **270** 223–6

[9] Haeberle H S, Helm J M, Navarro S M, Karnuta J M, Schaffer J L, Callaghan J J, Mont M A, Kamath A F, Krebs V E and Ramkumar P N 2019 Artificial intelligence and machine learning in lower extremity arthroplasty: a review *J. Arthroplasty* **34** 2201–3

[10] Myers T G, Ramkumar P N, Ricciardi B F, Urish K L, Kipper J and Ketonis C 2020 Artificial intelligence and orthopaedics: an introduction for clinicians *J. Bone Joint Surg. Am.* **102** 830–40

[11] Yu K H, Beam A L and Kohane I S 2018 Artificial intelligence in healthcare *Nat. Biomed. Eng.* **2** 719–31

[12] Ward T M, Mascagni P, Ban Y, Rosman G, Padoy N, Meireles O and Hashimoto D A 2021 Computer vision in surgery *Surgery* **169** 1253–6

[13] Nagami Y, Tominaga K, Machida H, Nakatani M, Kameda N, Sugimori S, Okazaki H, Tanigawa T, Yamagami H and Kubo N *et al* 2014 Usefulness of non-magnifying narrow-band imaging in screening of early esophageal squamous cell carcinoma: a prospective comparative study using propensity score matching *Am. J. Gastroenterol.* **109** 845–54

[14] Muto M, Minashi K, Yano T, Saito Y, Oda I, Nonaka S, Omori T, Sugiura H, Goda K and Kaise M *et al* 2010 Early detection of superficial squamous cell carcinoma in the head and neck region and esophagus by narrow band imaging: a multicenter randomized controlled trial *J. Clin. Oncol.* **28** 1566–72

[15] Neumann H and Bisschops R 2019 Artificial intelligence and the future of endoscopy *Dig. Endosc.* **31** 389–90

[16] Wang P, Berzin T M, Glissen B J, Bharadwaj S, Becq A, Xiao X, Liu P, Li L, Song Y and Zhang D *et al* 2019 Real-time automatic detection system increases colonoscopic polyp and adenoma detection rates: a prospective randomised controlled study *Gut* **68** 1813–9

[17] Ahmad O F, Soares A S, Mazomenos E, Brandao P, Vega R, Seward E, Stoyanov D, Chand M and Lovat L B 2019 Artificial intelligence and computer-aided diagnosis in colonoscopy: current evidence and future directions *Lancet. Gastroenterol. Hepatol.* **4** 71

[18] Wu L, He X, Liu M, Xie H, An P, Zhang J, Zhang H, Ai Y, Tong Q and Guo M *et al* 2021 Evaluation of the effects of an artificial intelligence system on endoscopy quality and preliminary testing of its performance in detecting early gastric cancer: a randomized controlled trial *Endoscopy* **53** 1199–207

[19] Qadir H A, Balasingham I, Solhusvik J, Bergsland J, Aabakken L and Shin Y 2020 Improving automatic polyp detection using CNN by exploiting temporal dependency in colonoscopy video *IEEE J. Biomed. Health Inform.* **24** 180–93.

[20] Than T D, Alici G, Zhou H and Li W 2012 A review of localization systems for robotic endoscopic capsules *IEEE Trans. Biomed. Eng.* **59** 2387–99

[21] Mori Y, Kudo S E and Mori K 2018 Potential of artificial intelligence-assisted colonoscopy using an endocytoscope (with video) *Dig. Endosc.* **30** 52–3

[22] Kwoh Y S, Hou J, Jonckheere E A and Hayati S 1988 A robot with improved absolute positioning accuracy for CT guided stereotactic brain surgery *IEEE Trans. Biomed. Eng.* **35** 153–60

[23] Autorino R, Porpiglia F, Dasgupta P, Rassweiler J, Catto J W, Hampton L J, Lima E, Mirone V, Derweesh I H and Debruyne F 2017 Precision surgery and genitourinary cancers *Eur. J. Surg. Oncol.* **43** 893–908

[24] St Mart J P, Goh E L and Shah Z 2020 Robotics in total hip arthroplasty: a review of the evolution, application and evidence base *EFORT Open Rev.* **5** 866–73

[25] Reismann J, Romualdi A, Kiss N, Minderjahn M I, Kallarackal J, Schad M and Reismann M 2019 Diagnosis and classification of pediatric acute appendicitis by artificial intelligence methods: an investigator-independent approach *PLoS One* **14** e222030

[26] Ryu B, Kim N, Heo E, Yoo S, Lee K, Hwang H, Kim J W, Kim Y, Lee J and Jung S Y 2017 Impact of an electronic health Record-Integrated personal health record on patient participation in health care: development and randomized controlled trial of MyHealthKeeper *J. Med. Internet Res.* **19** e401

[27] Ladas J, Ladas D, Lin S R, Devgan U, Siddiqui A A and Jun A S 2021 Improvement of multiple generations of intraocular lens calculation formulae with a novel approach using artificial intelligence *Transl. Vis. Sci. Technol.* **10** 7

[28] Pietrabissa A, Marconi S, Negrello E, Mauri V, Peri A, Pugliese L, Marone E M and Auricchio F 2020 An overview on 3D printing for abdominal surgery *Surg. Endosc.* **34** 1–13

[29] Shafi K A, Pompeu Y A, Vaishnav A S, Mai E, Sivaganesan A, Shahi P and Qureshi S A 2022 Does robot-assisted navigation influence pedicle screw selection and accuracy in minimally invasive spine surgery? *Neurosurg. Focus* **52** E4

[30] Shademan A, Decker R S, Opfermann J D, Leonard S, Krieger A and Kim P C 2016 Supervised autonomous robotic soft tissue surgery *Sci. Transl. Med.* **8** 337r–64r

[31] Saeidi H, Opfermann J D, Kam M, Wei S, Leonard S, Hsieh M H, Kang J U and Krieger A 2022 Autonomous robotic laparoscopic surgery for intestinal anastomosis *Sci. Robot* **7** j2908

[32] Fruscione M, Pickens R, Baker E H, Cochran A, Khan A, Ocuin L, Iannitti D A, Vrochides D and Martinie J B 2019 Robotic-assisted versus laparoscopic major liver resection: analysis of outcomes from a single center *HPB (Oxford)* **21** 906–11

[33] Loftus T J, Tighe P J, Filiberto A C, Efron P A, Brakenridge S C, Mohr A M, Rashidi P, Upchurch G J and Bihorac A 2020 Artificial intelligence and surgical decision-making *JAMA Surg.* **155** 148–58

[34] Vohs K D, Baumeister R F, Schmeichel B J, Twenge J M, Nelson N M and Tice D M 2008 Making choices impairs subsequent self-control: a limited-resource account of decision making, self-regulation, and active initiative *J. Pers. Soc. Psychol.* **94** 883–98

[35] Andras I, Mazzone E, van Leeuwen F, De Naeyer G, van Oosterom M N, Beato S, Buckle T, O'Sullivan S, van Leeuwen P J and Beulens A *et al* 2020 Artificial intelligence and robotics: a combination that is changing the operating room *World J. Urol.* **38** 2359–66

[36] Gutierrez G 2020 Artificial intelligence in the intensive care unit *Crit. Care* **24** 101

[37] Churpek M M, Yuen T C, Winslow C, Robicsek A A, Meltzer D O, Gibbons R D and Edelson D P 2014 Multicenter development and validation of a risk stratification tool for ward patients *Am. J. Respir. Crit. Care Med.* **190** 649–55

[38] Satava R M, Stefanidis D, Levy J S, Smith R, Martin J R, Monfared S, Timsina L R, Darzi A W, Moglia A and Brand T C *et al* 2020 Proving the effectiveness of the fundamentals of robotic surgery (FRS) skills curriculum: a single-blinded, multispecialty, multi-institutional randomized control trial *Ann. Surg.* **272** 384–92

[39] Shen Y T, Chen L, Yue W W and Xu H X 2021 Digital technology-based telemedicine for the COVID-19 pandemic *Front. Med. (Lausanne)* **8** 646506

[40] Shonaka T, Tani C, Iwata H, Otani M, Hasegawa K, Matsuno N, Furukawa H, Yoshida A and Sumi Y 2021 A comparison of laparoscopic procedures performed by novice medical students using 8K ultra-high-definition/two-dimensional and 2K high-definition/three-dimensional monitors *Surg. Today* **51** 1397–403

[41] Smart operating rooms 2020 https://etkho.com/en/smart-operating-rooms/

[42] Hashimoto D A, Rosman G, Rus D and Meireles O R 2018 Artificial intelligence in surgery: promises and perils *Ann. Surg.* **268** 70–6

[43] Balch J, Upchurch G R, Bihorac A and Loftus T J 2021 Bridging the artificial intelligence valley of death in surgical decision-making *Surgery* **169** 746–8

[44] Harish V, Morgado F, Stern A D and Das S 2020 Artificial intelligence and clinical decision making: the new nature of medical uncertainty *Acad. Med.* **96** 31

[45] O'Sullivan S, Nevejans N, Allen C, Blyth A, Leonard S, Pagallo U, Holzinger K, Holzinger A, Sajid M I and Ashrafian H 2019 Legal, regulatory, and ethical frameworks for development of standards in artificial intelligence (AI) and autonomous robotic surgery *Int. J. Med. Robot* **15** e1968

[46] Pesapane F, Volonté C, Codari M and Sardanelli F 2018 Artificial intelligence as a medical device in radiology: ethical and regulatory issues in Europe and the United States *Insights Imaging* **9** 745–53.

[47] Cominelli L, Feri F, Garofalo R, Giannetti C, Meléndez-Jiménez M A, Greco A, Nardelli M, Scilingo E P and Kirchkamp O 2021 Promises and trust in human-robot interaction *Sci. Rep.* **11** 9687

Chapter 9

Technical innovations to improve artificial intelligence generalizability of automated medical image diagnosis for clinical practice

Meirui Jiang, Cheng Chen, Quande Liu, Pheng-Ann Heng and Qi Dou

Model generalizability has increasingly been an important topic to tackle the data heterogeneity when deploying artificial intelligence (AI) models in the wild for intelligent medical image diagnosis. Data heterogeneity is ubiquitous in medical images, severely hindering large-scale adoption of AI models in real-world clinical practice. This chapter briefly reviews the current clinical applications and technical solutions on model generalizability and shows two example methods under the recent federated learning paradigm to handle data heterogeneity. The first is an effective and efficient learning strategy, called FedBN, to improve the convergence behaviors of training medical clients under feature shift. The second focuses on model generalizability when deploying federated models to external unseen medical clients, under the identified new problem setting, called FedDG. Despite significant progress in model generalizability that has been made by the medical image computing community, continuous advancement is in high demand to promote the wide application of intelligent models in clinical scenarios.

9.1 Introduction

?Model generalizability combating data heterogeneity is an important topic for intelligent medical image diagnosis, which aims to use smart machines to automatically detect abnormalities, characterize cancers, quantify tumors, suggest treatments, and predict prognosis in the wild [1–3]. Model generalization is a long-standing key problem in machine learning [4]. Typically, improving generalizability means alleviating overfitting, such that the model can learn general patterns (discard noisy specifics) in training data and yield a high performance on data it has not seen before (a.k.a. held-out testing data). Nowadays, popular AI techniques are based on deep neural networks, which essentially belong to a type of

doi:10.1088/978-0-7503-4637-5ch9

data-driven approach. This makes existing AI models unprecedentedly sensitive to data changes in terms of statistical distributions. The consequence is that a model may suffer from severe performance drop when being trained on one data source but applied to another [5].

Such a problem is very challenging, or even a bottleneck, for current AI-powered medical image diagnosis applications in the real world. The cross-dataset distribution discrepancy (i.e. data heterogeneity) is ubiquitous in medical imaging clinical practice. Pooling medical images from different sites and previous studies is very common in this field for building sufficiently large cohorts. Data from each hospital, or even data from each single scanner in the same hospital, present heterogeneity due to differences in vendors, acquisition protocols, population demographics, and other factors. For example, the choice of scanner manufacturer (e.g. Siemens, GE HealthCare, Philips, UI), the setting of imaging protocols (e.g. MRI pulse sequences of T1-weighted, T2-weighter), parameters within the same protocol (e.g. echo time, repetition time, flip angle), signal-to-noise ratio over time for the scanner, and regional disease characteristics can respectively or jointly cause data heterogeneity [6, 7]. Although scanner effects seem subtle, sometimes not even appreciable by human eyes, they can still significantly affect the properties of AI models. Recent studies [8–10] also revealed that such heterogeneity is somewhat inherent to the data itself and cannot be removed by classical image pre-processing techniques such as bias field correction, intensity normalization, percentile matching, and histogram standardization. Therefore, it is crucial to explore novel techniques for improving model generalizability, in order to apply intelligent medical image diagnosis systems at scale for clinical practice.

To date, tackling the heterogeneous data for generalizable medical image analysis has been extensively investigated. A wide set of applications such as brain, eye, chest, heart, abdomen, and histopathological scenarios were studied in the literature. Different image computing tasks including segmentation, classification, detection, registration, image quality assessment, and depth estimation were addressed for heterogeneous data. From a technical perspective, existing approaches can be broadly divided into two groups, i.e. domain adaptation and domain generalization, depending on whether the targeted testing data are used for training or not. By default, these techniques are developed on multi-center data, i.e. teaching the AI models by aggregating images from different medical institutions. This works in principle; however, concerns are increasingly being raised regarding privacy issues upon data sharing. Decentralized AI paradigms, e.g. federated learning (FL), emerge as a preferred solution in which a global model can be obtained while individual centers' data are held locally. But the flip side of the coin is it becomes harder to tackle the data heterogeneity and model generalization challenges. New ideas should be further explored to keep up with this trend.

In this chapter, we first briefly review the clinical application areas and medical image analysis tasks that encounter data heterogeneity and require model generalizability. Next, we explain the current technical solutions on domain adaptation and domain generalization. Then, we show two example methods under the recent FL scenario to handle data heterogeneity and improve generalizability on unseen data.

Finally, we discuss the current and future techniques on this topic prior to concluding remarks.

9.2 Clinical application areas of model generalizability in current literature

In the following, we briefly overview the existing application areas, which are categorized by different clinical scenarios, and list popular public datasets of model generalizability in current literature.

Brain image analysis is an active application area of model generalization due to the widely existing data heterogeneity caused by the various sequences and acquisition parameters of MRI. Usually, brain MRI images acquired from different cohorts have no standardized intensity values and present diverse histograms. Deep model generalization approaches have been studied in mainly three scenarios in brain image analysis: tumor/lesion segmentation [11–13], anatomical substructure segmentation [14], and brain states classification with functional MRI [15]. There are some public datasets that can be leveraged for cross-domain brain image analysis, such as the WMH Challenge dataset [16] for white matter hyperintensities segmentation consisting of images from five scanners in three different institutes, the Cam-CAN [17] and MRBrainS18[1] for brain structure segmentation, and iSeg-2019 [18] providing 6-month infant subjects from multiple sites with different protocols, scanners, etc.

Cardiac imaging is another hot application scenario for model generalization. Cross-modality domain adaptation has been intensively explored based on cardiac images, because of the well-organized, publicly available MRI and CT datasets for the heart, such as Multi-Modality Whole Heart Segmentation Challenge data [19]. In cross-modality adaptation, substructure segmentation networks were trained on MRI and adapted to CT, or vice versa. Although there is not very strong clinical relevance in such a setting, it could represent the most severe distribution shift of heterogeneous medical images, as MRI and CT images look distinct. This scenario can reflect methodological utmost efficacy in such extreme settings [20–24]. Recently, the cross-modality domain adaptation problem setting is adopted by Medical Image Computing and Computer Assisted Intervention Societygrand challenges such as MS-CMRSeg Challenge [25, 26] and crossMoDA2021 [27] to further explore and encourage technical novelties.

Eye disease diagnosis with retinal fundus images or optical coherence tomography (OCT) images are often influenced by the data heterogeneity resulting from different imaging devices and vendors. Current works mainly focus on tackling distribution shifts in segmentation tasks across different retinal fundus image datasets [28–31] or OCT datasets [32]. Some popular benchmark datasets include REFUGE [33], Drishti-GS [34] and RIM-ONE-r3 [35] retinal fundus datasets for optic disc and cup segmentation, two OCT datasets released from [32, 36] for retinal layer segmentation, etc.

[1] http://mrbrains18.isi.uu.nl/

Chest disease diagnosis has been studied under data heterogeneity with cross-domain x-ray datasets and CT datasets for a variety of tasks including thoracic organ/lung tumor segmentation [37–40], pneumonia diagnosis [41], multi-class chest disease recognition [42], COVID-19 assessment [43–45], etc. Available public datasets used in previous works include the Montgomery [46] dataset and Japanese Society of Radiological Technology [47] dataset for lung and heart segmentation, the Radiological Society of North America Pneumonia Detection Challenge dataset[2] and a pediatric chest x-ray dataset[3] for pneumonia diagnosis, and the National Institutes of HealthChest x-ray 14 dataset [48] and MIMIC Chest X-Ray dataset [49] for lung disease classification.

Abdomen multi-organ segmentation for liver, kidney, and spleen regions is also a popular application for model generalization under the severe distribution shift between MRI and CT data [50, 51]. The CHAOS [52] Challenge dataset with MRI images and the multi-atlas labeling beyond the CranialVault [53] dataset with CT images are commonly used for cross-modality abdominal multi-organ segmentation. Because of the availability of multiple public prostate MRI datasets collected from different sources, prostate segmentation across MRI datasets is a favorable application in previous domain generalization works [29, 54, 55]. The NIC-ISBI13 dataset [56], I2CVB dataset [57], and PROMISE12 [58] dataset are popular benchmarks for multi-site prostate segmentation.

Histopathology images usually present large appearance changes due to different staining processes. Cross-dataset adaptation with histopathology slides acquired from different stains is common in cancer classification [59, 60]. There are also works on cross-modality adaptation between histopathological images and microscopy images for nuclei segmentation [61] and cancer classification [62]. For histopathology image classification, popular datasets include Netherlands Cancer Institute and Vancouver General Hospital datasets [63] independently collected from two clinical sites and the Camelyon17 [64, 65] dataset with images acquired from five hospitals. For segmentation tasks, the MoNuSeg [66], TNBC [67], and BBBC039V1 [68] datasets are often used for cross-domain nucleus segmentation.

9.3 Technical tasks in medical image analysis prone to data heterogeneity

In the following, we describe different image computing tasks, including segmentation, classification, detection, registration, and depth estimation, that encounter generalization issues in clinical practice.

Segmentation of medical image data is a pixel/voxel-wise prediction task to assign a semantic label to every location for the region of interest in an image. This is a conventional, well-defined task in medical imaging and is widely used for lesion quantification assessment in radiology and tumor radiotherapy treatment planning in oncology. Due to data heterogeneity, the performance of deep neural networks

[2] https://www.kaggle.com/c/rsna-pneumonia-detection-challenge/data
[3] https://doi.org/10.17632/rscbjbr9sj.

degrades severely for cross-domain medical image segmentation. However, obtaining pixel-wise annotation for each new domain to train a segmentation model with supervised learning is infeasible in practice. Extensive domain adaptation and domain generalization methods have been proposed for segmentation tasks. These methods greatly contribute to reduce the expensive cost and time-consuming effort of per-pixel annotation. To achieve fine-grained pixel-level adaptation for the segmentation task, the per-pixel image appearance translation with the generative adversarial networks (GAN) is an effective solution and has been widely adopted in previous works [21, 38–40, 69–71]. To preserve the semantic structure during image translation, which is crucial for segmentation tasks, many image-to-image-translation–based model generalization methods introduce additional semantic-aware regularization into the GAN framework [38–40, 71]. For segmentation tasks, it is observed that the cross-domain distribution shift often leads to difficulty in predicting the complete shape of anatomies. In this regard, some methods achieve good model generalization by applying adversarial learning in the output space to regularize the shape of predictions on target images to be similar to the source predictions [28, 37, 50]. Again, due to considerable annotation cost, model adaptation, and generalization for segmentation, these tasks are mostly conducted in semi-supervised or unsupervised ways.

Classification is a common task for computer-aided medical image diagnosis and achieves great progress by adopting deep neural networks. Given an image, the classification model predicts the one-hot output for which category it belongs to, e.g. the characterization of lesion, sub-type of disease, stage of cancer, etc. However, the learned decision boundary of deep classifier lacks generalization capability when there exists a distribution shift between the training and test data, especially when the training datasets are limited. Model adaptation and generalization for classification task seem easier, because the model yields only a single overall prediction for the image as a whole. The key is to extract general, discriminative, robust, and sometimes compact representations in the latent space from a higher level. In the current field, available public datasets for cross-domain image classifications are relatively fewer, compared with the segmentation task. Early efforts focus on model generalization in histopathological image classification [59, 60, 72, 73], motivated by the common data heterogeneity caused by the staining process. There are also works on tackling distribution shifts in skin lesion classification [74, 75], brain activity classification [15], fundus image quality assessment [76], and vertebra ultrasound classification [77]. To generalize classification models across domains, the mainstream methods use feature-level alignment via either adversarial learning or discrepancy minimization in the latent space, so as to improve model performance on predicting new images.

Data heterogeneity has also been tackled in other medical image analysis tasks, but those are less often studied in the field. Here, we list some related works for brief examples. **Cell detection** from microscopy images aims to predict the location of each cell in an image. Domain adaptation method is developed to generalize cell detection models across different microscopy image datasets [78]. **Image registration** is the process of transforming a pair of images into a common coordinate system.

Generalizing image registration models across datasets of different image types is investigated in [79]. **Depth estimation** is a task of estimating a dense depth map for an image. There is prior effort in adapting depth estimation models between synthetic and real endoscopy images [80].

9.4 Technical approaches for AI model adaptation and generalization

In the following, we describe the current methods of domain adaptation and domain generalization that combat data heterogeneity in medical imaging.

As for terminology, the source domain means the original dataset with annotations being used to train the model. There can be one single source domain, as well as multiple source domains, depending on the number of available sites in practice. The target domain is the dataset for which the AI model is to be adapted or generalized to. Achieving a good performance on the target domain is the final goal. For domain adaptation methods, both source domain and target domain data are available. For domain generalization, only source domains are available; the target domain is unseen. It aims to train a model using multi-domain source data, such that the model can directly generalize to unseen data without the need of retraining on arbitrary target domains.

Domain adaptation has been an active research field to transfer knowledge learned from the source domain to the target data by aligning distributions across domains or adjusting decision boundaries. Early works employ pre-trained based transfer learning to reduce the required amounts of annotations in the target domain for segmentation tasks [12, 81, 82]. But these methods require additional labeled target data. Instead, unsupervised domain adaptation (UDA) without using target domain labels is more desirable, and many approaches have been proposed with different strategies. Adversarial learning is the most popular technique for UDA, by narrowing the domain shift between the target and source either in input space, feature space, or output space. With the use of GAN [83], especially CycleGAN [84], input-space domain alignment methods have been developed to transform the source images to appear like the target ones, or vice versa [38–40, 69–71, 85]. Another stream of methods focuses on feature-space alignment, aiming to extract domain-invariant features of deep neural networks through adversarial learning [11, 20, 60, 86, 87]. For domain adaptation in segmentation task, there are also works adopting adversarial learning in the output space, motivated by the observation that the semantic structure of segmentation target in medical images is usually consistent across domains [28, 37, 88, 89]. Image-, feature-, and output-space alignments have no conflict with each other and thus can be leveraged simultaneously to achieve strong domain adaptation [21, 50, 90, 91]. Besides adversarial learning, domain-invariant features can also be learned by directly minimizing the maximum mean discrepancy [14]. Pseudo-labeling is yet another effective technique to achieve domain adaptation with model self-training [78]. Moreover, there are other works leveraging semi-supervised learning approaches such as self-ensembling [92] and co-training [93] for UDA.

Domain generalization aims to generalize models to unseen domains without knowledge about the target distribution during training. Different methods have been proposed for learning generalizable and transferable representations. Several studies add data augmentation techniques to improve the model generalizability [94, 95], assuming that the domain shift could be simulated by conducting extensive transformations to data of source domains. Another promising direction is to develop domain generalization methods based on meta-learning [54, 73, 96–98], which is agnostic to the network and fully makes use of the gradient process. In [96], the meta-learning is guided by two complementary losses to explicitly regularize the semantic structure of the feature space. In [54], the shape compactness and shape smoothness are particularly enhanced to enhance the metaoptimization for segmentation tasks. A set of approaches [74, 99, 100] try to learn domain-invariant representations with feature-space regularization with linear-dependency modeling [74] or adversarial neural networks [99]. Instead of extracting domain-invariant features, there is also work aiming to find a feature space from the multiple source domains that are most similar to the current target test image [31]. To handle domain discrepancy, [101] develops an unsupervised Bayesian model to interpret the tissue information prior to the generalization in brain tissue segmentation. Most domain generalization methods require to access multiple-source domain data simultaneously. Instead, the latest single domain generalization (SDG) methods try to learn a model under the worst-case scenario with only one source domain to directly generalize to different unseen target domains. Early attempts try to achieve SDG by extracting domain-invariant semantic shape [29] or conducting data or feature augmentation [51, 102].

9.5 Distributed privacy-preserving techniques with data heterogeneity

The above techniques witness great success; however, as mentioned earlier, the need of gathering multi-center data risks patient privacy. FL presents a new trend to allow multi-center learning without aggregating data in one place. A standard FL paradigm is FedAvg [103], in which each local client (e.g. hospital) trains on their own data and uploads their model parameters only at a certain frequency to a global server. This central server aggregates all client models and produces a new global model, which is distributed back to each local client for a new round of FL training. This process is iteratively performed until model convergence, and all data are kept at each local client throughout training. Although FL has demonstrated some pilot progress on medical image analysis [45, 104–107], the heterogeneous data distributions propose a new challenge under the distributed scenario.

At least two issues are immediately noticeable. First, in distributed training, data heterogeneity can slow down the model convergence, making training clients suffer from the performance degradation, or even diverge the model. Second, for testing the model on a client from an unseen target domain, how to improve the domain generalization by utilizing distributed data is more challenging than the previous centralized paradigm. In other words, these two aspects raise questions on overcoming the internal data heterogeneity and external data heterogeneity regarding multi-center FL.

9.5.1 Federated model training under internal data heterogeneity

9.5.1.1 Federated averaging with local batch normalization

We show an effective and efficient learning strategy, called *FedBN*[4] [108]. Similar to FedAvg, FedBN performs local updates and averages local models. Moreover, FedBN assumes local models have batch normalization (BN) layers and excludes their parameters from the global averaging step. This simple modification achieves significant empirical improvements on heterogeneous data in experiments. We also present a theoretical analysis of FedBN improving the convergence behaviors under feature shift.

Problem setup. We assume $N \in \mathbb{N}$ clients to jointly train for $T \in \mathbb{N}$ epochs and to communicate after $E \in \mathbb{N}$ local iterations. Thus, the system has T/E communication rounds over the T epochs. For simplicity, we assume all clients to have $M \in \mathbb{N}$ training examples (a difference in training examples can be accounted for by weighted averaging [103]) for a regression task, i.e. each client $i \in [N]$ ($[N] = \{1, \dots, N\}$) has training examples $\left\{\left(x_j^i, y_j^i\right) \in \mathbb{R}^d \times \mathbb{R}: j \in [M]\right\}$. Furthermore, we assume a two-layer neural network with rectified linear unit (ReLU) activations trained by gradient descent. Let $v_k \in \mathbb{R}^d$ denote the parameters of the first layer, where $k \in [m]$ and m is the width of the hidden layer. Let $\left\|v\right\|_S \triangleq \sqrt{v^\top S v}$ denote the induced vector norm for a positive definite matrix S. We make the assumption of data heterogeneity in a more precise way in the following.

Assumption 9.1. *(Data distribution). For each client $i \in [N]$ the inputs x_j^i are centered ($\mathbb{E}x^i = 0$) with covariance matrix $S_i = \mathbb{E}x^i x^{i\top}$, where S_i is independent from the label y and may differ for each $i \in [N]$, e.g. $\boldsymbol{S}_i$ are not all identity matrices, and for each index pair $p \neq q$, $x_p \neq \kappa \cdot x_q$* for all $\kappa \in \mathbb{R}\setminus\{0\}$.

With assumption 9.1, the normalization of the first layer for client i is $\frac{v_k^\top x^i}{\| v_k \|_{S_i}}$. FedBN with client-specified BN parameters trains a model $f^*{:}\mathbb{R}^d \to \mathbb{R}$ parameterized by $(\boldsymbol{V}, \gamma, \boldsymbol{c}) \in \mathbb{R}^{m\times d} \times \mathbb{R}^{m\times N} \times \mathbb{R}^m$, i.e.

$$f^*(x; V, \gamma, c) = \frac{1}{\sqrt{m}} \sum_{k=1}^{m} c_k \sum_{i=1}^{N} \sigma\left(\gamma_{k,i} \cdot \frac{v_k^\top x}{\|v_k\|_{S_i}}\right) \cdot 1\{x \in \text{client}i\}, \tag{9.1}$$

where γ is the scaling parameter of BN, $\sigma(s) = \max\{s, 0\}$ is the ReLU activation function, and c is the top layer parameters of the network. FedAvg instead trains a function $f: \mathbb{R}^d \to \mathbb{R}$, which is a special case of equation (9.1) with $\gamma_{k,i} = \gamma_k$ for $\forall\, i \in [N]$. We take a random initialization of the parameters [109] in our analysis:

[4] https://github.com/med-air/FedBN

$$v_k(0) \sim N\left(0, \alpha^2 I\right), \quad c_k \sim U\{-1, 1\}, \text{ and } \quad \gamma_k = \gamma_{k,i} = \|v_k(0)\|_2/\alpha, \tag{9.2}$$

where α^2 controls the magnitude of v_k at initialization. The initialization of the BN parameters γ_k and $\gamma_{k,i}$ are independent of α. The parameters of the network $f^*(x; V, \gamma, c)$ are obtained by minimizing the empirical risk with respect to the squared loss using gradient descent:

$$L(f^*) = \frac{1}{NM}\sum_{i=1}^{N}\sum_{j=1}^{M}\left(f^*\left(x_j^i\right) - y_j^i\right)^2. \tag{9.3}$$

9.5.1.2 Convergence analysis

Here we study the trajectory of networks FedAvg (f) and FedBN (f^*)'s prediction through the neural tangent kernel (NTK) introduced by [110]. Recent machine learning theory studies [111–115] have shown that for finite-width, over-parameterized networks, the convergence rate is controlled by the least eigenvalue of the induced kernel in the training evolution.

To simplify tracing the optimization dynamics, we consider the case that the number of local updates E is 1. We can decompose the NTK into a magnitude component $\boldsymbol{G}(t)$ and direction component $\boldsymbol{V}(t)/\alpha^2$ following [115]:

$$\frac{\mathrm{d}f}{\mathrm{d}t} = -\Lambda(t)(f(t) - \boldsymbol{y}), \text{ where } \Lambda(t) := \frac{V(t)}{\alpha^2} + G(t).$$

Let $\lambda_{\min}(A)$ denote the minimal eigenvalue of matrix A. The matrices $V(t)$ and $G(t)$ are positive semi-definite, since they can be viewed as covariance matrices. This gives $\lambda_{\min}(\Lambda(t)) \geqslant \max\{\lambda_{\min}(V(t))/\alpha^2, \lambda_{\min}(G(t))\}$. According to NTK, the convergence rate is controlled by $\lambda_{\min}(\Lambda(t))$. Then, for $\alpha > 1$, convergence is dominated by $\boldsymbol{G}(t)$. Let $\Lambda(t)$ and $\Lambda^*(t)$ denote the evolution dynamics of FedAvg and FedBN, and let $G(t)$ and $G^*(t)$ denote the magnitude component in the evolution dynamics of FedAvg and FedBN. For the convergence analysis, we use the auxiliary version of the Gram matrices, which is defined as follows:

Definition 9.2. *Given sample points* $\left\{\boldsymbol{x}_p\right\}_{p=1}^{NM}$, *we define the auxiliary Gram matrices* $G^\infty \in \mathbb{R}^{NM\times NM}$ *and* $G^{*\infty} \in \mathscr{R}^{NM\times NM}$ *as*

$$\boldsymbol{G}_{pq}^{\infty}\& := \mathbb{E}_{v\sim N(0,\alpha^2 I)}\sigma\left(\boldsymbol{v}^\top \boldsymbol{x}_p\right)\sigma\left(\boldsymbol{v}^\top \boldsymbol{x}_q\right), \quad (\mathit{FedAvg}) \tag{9.4}$$

$$\boldsymbol{G}_{pq}^{*\infty}\& := \mathbb{E}_{\boldsymbol{v}\sim N(0,\alpha^2 I)}\sigma\left(\boldsymbol{v}^\top \boldsymbol{x}_p\right)\sigma\left(\boldsymbol{v}^\top \boldsymbol{x}_q\right)\mathbf{1}\left\{i_p = i_q\right\}. \quad (\text{FedBN}) \tag{9.5}$$

Given assumption 9.1, we use the key results in [115] to show that G^∞ is positive definite. Further, we show that $G^{*\infty}$ is positive definite. We use the fact that the distance between $G(t)$ and its auxiliary version is small in over-parameterized neural networks, such that $\boldsymbol{G}(t)$ remains positive definite.

Lemma 9.3. *Fix points* $\{x_p\}_{p=1}^{NM}$ *satisfying assumption 9.1. Then Gram matrices* $\boldsymbol{G}^{\infty}$ *and* $\boldsymbol{G}^{*\infty}$ *defined as in equations (9.4) and (9.5) are strictly positive definite. Let the least eigenvalues be* $\lambda_{\min}(G^{\infty}) = :\mu_0$ *and* $\lambda_{\min}(G^{*\infty}) = :\mu_0^*$, where $\mu_0, \mu_0^* > 0$.

Based on our formulation, the convergence rate of FedAvg (theorem 9.4) can be derived from [115] by considering non-identical covariance matrices. We derive the convergence rate of FedBN in corollary 9.5. Our key result of comparing the convergence rates between FedAvg and FedBN is culminated in corollary 9.6.

Theorem 9.4 *(G-dominated convergence for FedAvg [115]). Suppose network (4) is initialized as in (2) with* $\alpha > 1$ *and trained using gradient descent and assumption 9.1 holds. Given the loss function of training the neural network is the square loss with targets y satisfying* $\|y\|_{\infty} = O(1)$. *If* $m = \Omega\left(\max\left\{N^4M^4 \log(NM/\delta)/\alpha^4\mu_0^4,\ N^2M^2 \log(NM/\delta)/\mu_0^2\right\}\right)$, *then with probability* $1 - \delta$,

1. *For iterations* $t = 0, 1, \ldots,$ *the evolution matrix* $\Lambda(t)$ *satisfies* $\lambda_{\min}(\Lambda(t)) \geqslant \frac{\mu_0}{2}$.
2. *Training with gradient descent of step-size* $\eta = O\left(\frac{1}{\|\Lambda(t)\|}\right)$ *converges linearly as*

$$\|f(t) - y\|_2^2 \leqslant \left(1 - \frac{\eta\mu_0}{2}\right)^t \|f(0) - y\|_2^2.$$

Following the key ideas in [115], here we further characterize the convergence for FedBN.

Corollary 9.5 *(G-dominated convergence for FedBN). Suppose network (5) and all other conditions in theorem 9.4. With probability* $1 - \delta$, *for iterations* $t = 0, 1, \ldots,$ *the evolution matrix* $\Lambda^*(t)$ *satisfies* $\lambda_{\min}(\Lambda^*(t)) \geqslant \frac{\mu_0^*}{2}$ *and training with gradient descent of step-size* $\eta = O\left(\frac{1}{\|\Lambda^*(t)\|}\right)$ *converges linearly as* $\|f^*(t) - y\|_2^2 \leqslant \left(1 - \frac{\eta\mu_0^*}{2}\right)^t \|f^*(0) - y\|_2^2$.

The exponential factor of convergence for FedAvg $(1 - \eta\mu_0/2)$ and FedBN $\left(1 - \eta\mu_0^*/2\right)$ are controlled by the smallest eigenvalue of $G(t)$, respectively $G^*(t)$. Then we can analyze the convergence performance of FedAvg and FedBN by comparing $\lambda_{\min}(G^{\infty})$ and $\lambda_{\min}(G^{*\infty})$.

Corollary 9.6 *(Convergence rate comparison between FedAvg and FedBN). For the G-dominated convergence, the convergence rate of FedBN is faster than that of FedAvg.*

More details of the proof please refer to the original FedBN paper [108].

9.5.1.3 Experimental results

To better understand how our proposed algorithm can be beneficial in real-world data heterogeneity, we have extensively validated the effectiveness of FedBN in comparison with other methods on two different tasks: breast cancer histology image classification and prostate MRI segmentation. We run three trials and report the average results with standard deviation.

Datasets and setup. For the **breast cancer histology image classification** task, we use the public tumor dataset Camelyon17, which contains 450 000 histology images with different stains from five different hospitals [65]. As shown in figure 9.1, we take each hospital as a single client, and images from different clients have heterogeneous appearances but share the same label distribution (i.e. normal and tumor tissues). We use a deep network of DenseNet121 [120] and train the model for 100 epochs at the client-side with different communication frequencies. We use cross-entropy loss and SDG optimizer with a learning rate of 1e−3. For the **prostate MRI segmentation** task, we use a multi-site prostate segmentation dataset [8], which contains six different data sources from three public datasets [56–58]. We regard each data source as a client and train the U-Net using Adam optimizer with a learning rate of 1e−4, momentum of 0.9 and 0.99.

We report the performance of global models, i.e. the final results of our overall framework. The model was selected using the separate validation set and evaluated on the testing set. If not specified, our default setting for the local update epoch is 1. We use the momentum of 0.9 and weight decay of 1e−4 for all optimizers.

Results and analysis. We compare our approach with recent state-of-the-art (SOTA) FL methods towards solving the data heterogeneity problem. Both FedProx [116] and a recent method MOON [119] tackle the data heterogeneity problem by constraining the dissimilarity between local and global models to reduce global aggregation shifts. FedAdam [118] and FedNova [117] are proposed as general methods to tackle global drifts. For the breast cancer histology image classification shown in table 9.1, we report the testing accuracy on five different clients and the

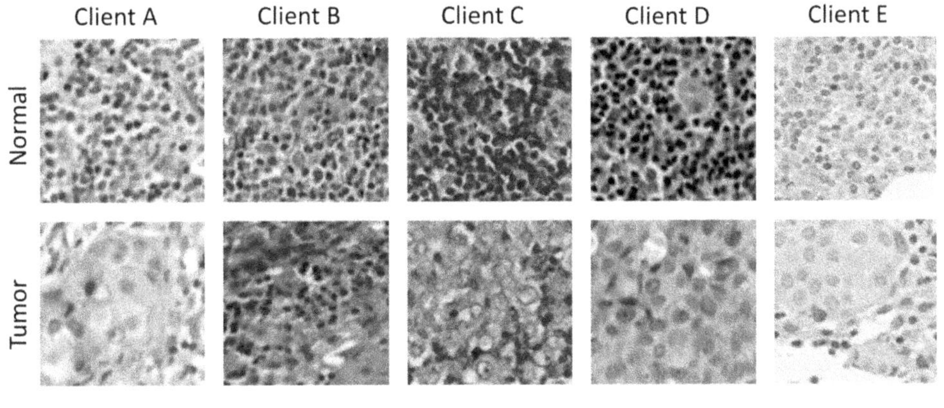

Figure 9.1. Examples of breast histology images of normal and tumor tissues from five clients, showing large heterogeneity. Reproduced from [107], Copyright © Association for the Advancement of Artificial Intelligence. All rights reserved.

Table 9.1. Results for histology nuclei segmentation and prostate MRI segmentation. The results of the Dice coefficient are reported. Each column represents one client, and Avg. refers to the average Dice.

	Breast cancer histology image classification (accuracy %)						Prostate MRI segmentation (Dice %)						
	A	B	C	D	E	Avg.	A	B	C	D	E	F	Avg.
FedAvg	**91.10**	83.12	82.06	87.49	74.78	83.71	90.04	94.31	92.60	92.21	90.14	89.36	91.44
	< 0.001	< 0.001	< 0.001	< 0.001	< 0.001	< 0.001	< 0.001	0.087	< 0.001	0.008	< 0.001	0.004	< 0.001
[103]	(0.46)	(1.58)	(8.52)	(2.49)	(3.19)	(6.16)	(1.27)	(0.28)	(0.66)	(0.71)	(0.27)	(1.76)	(1.91)
FedProx	91.03	82.88	82.78	87.07	74.93	83.74	90.65	94.60	92.64	92.19	89.36	87.07	91.08
	0.073	< 0.001	< 0.001	< 0.001	< 0.001	< 0.001	< 0.001	0.063	< 0.001	0.021	< 0.001	< 0.001	< 0.001
[116]	(0.50)	(1.63)	(8.56)	(1.76)	(3.05)	(5.99)	(1.95)	(0.30)	(1.03)	(0.15)	(0.97)	(1.53)	(2.66)
FedNova	90.99	82.97	82.40	86.93	74.86	83.61	90.73	94.26	92.73	91.91	90.01	89.94	91.60
	0.152	< 0.001	< 0.001	< 0.001	< 0.001	< 0.001	< 0.001	0.049	< 0.001	< 0.001	< 0.001	0.015	< 0.001
[117]	(0.54)	(1.76)	(9.21)	(1.58)	(3.12)	(6.00)	(0.41)	(0.08)	(1.29)	(0.61)	(0.87)	(1.54)	(1.70)
FedAdam	87.45	80.38	76.89	89.27	**77.86**	82.37	90.02	**94.84**	93.30	91.70	90.17	87.77	91.30
	< 0.001	< 0.001	< 0.001	< 0.001	< 0.001	< 0.001	< 0.001	0.172	0.036	< 0.001	< 0.001	< 0.001	< 0.001
[118]	(0.77)	(2.03)	(14.03)	(1.28)	(2.68)	(5.65)	(0.29)	(0.11)	(0.79)	(0.16)	(1.46)	(1.35)	(2.53)
MOON	88.92	83.52	84.71	90.02	67.79	82.99	91.79	93.63	93.01	**92.61**	91.22	91.14	92.23
	< 0.001	< 0.001	< 0.001	< 0.001	< 0.001	< 0.001	0.008	0.017	< 0.001	0.023	< 0.001	0.057	< 0.001
[119]	(1.54)	(0.31)	(5.14)	(1.56)	(2.06)	(8.93)	(1.64)	(0.21)	(0.75)	(0.53)	(0.61)	(0.88)	(1.01)
FedBN	89.35	**90.25**	**94.16**	**94.04**	68.87	**87.33**	**92.68**	94.83	**93.77**	92.32	**93.20**	89.68	**92.75**
(Ours)	(8.50)	(1.66)	(LOO)	(2.32)	(22.14)	(10.55)	(0.52)	(0.47)	(0.41)	(0.19)	(0.45)	(0.60)	(1.74)

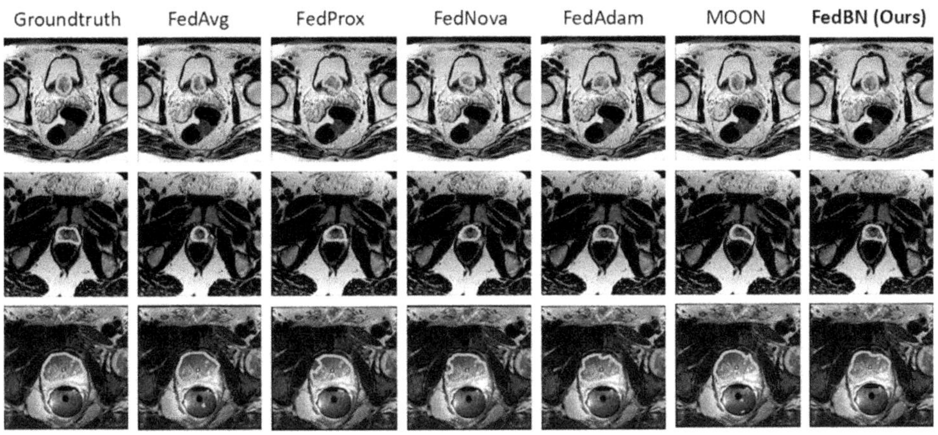

Figure 9.2. Qualitative comparison on segmentation results with our method and other state-of-the-art methods. The top two rows are for the task of prostate MRI segmentation, and the bottom two rows are for the task of histology nuclei segmentation.

average results. It can be observed that alternative methods only achieve minor improvements than FedAvg on certain clients. Our method FedBN exceeds by a non-negligible margin on four clients significantly, reaching an accuracy of 87.33% on average. Interestingly, we found the standard deviation on client E is large. The reason may come from that images in client E appear differently as shown in figure 9.1, making the training procedure not as stable as other clients.

For segmentation tasks, the experimental results of Dice are shown in table 9.1 in the form of a single client and average performance. As MRI images show fewer domain shifts than histology images, the performance gap of each client is not as large as histology image classification. Our method still achieves the highest Dice of 92.75% regarding the average performance. Besides, we visualize the segmentation results to demonstrate a qualitative comparison, as shown in figure 9.2. Compared with the first ground-truth column, due to the heterogeneous features, other FL methods either cover more or fewer areas. As can be observed from the second column, the heterogeneity in features also makes FedAvg fail to obtain an accurate boundary, while our approach shows more accurate boundaries. The results are inspiring and bring the hope of deploying FedBN to the healthcare field, where data are often limited, isolated, and heterogeneous on features.

9.5.2 Federated domain generalization for testing under external data heterogeneity

9.5.2.1 Method

To further tackle the data heterogeneity issues when deploying the federated models to external unseen medical centers, we identify the problem setting of *Federated Domain Generalization* (FedDG)[5] [121], which aims to learn a federated model from multiple decentralized source domains such that it can directly generalize to

[5] https://github.com/liuquande/FedDG-ELCFS

completely unseen domains. In FedDG, we denote $(\mathscr{X}, \mathscr{Y})$ as the joint image and label space of a task and $\mathscr{S} = \{\mathscr{S}^1, \mathscr{S}^2, \dots, \mathscr{S}^K\}$ as the set of K distributed source domains involved in FL. Each domain contains data and label pairs of $\mathscr{S}^k = \left\{\left(x_i^k, y_i^k\right)\right\}_{i=1}^{N^k}$, which are sampled from a domain-specific distribution $(\mathscr{X}^k, \mathscr{Y})$. The goal of FedDG is to learn a model $f_\theta: \mathscr{X} \to \mathscr{Y}$ using the K distributed source domains, such that it can directly generalize to a completely unseen testing domain $\mathscr{T}$ with a high performance. An overview of our proposed method is shown in figure 9.3.

Continuous frequency space interpolation. To address the restriction of decentralized datasets, the foundation of our solution is to exchange the distribution information across clients, such that each local client can get access to multi-source data distributions for learning generalizable parameters. Considering that sharing raw images is forbidden, we propose to exploit the information inherent in the frequency space, which enables the separation of the distribution (i.e. style) information from the original images to be shared between clients without privacy leakage.

Specifically, given a sample $x_i^k \in \mathbb{R}^{H\times W\times C}$ ($C = 3$ for RGB image and $C = 1$ for gray-scale image) from the kth client, we can obtain its frequency space signal through fast Fourier transform [122] as

$$\mathscr{F}(x_i^k)(u, v, c) = \sum_{h=0}^{H-1}\sum_{w=0}^{W-1} x_i^k(h, w, c)e^{-j2\pi\left(\frac{h}{H}u+\frac{w}{W}v\right)}. \tag{9.6}$$

This frequency space signal $\mathscr{F}(x_i^k)$ can be further decomposed to an amplitude spectrum $\mathscr{A}_i^k \in \mathbb{R}^{H\times W\times C}$ and a phase spectrum $\mathscr{P}_i^k \in \mathbb{R}^{H\times W\times C}$, which respectively reflect the low-level distributions (e.g. style) and high-level semantics (e.g. object) of the image. To exchange the distribution information across clients, we first construct a distribution bank $\mathscr{A} = [\mathscr{A}^1, \dots, \mathscr{A}^K]$, where each $\mathscr{A}^k = \{\mathscr{A}_i^k\}_{i=1}^{N^k}$ contains all

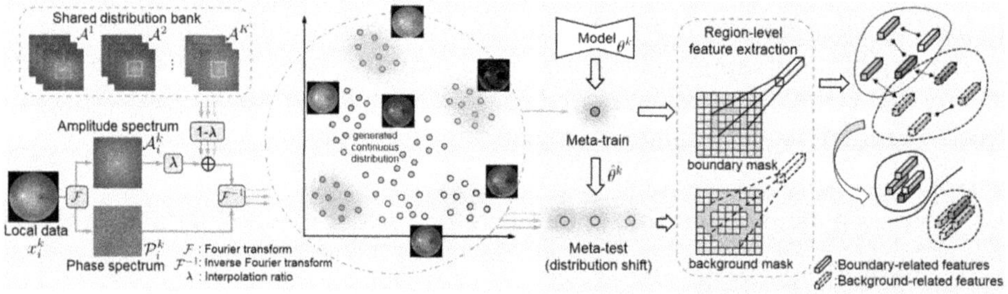

Figure 9.3. Overview of our proposed episodic learning in continuous frequency space. The distribution information is exchanged across clients from frequency space with a continuous interpolation mechanism, enabling each local client to access the multi-source distributions. An episodic training paradigm is then established to expose the local optimization to domain shift, with explicit regularization to promote domain-independent feature cohesion and separation at the ambiguous boundary region for improving generalizability. © 2021 IEEE. Reprinted, with permission, from [121].

amplitude spectrum of images from the kth client, representing the distribution of $\mathcal{X}^k$. This bank is then made accessible to all clients as shared distribution knowledge.

Next, we design a continuous interpolation mechanism within the frequency space, aiming to transmit multi-source distribution information to a local client leveraging the distribution bank. As shown in the left part of figure 9.3, given a local image x_i^k at client k, we can replace some low-frequency components of its amplitude spectrum with the ones in distribution bank $\mathcal{A}$, while its phase spectrum is unaffected to preserve the semantic content. As an outcome, we can generate images with transformed appearances exhibiting distribution characteristics of other clients. More importantly, we continuously interpolate between the amplitude spectrum of local data and the transferred amplitude spectrum of other domains. In this way, we can enrich the established multi-domain distributions for each local client, benefiting from a dedicated dense space with smooth distribution changes. Formally, this is achieved by randomly sampling an amplitude spectrum item $\mathcal{A}_j^n (n \neq k)$ from the distribution bank and then synthesizing a new amplitude spectrum by interpolating between $\mathcal{A}_i^k$ and $\mathcal{A}_j^n$. Let $\mathcal{M} = \mathbb{1}_{(h,\, w) \in [-\alpha H:\alpha H,\, -\alpha W:\alpha W]}$ be a binary mask which controls the scale of low-frequency component within amplitude spectrum to be exchanged and whose value is 1 at the central region and 0 elsewhere. Denote λ as the interpolation ratio adjusting the amount of distribution information contributed by $\mathcal{A}_i^k$ and $\mathcal{A}_j^n$, the generated new amplitude spectrum interacting distributions for local client k and external client n is represented as

$$\mathcal{A}_{i,\lambda}^{k \to n} = \left((1 - \lambda)\mathcal{A}_i^k + \lambda \mathcal{A}_j^n\right) \times \mathcal{M} + \mathcal{A}_i^k \times (1 - \mathcal{M}). \tag{9.7}$$

After obtaining the interpolated amplitude spectrum $\mathcal{A}_{i,\lambda}^{k \to n}$, we then combine it with the original phase spectrum to generate the transformed image via inverse Fourier transform $\mathcal{F}^{-1}$ as $x_{i,\lambda}^{k \to n} = \mathcal{F}^{-1}\left(\mathcal{A}_{i,\lambda}^{k \to n}, \mathcal{P}_i^k\right)$, where the generated image $x_{i,\lambda}^{k \to n}$ preserves the original semantics of x_i^k while carrying a new distribution interacted between $\mathcal{X}^k$ and $\mathcal{X}^n$. In our implementation, the interpolation ratio λ will be dynamically sampled from [0.0, 1.0] to generate images via a continuous distribution space. Note that the method described above does not require heavy computations and thus can be performed online as the local learning goes on. Practically, for each input x_i^k, we will sample an amplitude spectrum A_j^n from the distribution bank for each external client $n \neq k$ and transform its image appearance as equation (9.7). Through this, we obtain $K - 1$ transformed images $\left\{x_{i,\lambda}^{k \to n}\right\}_{n \neq k}$ of different distributions, which share the same semantic label as x_i^k. For ease of denotation, we represent these transformed images as t_i^k hereafter, i.e. $t_i^k = \left\{x_{i,\lambda}^{k \to n}\right\}_{n \neq k}$.

Boundary-oriented episodic learning. In the following, we carefully design a boundary-oriented episodic learning scheme for local training, by particularly meeting challenges of model generalization in medical image segmentation scenarios. We establish the local training as an episodic meta-learning scheme, which learns generalizable model parameters by simulating train/test domain shift explicitly. Note that in our case, the domain shift at a local client comes from the data generated from frequency space with different distributions. Specifically, in each iteration, we consider the raw input x_i^k as meta-train and its counterparts t_i^k generated from frequency space as meta-test presenting distribution shift (cf figure 9.3). The meta-learning scheme can then be decoupled to two steps. First, the model parameters θ^k are updated on meta-train with segmentation Dice loss $\mathcal{L}_{seg}$:

$$\hat{\theta}^k = \theta^k - \beta \nabla_{\theta^k} \mathcal{L}_{\text{seg}}\left(x_i^k; \theta^k\right), \tag{9.8}$$

where β denotes the learning rate for the inner-loop update. Second, a meta-update is performed to virtually evaluate the updated parameters $\hat{\theta}^k$ on the held-out meta-test data t_i^k with a meta-objective $\mathcal{L}_{\text{meta}}$. Crucially, this objective is computed with the updated parameters $\hat{\theta}^k$ but optimized w.r.t. the original parameters θ^k. Such optimization paradigm aims make the learning on source domains able to further fulfill certain properties desired in unseen domains, which are quantified by $\mathcal{L}_{\text{meta}}$.

In our case, we define the $\mathcal{L}_{\text{meta}}$ with considering specific challenges in medical image segmentation. Particularly, we design a new boundary-oriented objective to enhance the domain-invariant boundary delineation, by carefully learning from the local data x_i^k and the corresponding t_i^k generated from frequency space with multi-source distributions. The boundary-oriented objective helps the model avoid suffering from ambiguous decision boundaries and be robust to the distribution shift when deployed to unseen domains outside federation.

Specifically, we first extract the boundary-related and background-related features for the input samples. Given image x_i^k with segmentation label y_i^k, we can extract its binary boundary mask $y_{i\_bd}^k$ and background mask $y_{i\_bg}^k$ with morphological operations on y_i^k. Here, the mask $y_{i\_bg}^k$ only contains background pixels around the anatomy boundary instead of from the whole image, as we expect to enhance the discriminability for features around the boundary region. Let Z_i^k denote the activation map extracted from layer l, which is interpolated with bilinear interpolation to keep consistent dimensions as y_i^k. Then the boundary-related and background-related features of x_i^k can be extracted from Z_i^k with masked average pooling over $y_{i\_bd}^k$ and $y_{i\_bg}^k$ as

$$h_{i\_bd}^k = \frac{\sum_{h,w} Z_i^k * y_{i\_bd}^k}{\sum_{h,w} y_{i\_bd}^k}; h_{i\_bg}^k = \frac{\sum_{h,w} Z_i^k * y_{i\_bg}^k}{\sum_{h,w} y_{i\_bg}^k}, \tag{9.9}$$

where $*$ denotes element-wise product. The produced $h_{i\_bd}^k$ and $h_{i\_bg}^k$ are single-dimensional vectors, representing the averaged region-level features of the boundary and background pixels. By further performing the same operation for $K - 1$ transformed images t_i^k with different distributions transferred from the frequency space, we accordingly obtain together K boundary-related and K background-related features.

Next, we enhance the domain-invariance and discriminability of these features by regularizing their intra-class cohesion and inter-class separation regardless of distributions. Here, we employ the well-established InfoNCE [123] objective to impose such regularization. Denote (h_m, h_p) as a pair of features, which is a positive pair if h_m and h_p are of the same class (both boundary-related or background-related) and otherwise negative pair. In our case, the InfoNCE loss is defined over each positive pair (h_m, h_p) within the $2 \times K$ region-level features as

$$\ell(h_m, h_p) = -\log \frac{\exp(h_m \odot h_p/\tau)}{\sum_{q=1,\, q \neq m}^{2K} \mathbb{F}(h_m, h_q) \cdot \exp(h_m \odot h_q/\tau)}, \tag{9.10}$$

where $\odot$ denotes the cosine similarity: $a \odot b = \frac{\langle a, b \rangle}{\| a \|_2 \| b \|_2}$; the value of $\mathbb{F}(h_m, h_q)$ is 0 and 1 for positive and negative pair, respectively; and τ denotes the temperature parameter. The final loss $\mathcal{L}_{\text{boundary}}$ is the average of ℓ over all positive pairs:

$$\mathcal{L}_{\text{boundary}} = \sum_{m=1}^{2K} \sum_{p=m+1}^{2K} \frac{(1 - \mathbb{F}(h_m, h_p)) \cdot \ell(h_m, h_p)}{B(K, 2) \times 2}, \tag{9.11}$$

where $B(K, 2)$ is the number of combinations.

Overall local learning objective. The overall meta-objective is composed of the segmentation Dice loss $\mathcal{L}_{\text{seg}}$ and the boundary-oriented objective $\mathcal{L}_{\text{boundary}}$ as

$$\mathcal{L}_{\text{meta}} = \mathcal{L}_{\text{seg}}(t_i^k; \hat{\theta}^k) + \gamma \mathcal{L}_{\text{boundary}}(x_i^k, t_i^k; \hat{\theta}^k), \tag{9.12}$$

where $\hat{\theta}^k$ is the updated parameter from equation (9.8) and γ is a balancing hyper-parameter. Finally, both the inner-loop and meta-objective will be optimized together with respect to the original parameter θ^k as $\arg\min_{\theta^k} \mathcal{L}_{\text{seg}}(x_i^k; \theta^k) + \mathcal{L}_{\text{meta}}(x_i^k, t_i^k; \hat{\theta}^k)$. In a federated round, once the local learning is finished, the local parameters θ^k from all clients will be aggregated at the server to update the global model.

9.5.2.2 *Experimental results*

We evaluate our method on two medical image segmentation tasks, i.e. the optic disc and cup segmentation on retinal fundus images [33] and the prostate segmentation on T2-weighted MRI [58], by conducting comparison with DG methods that can be incorporated in the federated paradigm.

Datasets and evaluation metrics. We employ **retinal fundus images from four different clinical centers** of public datasets [33–35] for optic disc and cup segmentation. For pre-processing, we center-crop a 800×800 disc region for these data uniformly and then resize the cropped region to 384×384 as network input. We further collect **prostate T2-weighted MRI images from six different data sources** partitioned from the public datasets [8, 56–58] for the prostate MRI segmentation task. All the data are pre-processed to have a similar field of view for the prostate region and resized to 384×384 in axial plane. We then normalize the data

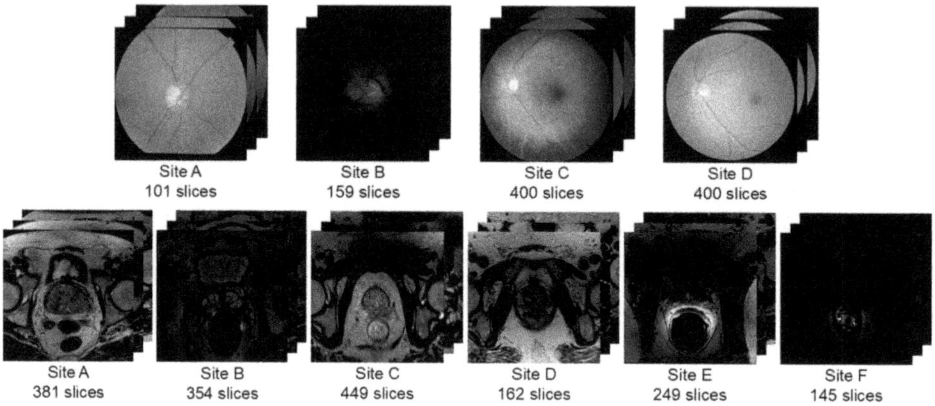

Figure 9.4. Example cases and slice number of each data source in fundus image segmentation and prostate MRI segmentation tasks. © 2021 IEEE. Reprinted, with permission, from [121].

individually to zero mean and unit variance in intensity values. The example cases and sample numbers of each data source are presented in figure 9.4. For evaluation, we adopt two commonly used metrics of Dice coefficient (Dice) and Hausdorff distance (HD), to quantitatively evaluate the segmentation results.

Results and analysis. In our experiments, we follow the practice in domain generalization literature to adopt the leave-one-domain-out strategy, i.e. training on $K - 1$ distributed source domains and testing on the one left-out unseen target domain.

We compare with recent SOTA DG methods that are free from data centralization and can be incorporated into the local learning process in federated paradigm, including: JiGen [124], an effective self-supervised learning approach to learn general representations by solving jigsaw puzzles; BigAug [94], a method that performs extensive data transformations to regularize general representation learning; Epi-FCR [125], a scheme to periodically exchange partial model (classifier or feature extractor) across domains to expose model learning to domain shift; and RSC [126], a method that randomly discards the dominating features to promote robust model optimization. For the implementation, we follow their public code or paper and establish them in the federated setting.

Table 9.2 presents the quantitative results for retinal fundus segmentation. We see that different DG methods can improve the overall generalization performance more or less over FedAvg. This attributes to their regularization effect on the local learning to extract general representations. Compared with these methods, our episodic learning in continuous frequency space (ELCFS) achieves higher overall performance and obtains improvements on most unseen sites in terms of Dice and HD for both optic disc and cup segmentation. This benefits from our frequency space interpolation mechanism, which presents multi-domain distributions to the local client. For prostate MRI segmentation in table 9.3, the comparison DG methods generally perform better than FedAvg, but the improvements are relatively marginal. Our ELCFS obtains the highest Dice across all the six unseen sites and HD on most sites. Overall, our method

Table 9.2. Comparison of federated domain generalization results on optic disc/cup segmentation from fundus images.

Task	Optic disc segmentation					Optic disc segmentation						Optic disc segmentation					Optic disc segmentation				
Unseen site	A	B	C	D	Avg.	A	B	C	D	Avg.	Overall	A	B	C	D	Avg.	A	B	C	D	Avg.	Overall
	Dice coefficient (Dice)↑											Hausdorff distance (HD)↓										
JiGen [124]	93.92	85.91	92.63	94.03	91.62	82.26	70.68	83.32	**85.70**	80.47	86.06	13.12	20.18	11.29	8.15	13.19	20.88	23.21	11.55	9.23	16.22	14.71
	< 0.001	< 0.001	< 0.001	< 0.001	< 0.001	< 0.001	< 0.001	< 0.001	0.005	< 0.001	< 0.001	< 0.001	< 0.001	< 0.001	< 0.001	< 0.001	< 0.001	< 0.001	< 0.001	< 0.001	< 0.001	< 0.001
BigAug [94]	91.49	86.18	92.09	91.67	91.36	81.62	69.46	82.64	84.51	79.56	85.46	16.91	19.01	11.51	8.76	14.05	21.21	21.10	12.02	10.47	16.70	15.19
	< 0.001	< 0.001	< 0.001	< 0.001	< 0.001	< 0.001	< 0.001	< 0.001	< 0.001	< 0.001	< 0.001	< 0.001	< 0.001	< 0.001	< 0.001	< 0.001	< 0.001	< 0.001	< 0.001	< 0.001	< 0.001	< 0.001
Epi-FCR [125]	94.34	86.22	92.88	93.73	91.79	83.06	70.25	83.68	83.14	80.03	85.91	13.02	18.97	**10.67**	8.47	12.78	19.12	21.94	11.50	10.86	15.86	14.32
	< 0.001	< 0.001	< 0.001	< 0.001	< 0.001	< 0.001	< 0.001	< 0.001	< 0.001	< 0.001	< 0.001	< 0.001	< 0.001	0.005	< 0.001	< 0.001	< 0.001	< 0.001	< 0.001	< 0.001	< 0.001	< 0.001
RSC [126]	94.50	86.21	92.23	94.15	91.77	81.77	69.37	83.40	84.82	79.84	85.80	19.44	19.26	13.47	8.14	15.08	23.85	24.01	11.38	9.79	17.25	16.16
	< 0.001	< 0.001	< 0.001	< 0.001	< 0.001	< 0.001	< 0.001	< 0.001	< 0.001	< 0.001	< 0.001	< 0.001	< 0.001	< 0.001	< 0.001	< 0.001	< 0.001	< 0.001	< 0.001	< 0.001	< 0.001	< 0.001
FedAvg [103]	92.88	85.73	92.07	93.21	90.97	80.84	69.71	82.28	83.35	79.05	85.01	17.01	20.68	11.70	9.33	14.68	20.77	26.01	11.85	10.03	17.17	15.93
	< 0.001	< 0.001	< 0.001	< 0.001	< 0.001	< 0.001	< 0.001	< 0.001	< 0.001	< 0.001	< 0.001	< 0.001	< 0.001	< 0.001	< 0.001	< 0.001	< 0.001	< 0.001	< 0.001	< 0.001	< 0.001	< 0.001
ELCFS (Ours)	**95.37**	**87.52**	**93.37**	**94.50**	**92.69**	**84.13**	**71.88**	**83.94**	85.51	**81.37**	**87.03**	**11.36**	**17.10**	10.83	**7.24**	**11.63**	**19.36**	**11.17**	**8.91**	**14.52**	**13.07**	

Table 9.3. Comparison of federated domain generalization results on prostate MRI segmentation.

Unseen site	A	B	C	D	E	F	Average	A	B	C	D	E	F	Average
			Dice coefficient (Dice)↑							Dice coefficient (Dice)↓				
JiGen [124]	89.95	85.81	84.06	87.34	81.32	89.11	86.26	10.51	11.53	11.70	11.49	14.80	9.02	11.51
	< 0.001	< 0.001	< 0.001	< 0.001	< 0.001	< 0.001	< 0.001	< 0.001	< 0.001	0.002	< 0.001	< 0.001	< 0.001	< 0.001
BigAug [94]	89.63	84.62	83.86	87.66	81.20	88.96	85.99	10.68	11.78	12.07	**10.66**	13.98	9.73	11.48
	< 0.001	< 0.001	< 0.001	< 0.001	< 0.001	< 0.001	< 0.001	< 0.001	< 0.001	< 0.001	< 0.001	< 0.001	< 0.001	< 0.001
Epi-FCR [125]	89.72	85.39	84.97	86.55	80.63	89.76	86.17	10.60	12.31	12.29	12.00	15.68	8.81	11.95
	< 0.001	< 0.001	< 0.001	< 0.001	< 0.001	< 0.001	< 0.001	< 0.001	< 0.001	< 0.001	< 0.001	< 0.001	< 0.001	< 0.001
RSC [126]	88.86	85.56	84.36	86.21	79.97	89.80	85.80	10.57	11.84	14.76	13.07	14.79	8.83	12.31
	< 0.001	< 0.001	< 0.001	< 0.001	< 0.001	< 0.001	< 0.001	< 0.001	< 0.001	< 0.001	< 0.001	< 0.001	< 0.001	< 0.001
FedAvg [103]	89.02	84.48	84.11	86.30	80.38	89.15	85.57	11.64	12.01	14.86	11.80	14.90	9.30	12.42
	< 0.001	< 0.001	< 0.001	< 0.001	< 0.001	< 0.001	< 0.001	< 0.001	< 0.001	< 0.001	< 0.001	< 0.001	< 0.001	< 0.001
ELCFS (Ours)	**90.19**	**87.17**	**85.26**	**88.23**	**83.02**	**90.47**	**87.39**	**10.30**	**11.49**	**11.50**	11.57	**11.08**	**8.31**	**10.88**

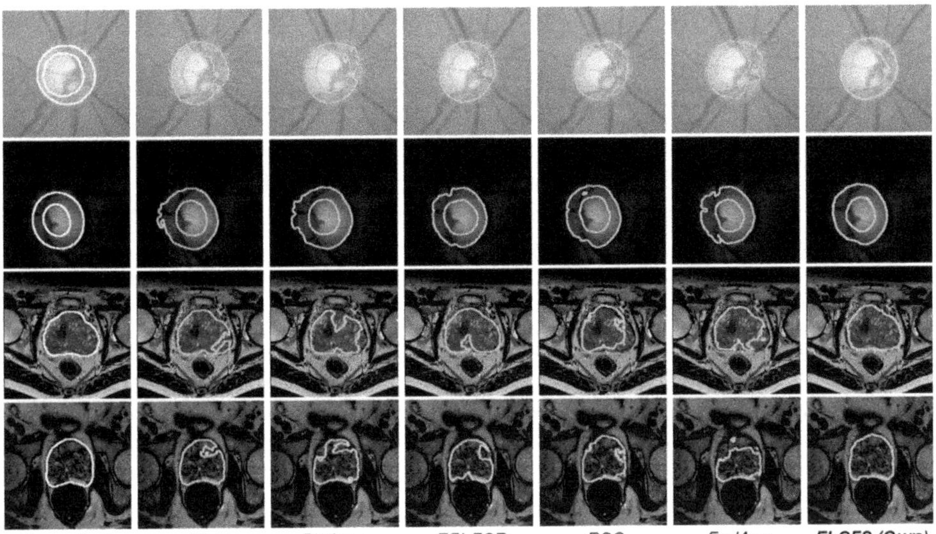

Figure 9.5. Qualitative comparison on the generalization results of different methods in fundus image segmentation (top two rows) and prostate MRI segmentation (bottom two tows). © 2021 IEEE. Reprinted, with permission, from [121].

improves over FedAvg for Dice from 85.57% to 87.39% and HD from 12.42 to 10.88, outperforming other DG methods. Figure 9.5 shows the segmentation results with two cases from unseen domains for each task. It is observed that our method accurately segments the structure and delineates the boundary in images of unknown distributions, whereas other methods sometimes fail to do so.

9.6 Discussion and summary

Existing adaptation- and generalization-based methods have been active research fields already with solutions to overcome such domain distribution shifts under the centralized data. Domain adaptation methods aim to align distributions across domains, and domain generalization mainly focuses on learning generalizable and transferable representations. However, these well-formulated algorithms are mainly designed under the assumption of gathering data together. Collecting a sufficiently large amount of data itself is a challenging issue given the concern on patients' privacy and data collection protocols. FL methods are more appealing and practical in the long-run for real-world clinical applications. It is therefore urgent to develop techniques for combating data heterogeneity in such a new distributed paradigm. Extending some existing domain adaptation/generalization methods to FL frameworks is a short-term solution. Designing and developing novel techniques that better suit the characteristics of FL paradigm is more important. Besides our illustrated two example methods in section 9.5, some other self-training [78], self-ensembling [92] and augmentation-based methods [51, 102] have also been investigated on federated data heterogeneity.

Recently, the test-time adaptation has been an emerging topic to efficiently tackle the cross-domain distribution shift at test time for medical images from different institutions. Unlike methods mentioned above, test-time adaptation methods are able to continuously update a model with the distributional information provided by a single test sample. For example, the method Denoising Test-Time Adaptation (DTTA) [127] employs denoising auto-encoders to learn shape priors in the source domain, which are leveraged for adaptation at test time. Similarly, Valvano *et al* [128] keep mask discriminators to provide prior knowledge of shape and fine-tune the segmentor on each individual test instance to optimize the learned prior knowledge. Zhu *et al* [129] try to fine-tune the learned model with test-time training on each test image pair to improve the generalization accuracy of learning-based registration. The method Autoencoder Test-Time Adaptation (ATTA) [32] trains a set of auto-encoders on the source dataset and updates a set of adaptors at test time to minimize the distribution shift indicated by the auto-encoders' reconstruction loss. Since the test-time adaptation methods [32, 127–129] have no restriction on the training process, combining the test-time techniques with FL models can further boost the model generalizability. To date, limited investigations with test-time adaptation methods have been conducted on medical images; however, we foresee a surge in this topic owing to its accuracy, efficiency, scalability, and privacy protection.

In summary, this chapter focuses on the problem of data heterogeneity to improve model generalizability towards clinical practice. This is an essential and immediate topic for AI-enabled automated medical image diagnosis. Significant progress has been achieved by the medical image computing community in recent years. Resolving the issue will facilitate to promote deep learning applications on large-scale real-world clinical datasets from different medical institutions.

Acknowledgments

We sincerely thank our colleagues Dr Xiaoxiao Li, Dr Xiaofei Zhang, Dr Michael Kamp, and Dr Jing Qin, for their valuable works in original papers of FedBN and FedDG, which are essential for the contents of section 9.5 in this chapter.

References

[1] Castro D C, Walker I and Glocker B 2020 Causality matters in medical imaging *Nat. Commun.* **11** 1–10

[2] Esteva A, Kuprel B, Novoa R A, Ko J, Swetter S M, Blau H M and Thrun S 2017 Dermatologist-level classification of skin cancer with deep neural networks *Nature* **542** 115–8

[3] Menze B H, Jakab A, Bauer S, Kalpathy-Cramer J, Farahani K, Kirby J, Burren Y, Porz N, Slotboom J and Wiest R *et al* 2014 The multimodal brain tumor image segmentation benchmark (BRATS) *IEEE Trans. Med. Imaging* **34** 1993–2024

[4] Olivier B and André E 2002 Stability and generalization *J. Mach. Learn. Res.* **2** 499–526

[5] Mårtensson G, Ferreira D, Granberg T, Cavallin L, Oppedal K, Padovani A, Rektorova I, Bonanni L, Pardini M and Kramberger M G *et al* 2020 The reliability of a deep learning

model in clinical out-of-distribution MRI data: a multicohort study *Med. Image Anal.* **66** 101714

[6] Weese J and Lorenz C 2016 Four challenges in medical image analysis from an industrial perspective *Med. Image Anal.* **33** 44–9

[7] Aubreville M, Bertram C A, Donovan T A, Marzahl C, Maier A and Klopfleisch R 2020 A completely annotated whole slide image dataset of canine breast cancer to aid human breast cancer research *Sci. Data* **7** 1–10

[8] Liu Q, Dou Q, Yu L and Heng P A 2020 MS-Net: multi-site network for improving prostate segmentation with heterogeneous MRI data *IEEE Trans. Med. Imaging* **39** 2713–24

[9] Glocker B, Robinson R, Castro D C, Dou Q and Konukoglu E 2019 Machine learning with multi-site imaging data: an empirical study on the impact of scanner effects *Medical Imaging Meets NeurIPS (MedNeurIPS) Workshop*

[10] Wachinger C, Becker B G, Rieckmann A and Pölsterl S 2019 Quantifying confounding bias in neuroimaging datasets with causal inference *Int. Conf. on Medical Image Computing and Computer-Assisted Intervention* (Berlin: Springer) pp 484–92

[11] Kamnitsas K, Baumgartner C, Ledig C, Newcombe V, Simpson J, Kane A, Menon D, Nori A, Criminisi A and Rueckert D *et al* 2017 Unsupervised domain adaptation in brain lesion segmentation with adversarial networks *Int. Conf. on Information Processing in Medical Imaging* (Berlin: Springer) pp 597–609

[12] Ghafoorian M, Mehrtash A, Kapur T, Karssemeijer N, Marchiori E, Pesteie M, Guttmann C R G, de Leeuw F-E, Tempany C M and van Ginneken B *et al* 2017 Transfer learning for domain adaptation in MRI: application in brain lesion segmentation *Int. Conf. on Medical Image Computing and Computer-Assisted Intervention* (Berlin: Springer) pp 516–24

[13] Valverde S, Salem M, Cabezas M, Pareto D, Vilanova J C, Ramió-Torrentà L, Rovira À, Salvi J, Oliver A and Lladó X 2019 One-shot domain adaptation in multiple sclerosis lesion segmentation using convolutional neural networks *NeuroImage: Clin* **21** 101638

[14] Pichler G, Dolz J, Ayed I B and Piantanida P 2020 On direct distribution matching for adapting segmentation networks *Medical Imaging with Deep Learning* (PMLR) pp 624–37

[15] Gao Y, Zhang Y, Cao Z, Guo X and Zhang J 2019 Decoding brain states from fMRI signals by using unsupervised domain adaptation *IEEE J. Biomed. Health Inf.* **24** 1677–85

[16] Kuijf H J, Matthijs Biesbroek J, De Bresser J, Heinen R, Andermatt S, Bento M, Berseth M, Belyaev M, Cardoso M J and Casamitjana A *et al* 2019 Standardized assessment of automatic segmentation of white matter hyperintensities and results of the WMH segmentation challenge *IEEE Trans. Med. Imaging* **38** 2556–68

[17] Shafto M A, Tyler L K, Dixon M, Taylor J R, Rowe J B, Cusack A J, Marslen-Wilson W D, Duncan J, Dalgleish T and Henson R N *et al* 2014 The Cambridge Centre for Ageing and Neuroscience (Cam-CAN) study protocol: a cross-sectional, lifespan, multidisciplinary examination of healthy cognitive ageing *BMC Neurol.* **14** 1–25

[18] Sun Y, Gao K, Wu Z, Li G, Zong X, Lei Z, Wei Y, Ma J, Yang X and Feng X *et al* 2021 Multi-site infant brain segmentation algorithms: the iSeg-2019 challenge *IEEE Trans. Med. Imaging* **40** 1363–76

[19] Zhuang X and Shen J 2016 Multi-scale patch and multi-modality atlases for whole heart segmentation of MRI *Med. Image Anal.* **31** 77–87

[20] Dou Q, Ouyang C, Chen C, Chen H and Heng P-A 2018 Unsupervised cross-modality domain adaptation of ConvNets for biomedical image segmentations with adversarial loss *Proc. of the 27th Int. Joint Conf. on Artificial Intelligence* pp 691–7

[21] Chen C, Dou Q, Chen H, Qin J and Heng P-A 2019 Synergistic image and feature adaptation: towards cross-modality domain adaptation for medical image segmentation *Proc. of the AAAI Conf. on Artificial Intelligence* 33 pp 865–72
[22] Wu F and Zhuang X 2020 CF distance: a new domain discrepancy metric and application to explicit domain adaptation for cross-modality cardiac image segmentation *IEEE Trans. Med. Imaging* **39** 4274–85
[23] Bian C, Yuan C, Wang J, Li M, Yang X, Yu S, Ma K, Yuan J and Zheng Y 2020 Uncertainty-aware domain alignment for anatomical structure segmentation *Med. Image Anal.* **64** 101732
[24] Pei C, Wu F, Huang L and Zhuang X 2021 Disentangle domain features for cross-modality cardiac image segmentation *Med. Image Anal.* **71** 102078
[25] Zhuang X 2018 Multivariate mixture model for myocardial segmentation combining multisource images *IEEE Trans. Pattern Anal. Mach. Intell.* **41** 2933–46
[26] Zhuang X 2016 Multivariate mixture model for cardiac segmentation from multi-sequence MRI *Int. Conf. on Medical Image Computing and Computer-Assisted Intervention* (Berlin: Springer) pp 581–8
[27] Dorent R, Kujawa A, Ivory M, Bakas S, Rieke N, Joutard S, Glocker B, Cardoso J, Modat M and Batmanghelich K *et al* 2022 CrossMoDA 2021 challenge: benchmark of cross-modality domain adaptation techniques for vestibular schwannoma and cochlea segmentation arXiv:2201.02831
[28] Wang S, Yu L, Yang X, Fu C-W and Heng P-A 2019 Patch-based output space adversarial learning for joint optic disc and cup segmentation *IEEE Trans. Med. Imaging* **38** 2485–95
[29] Liu Q, Chen C, Dou Q and Heng P-A 2022 Single-domain generalization in medical image segmentation via test-time adaptation from shape dictionary *36th AAAI Conf. on Artificial Intelligence* pp 1756–64
[30] Liu P, Kong B, Li Z, Zhang S and Fang R 2019 CFEA: collaborative feature ensembling adaptation for domain adaptation in unsupervised optic disc and cup segmentation *Int. Conf. on Medical Image Computing and Computer Assisted Intervention* (Berlin: Springer) pp 521–9
[31] Wang S, Yu L, Li K, Yang X, Fu C-W and Heng P-A 2020 DoFE: domain-oriented feature embedding for generalizable fundus image segmentation on unseen datasets *IEEE Trans. Med. Imaging* **39** 4237–48
[32] He Y, Carass A, Zuo L, Dewey B E and Prince J L 2021 Autoencoder based self-supervised test-time adaptation for medical image analysis *Med. Image Anal.* **72** 102136
[33] Orlando J I, Fu H, Barbosa Breda J, van Keer K, Bathula D R, Diaz-Pinto A, Fang R, Heng P-A, Kim J and Lee J H *et al* 2020 Refuge challenge: a unified framework for evaluating automated methods for glaucoma assessment from fundus photographs *Med. Image Anal.* **59** 101570
[34] Sivaswamy J, Krishnadas S R, Chakravarty A, Joshi G D, Ujjwal and Syed T A *et al* 2015 A comprehensive retinal image dataset for the assessment of glaucoma from the optic nerve head analysis *JSM Biomed. Imaging Data* **2** 1004
[35] Fumero F, Alayón S, Sanchez J L, Sigut J and Gonzalez-Hernandez M 2011 Rim-one: an open retinal image database for optic nerve evaluation *24th Int. Symp. on Computer-based Medical Systems (CBMS)* (Piscataway, NJ: IEEE) pp 1–6
[36] He Y, Carass A, Solomon S D, Saidha S, Calabresi P A and Prince J L 2019 Retinal layer parcellation of optical coherence tomography images: data resource for multiple sclerosis and healthy controls *Data Brief* **22** 601–4

[37] Dong N, Kampffmeyer M, Liang X, Wang Z, Dai W and Xing E 2018 Unsupervised domain adaptation for automatic estimation of cardiothoracic ratio *Int. Conference on Medical Image Computing and Computer-Assisted Intervention* (Berlin: Springer) pp 544–52

[38] Zhang Y, Miao S, Mansi T and Liao R 2018 Task driven generative modeling for unsupervised domain adaptation: application to x-ray image segmentation *Int. Conf. on Medical Image Computing and Computer-Assisted Intervention* (Berlin: Springer) pp 599–607

[39] Jiang J, Hu Y-C, Tyagi N, Zhang P, Rimner A, Mageras G S, Deasy J O and Veeraraghavan H 2018 Tumor-aware, adversarial domain adaptation from CT to MRI for lung cancer segmentation *Int. Conf. on Medical Image Computing and Computer-Assisted Intervention* (Berlin: Springer) pp 777–85

[40] Chen C, Dou Q, Chen H and Heng P-A 2018 Semantic-aware generative adversarial nets for unsupervised domain adaptation in chest x-ray segmentation *Int. Workshop on Machine Learning in Medical Imaging* (Berlin: Springer) pp 143–51

[41] Tang Y, Tang Y, Sandfort V, Xiao J and Summers R M 2019 TUNA-Net: task-oriented unsupervised adversarial network for disease recognition in cross-domain chest x-rays *Int. Conf. on Medical Image Computing and Computer-Assisted Intervention* (Springer) pp 431–40

[42] Lenga M, Schulz H and Saalbach A 2020 Continual learning for domain adaptation in chest x-ray classification *Medical Imaging with Deep Learning* (PMLR) pp 413–23

[43] Xu G-X, Liu C, Liu J, Ding Z, Shi F, Guo M, Zhao W, Li X, Wei Y and Gao Y *et al* 2021 Cross-site severity assessment of COVID-19 from CT images via domain adaptation *IEEE Trans. Med. Imaging* **41** 88–102

[44] Wang Z, Liu Q and Dou Q 2020 Contrastive cross-site learning with redesigned net for COVID-19 CT classification *IEEE J. Biomed. Health Inf.* **24** 2806–13

[45] Dou Q, So T Y, Jiang M, Liu Q, Vardhanabhuti V, Kaissis G, Li Z, Si W, Lee H H C and Yu K *et al* 2021 Federated deep learning for detecting COVID-19 lung abnormalities in CT: a privacy-preserving multinational validation study *NPJ Digit. Med.* **4** 1–11

[46] Jaeger S, Candemir S, Antani S, Wáng Y-X J, Lu P-X and Thoma G 2014 Two public chest x-ray datasets for computer-aided screening of pulmonary diseases *Quant. Imaging Med. Surg.* **4** 475

[47] Shiraishi J, Katsuragawa S, Ikezoe J, Matsumoto T, Kobayashi T, Komatsu K, Matsui M, Fujita H, Kodera Y and Doi K 2000 Development of a digital image database for chest radiographs with and without a lung nodule: receiver operating characteristic analysis of radiologists' detection of pulmonary nodules *Am. J. Roentgenol.* **174** 71–4

[48] Wang X, Peng Y, Lu L, Lu Z, Bagheri M and Summers R M 2017 Chestx-ray8: hospital-scale chest x-ray database and benchmarks on weakly supervised classification and localization of common thorax diseases *Proc. of the IEEE Conf. on Computer Vision and Pattern Recognition* pp 2097–106

[49] Johnson A E W, Pollard T J, Greenbaum N R, Lungreen M P, Deng C-Y, Peng Y, Lu Z, Mark R G, Berkowitz S J and Horng S 2019 MIMIC-CXR-JPG, a large publicly available database of labeled chest radiographs arXiv:1901.07042

[50] Chen C, Dou Q, Chen H, Qin J and Heng P A 2020 Unsupervised bidirectional cross-modality adaptation via deeply synergistic image and feature alignment for medical image segmentation *IEEE Trans. Med. Imaging* **39** 2494–505

[51] Ouyang C, Chen C, Li S, Li Z, Qin C, Bai W and Rueckert D 2021 Causality-inspired single-source domain generalization for medical image segmentation arXiv:2111.12525

[52] Kavur A E, Gezer N S, Barış M, Aslan S, Conze P-H, Groza V, Pham D D, Chatterjee S, Ernst P and Özkan S *et al* 2021 CHAOS challenge – combined (CT-MR) healthy abdominal organ segmentation *Med. Image Anal.* **69** 101950

[53] Landman B, Xu Z, Iglesias J E, Styner M, Langerak T R and Klein A 2017 Multi-atlas labeling beyond the cranial vault - workshop and challenge 10.7303/syn3193805

[54] Liu Q, Dou Q and Heng P-A 2020 Shape-aware meta-learning for generalizing prostate MRI segmentation to unseen domains *Int. Conf. on Medical Image Computing and Computer-Assisted Intervention* (Berlin: Springer) pp 475–85

[55] Gibson E, Hu Y, Ghavami N, Ahmed H U, Moore C, Emberton M, Huisman H J and Barratt D C 2018 Inter-site variability in prostate segmentation accuracy using deep learning *Int. Conf. on Medical Image Computing and Computer-Assisted Intervention* (Berlin: Springer) pp 506–14

[56] Bloch N, Madabhushi A, Huisman H, Freymann J, Kirby J, Grauer M, Enquobahrie A, Jaffe C, Clarke L and Farahani K 2015 NCI-ISBI 2013 challenge - automated segmentation of prostate structures 10.7937/K9/TCIA.2015.zF0vlOPv

[57] Lemaître G, Martí R, Freixenet J, Vilanova J C, Walker P M and Meriaudeau F 2015 Computer-aided detection and diagnosis for prostate cancer based on mono and multi-parametric MRI: a review *Comput. Biol. Med.* **60** 8–31

[58] Litjens G, Toth R, van de Ven W, Hoeks C, Kerkstra S, van Ginneken B, Vincent G, Guillard G, Birbeck N and Zhang J *et al* 2014 Evaluation of prostate segmentation algorithms for MRI: the promise12 challenge *Med. Image Anal.* **18** 359–73

[59] Sagawa S, Koh P W, Lee T, Gao I, Xie S M, Shen K, Kumar A, Hu W, Yasunaga M and Marklund H *et al* 2021 Extending the WILDS benchmark for unsupervised adaptation arXiv:2112.05090

[60] Ren J, Hacihaliloglu I, Singer E A, Foran D J and Qi X 2018 Adversarial domain adaptation for classification of prostate histopathology whole-slide images *Int. Conf. on Medical Image Computing and Computer-Assisted Intervention* (Berlin: Springer) pp 201–9

[61] Liu D, Zhang D, Song Y, Zhang F, O'Donnell L, Huang H, Chen M and Cai W 2020 Unsupervised instance segmentation in microscopy images via panoptic domain adaptation and task re-weighting *Proc. of the IEEE/CVF Conf. on Computer Vision and Pattern Recognition* pp 4243–52

[62] Zhang Y, Chen H, Wei Y, Zhao P, Cao J, Fan X, Lou X, Liu H, Hou J and Han X *et al* 2019 From whole slide imaging to microscopy: deep microscopy adaptation network for histopathology cancer image classification *Int. Conf. on Medical Image Computing and Computer-Assisted Intervention* (Berlin: Springer) pp 360–8

[63] Beck A H, Sangoi A R, Leung S, Marinelli R J, Nielson T O, van de Vijver M J, West R B, van de Rijin M and Koller D 2011 Systematic analysis of breast cancer morphology uncovers stromal features associated with survival *Sci. Transl. Med.* **3** 108ra113

[64] Koh P W, Sagawa S, Marklund H, Xie S M, Zhang M, Balsubramani A, Hu W, Yasunaga M, Phillips R L and Gao I *et al* 2021 Wilds: a benchmark of in-the-wild distribution shifts *Int. Conf. on Machine Learning* (PMLR) pp 5637–64

[65] Bandi P, Geessink O, Manson Q, Dijk M V, Balkenhol M, Hermsen M, Bejnordi B E, Lee B, Paeng K and Zhong A *et al* 2018 From detection of individual metastases to classification of lymph node status at the patient level: the CAMELYON17 challenge *IEEE Trans. Med. Imaging* **38** 550–60

[66] Kumar N, Verma R, Anand D, Zhou Y, Onder O F, Tsougenis E, Chen H, Heng P-A, Li J and Hu Z *et al* 2019 A multi-organ nucleus segmentation challenge *IEEE Trans. Med. Imaging* **39** 1380–91

[67] Naylor P, Laé M, Reyal F and Walter T 2018 Segmentation of nuclei in histopathology images by deep regression of the distance map *IEEE Trans. Med. Imaging* **38** 448–59

[68] Ljosa V, Sokolnicki K L and Carpenter A E 2012 Annotated high-throughput microscopy image sets for validation *Nat. Methods* **9** 637

[69] Zhao H, Li H, Maurer-Stroh S, Guo Y, Deng Q and Cheng L 2018 Supervised segmentation of un-annotated retinal fundus images by synthesis *IEEE Trans. Med. Imaging* **38** 46–56

[70] Huo Y, Xu Z, Moon H, Bao S, Assad A, Moyo T K, Savona M R, Abramson R G and Landman B A 2018 SynSeg-Net: synthetic segmentation without target modality ground truth *IEEE Trans. Med. Imaging* **38** 1016–25

[71] Zhang Z, Yang L and Zheng Y 2018 Translating and segmenting multimodal medical volumes with cycle-and shape-consistency generative adversarial network *Proc. of the IEEE Conf. on Computer Vision and Pattern Recognition* pp 9242–51

[72] Huang Y, Zheng H, Liu C, Ding X and Rohde G K 2017 Epithelium-stroma classification via convolutional neural networks and unsupervised domain adaptation in histopathological images *IEEE J. Biomed. health Inf.* **21** 1625–32

[73] Li C, Lin X, Mao Y, Lin W, Qi Q, Ding X, Huang Y, Liang D and Yu Y 2022 Domain generalization on medical imaging classification using episodic training with task augmentation *Comput. Biol. Med.* **141** 105144

[74] Li H, Wang Y F, Wan R, Wang S, Li T-Q and Kot A C 2020 Domain generalization for medical imaging classification with linear-dependency regularization *34th Conf. on Neural Information Processing Systems (NeurIPS)*

[75] Gu Y, Ge Z, Bonnington C P and Zhou J 2019 Progressive transfer learning and adversarial domain adaptation for cross-domain skin disease classification *IEEE J. Biomed. Health Inf.* **24** 1379–93

[76] Shen Y, Sheng B, Fang R, Li H, Dai L, Stolte S, Qin J, Jia W and Shen D 2020 Domain-invariant interpretable fundus image quality assessment *Med. Image Anal.* **61** 101654

[77] Zhang T, Cheng J, Fu H, Gu Z, Xiao Y, Zhou K, Gao S, Zheng R and Liu J 2019 Noise adaptation generative adversarial network for medical image analysis *IEEE Trans. Med. Imaging* **39** 1149–59

[78] Xing F, Bennett T and Ghosh D 2019 Adversarial domain adaptation and pseudolabeling for cross-modality microscopy image quantification *Int. Conf. on Medical Image Computing and Computer-Assisted Intervention* (Berlin: Springer) pp 740–9

[79] Mahapatra D and Ge Z 2020 Training data independent image registration using generative adversarial networks and domain adaptation *Pattern Recognit.* **100** 107109

[80] Mahmood F, Chen R and Durr N J 2018 Unsupervised reverse domain adaptation for synthetic medical images via adversarial training *IEEE Trans. Med. Imaging* **37** 2572–81

[81] Van Opbroek A, Arfan Ikram M, Vernooij M W and De Bruijne M 2014 Transfer learning improves supervised image segmentation across imaging protocols *IEEE Trans. Med. Imaging* **34** 1018–30

[82] Karani N, Chaitanya K, Baumgartner C and Konukoglu E 2018 A lifelong learning approach to brain MR segmentation across scanners and protocols *Int. Conf. on Medical Image Computing and Computer-Assisted Intervention* (Berlin: Springer) pp 476–84

[83] Goodfellow I, Pouget-Abadie J, Mirza M, Xu B, Warde-Farley D, Ozair S, Courville A and Bengio Y 2014 Generative adversarial nets *Advances in Neural Information Processing Systems*

[84] Zhu J-Y, Park T, Isola P and Efros A A 2017 Unpaired image-to-image translation using cycle-consistent adversarial networks *Proc. of the IEEE Int. Conf. on Computer Vision* pp 2223–32

[85] Yang X, Dou H, Li R, Wang X, Bian C, Li S, Ni D and Heng P-A 2018 Generalizing deep models for ultrasound image segmentation *Int. Conf. on Medical Image Computing and Computer-Assisted Intervention* (Berlin: Springer) pp 497–505

[86] Degel M A, Navab N and Albarqouni S 2018 Domain and geometry agnostic CNNs for left atrium segmentation in 3D ultrasound *Int. Conf. on Medical Image Computing and Computer-Assisted Intervention* (Berlin: Springer) pp 630–7

[87] Le Zhang M, Pereañez S K, Piechnik S, Neubauer S E, Petersen and Frangi A F 2018 Multi-input and dataset-invariant adversarial learning (MDAL) for left and right-ventricular coverage estimation in cardiac MRI *Int. Conf. on Medical Image Computing and Computer-Assisted Intervention* (Berlin: Springer) pp 481–9

[88] Joyce T, Chartsias A and Tsaftaris S A 2018 Deep multi-class segmentation without ground-truth labels *1st Conf. on Medical Imaging with Deep Learning (MIDL)*

[89] Wang S, Yu L, Li K, Yang X, Fu C-W and Heng P-A 2019 Boundary and entropy-driven adversarial learning for fundus image segmentation *Int. Conf. on Medical Image Computing and Computer-Assisted Intervention* (Berlin: Springer) pp 102–10

[90] Jia X, Wang S, Liang X, Balagopal A, Nguyen D, Yang M, Wang Z, Ji J X, Qian X and Jiang S 2019 Cone-beam computed tomography (CBCT) segmentation by adversarial learning domain adaptation *Int. Conf. on Medical Image Computing and Computer-Assisted Intervention* (Berlin: Springer) pp 567–75

[91] Dong J, Cong Y, Sun G, Zhong B and Xu X 2020 What can be transferred: unsupervised domain adaptation for endoscopic lesions segmentation *Proc. of the IEEE/CVF Conf. on Computer Vision and Pattern Recognition* pp 4023–32

[92] Perone C S, Ballester P, Barros R C and Cohen-Adad J 2019 Unsupervised domain adaptation for medical imaging segmentation with self-ensembling *NeuroImage* **194** 1–11

[93] Xia Y, Yang D, Yu Z, Liu F, Cai J, Yu L, Zhu Z, Xu D, Yuille A and Roth H 2020 Uncertainty-aware multi-view co-training for semi-supervised medical image segmentation and domain adaptation *Med. Image Anal.* **65** 101766

[94] Zhang L, Wang X, Yang D, Sanford T, Harmon S, Turkbey B, Wood B J, Roth H, Myronenko A and Xu D *et al* 2020 Generalizing deep learning for medical image segmentation to unseen domains via deep stacked transformation *IEEE Trans. Med. Imaging* **39** 2531–40

[95] Chen C, Bai W, Davies R H, Bhuva A N, Manisty C H, Augusto J B, Moon J C, Aung N, Lee A M and Sanghvi M M *et al* 2020 Improving the generalizability of convolutional neural network-based segmentation on CMR images *Front. Cardiovasc. Med.* **7** 105

[96] Dou Q, de Castro D C, Kamnitsas K and Glocker B 2019 Domain generalization via model-agnostic learning of semantic features *Advances in Neural Information Processing Systems* pp 6450–61

[97] Liu X, Thermos S, O'Neil A and Tsaftaris S A 2021 Semi-supervised meta-learning with disentanglement for domain-generalised medical image segmentation *Int. Conf. on Medical Image Computing and Computer-Assisted Intervention* (Berlin: Springer) pp 307–17

[98] Finn C, Abbeel P and Levine S 2017 Model-agnostic meta-learning for fast adaptation of deep networks arXiv:1703.03400
[99] Otálora S, Atzori M, Andrearczyk V, Khan A and Müller H 2019 Staining invariant features for improving generalization of deep convolutional neural networks in computational pathology *Front. Bioeng. Biotechnol.* **7** 198
[100] Aslani S, Murino V, Dayan M, Tam R, Sona D and Hamarneh G 2020 Scanner invariant multiple sclerosis lesion segmentation from MRI *IEEE 17th Int. Symp. on Biomedical Imaging (ISBI)* (Piscataway, NJ: IEEE) pp 781–5
[101] Kouw W M, Ørting S N, Petersen J, Pedersen K S and de Bruijne M 2019 A cross-center smoothness prior for variational Bayesian brain tissue segmentation *Int. Conf. on Information Processing in Medical Imaging* (Berlin: Springer) pp 360–71
[102] Chen C, Hammernik K, Ouyang C, Qin C, Bai W and Rueckert D 2021 Cooperative training and latent space data augmentation for robust medical image segmentation *Int. Conf. on Medical Image Computing and Computer-Assisted Intervention* (Berlin: Springer) pp 149–59
[103] McMahan B, Moore E, Ramage D, Hampson S and Agüera y Arcas B 2017 Communication-efficient learning of deep networks from decentralized data *Proc. of the 20th Int. Conf. on Artificial Intelligence and Statistics (AISTATS)* pp 1273–82
[104] Rieke N, Hancox J, Li W, Milletari F, Roth H R, Albarqouni S, Bakas S, Galtier M N, Landman B A and Maier-Hein K *et al* 2020 The future of digital health with federated learning *NPJ Digit. Med.* **3** 1–7
[105] Sheller M J, Edwards B, Anthony Reina G, Martin J, Pati S, Kotrotsou A, Milchenko M, Xu W, Marcus D and Colen R R *et al* 2020 Federated learning in medicine: facilitating multi-institutional collaborations without sharing patient data *Sci. Rep.* **10** 1–12
[106] Roth H R, Chang K, Singh P, Neumark N, Li W, Gupta V, Gupta S, Qu L, Ihsani A and Bizzo B C *et al* 2020 Federated learning for breast density classification: a real-world implementation *Domain Adaptation and Representation Transfer, and Distributed and Collaborative Learning* (Berlin: Springer) pp 181–91
[107] Jiang M, Wang Z and Dou Q 2022 HarmoFL: harmonizing local and global drifts in federated learning on heterogeneous medical images *36th AAAI Conf. on Artificial Intelligence*
[108] Li X, Jiang M, Zhang X, Kamp M and Dou Q 2021 FedBN: federated learning on non-IID features via local batch normalization *Int. Conf. on Learning Representations*
[109] Salimans T and Kingma D P 2016 Weight normalization: a simple reparameterization to accelerate training of deep neural networks *Advances in Neural Information Processing Systems* pp 901–9
[110] Jacot A, Gabriel F and Hongler C 2018 Neural tangent kernel: convergence and generalization in neural networks *Advances in Neural Information Processing Systems* pp 8571–80
[111] Arora S, Du S S, Hu W, Li Z and Wang R 2019 Fine-grained analysis of optimization and generalization for overparameterized two-layer neural networks arXiv:1901.08584
[112] Du S S, Zhai X, Poczos B and Singh A 2018 Gradient descent provably optimizes over-parameterized neural networks arXiv:1810.02054
[113] Allen-Zhu Z, Li Y and Song Z 2019 A convergence theory for deep learning via over-parameterization *Int. Conf. on Machine Learning* (PMLR) pp 242–52
[114] van den Brand J, Peng B, Song Z and Weinstein O 2020 Training (overparametrized) neural networks in near-linear time arXiv:2006.11648

[115] Dukler Y, Gu Q and Montúfar G 2020 Optimization theory for ReLU neural networks trained with normalization layers *Proc. of the 37th Int. Conf. on Machine Learning* (PMLR) pp 2751–60

[116] Li T, Sahu A K, Zaheer M, Sanjabi M, Talwalkar A and Smith V 2020 Federated optimization in heterogeneous networks *Conf. on Machine Learning and Systems*

[117] Wang J, Liu Q, Liang H, Joshi G and Poor H V 2020 Tackling the objective inconsistency problem in heterogeneous federated optimization *Advances in Neural Information Processing Systems*

[118] Reddi S J, Charles Z, Zaheer M, Garrett Z, Rush K, Konecný J, Kumar S and Brendan McMahan H 2021 Adaptive federated optimization *Int. Conf. on Learning Representations*

[119] Li Q, He B and Song D 2021 Model-contrastive federated learning *Proc. of the IEEE/CVF Conf. on Computer Vision and Pattern Recognition* pp 10713–22

[120] Huang G, Liu Z, Van Der Maaten L and Weinberger K Q 2017 Densely connected convolutional networks *Proc. of the IEEE Conf. on Computer Vision and Pattern Recognition* pp 4700–8

[121] Liu Q, Chen C, Qin J, Dou Q and Heng P-A 2021 FedDG: federated domain generalization on medical image segmentation via episodic learning in continuous frequency space *Proc. of the IEEE/CVF Conf. on Computer Vision and Pattern Recognition* pp 1013–23

[122] Nussbaumer H J 1981 The fast Fourier transform *Fast Fourier Transform and Convolution Algorithms* (Berlin: Springer) Springer Series in Information Sciences 2 pp 80–111

[123] Chen T, Kornblith S, Norouzi M and Hinton G 2020 A simple framework for contrastive learning of visual representations arXiv:2002.05709

[124] Carlucci F M, D'Innocente A, Bucci S, Caputo B and Tommasi T 2019 Domain generalization by solving jigsaw puzzles *Proc. of the IEEE Conf. on Computer Vision and Pattern Recognition* pp 2229–38

[125] Li D, Zhang J, Yang Y, Liu C, Song Y-Z and Hospedales T M 2019 Episodic training for domain generalization *Proc. of the IEEE Int. Conf. on Computer Vision* pp 1446–55

[126] Huang Z, Wang H, Xing E P and Huang D 2020 Self-challenging improves cross-domain generalization *Computer Vision – ECCV*

[127] Karani N, Erdil E, Chaitanya K and Konukoglu E 2021 Test-time adaptable neural networks for robust medical image segmentation *Med. Image Anal.* **68** 101907

[128] Valvano G, Leo A and Tsaftaris S A 2021 Stop throwing away discriminators! Re-using adversaries for test-time training *Domain Adaptation and Representation Transfer, and Affordable Healthcare and AI for Resource Diverse Global Health* (Berlin: Springer) pp 68–78

[129] Zhu W, Huang Y, Xu D, Qian Z, Fan W and Xie X 2021 Test-time training for deformable multi-scale image registration *IEEE Int. Conf. on Robotics and Automation (ICRA)*

www.ingramcontent.com/pod-product-compliance
Ingram Content Group UK Ltd.
Pitfield, Milton Keynes, MK11 3LW, UK
UKHW052039301026
9729IPUK00019B/308